PROGRESS IN CLINICAL AND BIOLOGICAL RESEARCH

RECENT TITLES

See pages following the index for previous titles in this series.

HORMONES AND CANCER

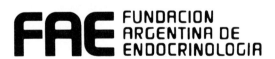

HORMONES AND CANCER

Proceedings of the International Symposium on Hormones
and Cancer held in Buenos Aires, Argentina May 9–13, 1983

Editors

ERLIO GURPIDE
Mt. Sinai School of Medicine
Mt. Sinai Hospital
New York, New York

RICARDO CALANDRA
Laboratorio de Esteroides
Instituto de Biología y Medicina Experimental
Buenos Aires, Argentina

CARLOS LEVY
División de Endocrinología
Hospital Ramos Mejía
Buenos Aires, Argentina

ROBERTO J. SOTO
Fundación Argentina de Endocrinología
Buenos Aires, Argentina

ALAN R. LISS, INC. • NEW YORK

Address all Inquiries to the Publisher
Alan R. Liss, Inc., 150 Fifth Avenue, New York, NY 10011

Library of Congress Cataloging in Publication Data

International Symposium on Hormones and Cancer (1983:
  Buenos Aires, Argentina)
  Hormones and Cancer

  Bibliography: p.
  Includes index.
  1. Cancer—Endocrine aspects—Congresses.
I. Gurpide, Erlio, 1927- . II. Title. [DNLM:
1. Hormones—Pharmacodynamics—Congresses. 2. Neoplasms,
Hormone-dependent—Congresses. W1 PR668E v.142 / QZ 200
I6123h 1983]
RC268.2.I58 1984   616.99′4071   83-24830
ISBN 0-8451-0142-0

Contents

Contributors

Alberto Baldi, Laboratorio de Esteroides, Instituto de Biología y Medicina Experimental, Buenos Aires, Argentina **[97]**

Etienne-Emile Baulieu, CNRS ER 125 and INSERM Unit 33, Lab Hormones, 94270 Bicêtre, France **[133, 167]**

Stephen B. Baylin, Department of Medicine and The Oncology Center, The Johns Hopkins Hospital, Baltimore, MD 21205 **[291]**

Nadine Binart, CNRS ER 125 and INSERM Unit 33, Lab Hormones, 94270 Bicêtre, France **[167]**

Clara D. Bloomfield, Department of Medicine, Section of Medical Oncology, University of Minnesota, Minneapolis, MN 55455 **[195, 223]**

Rosalyn Blumenthal, Department of Obstetrics, Gynecology, and Reproductive Science, Mount Sinai School of Medicine, New York, NY 10029 **[145]**

Jack E. Bodwell, Department of Physiology, Dartmouth Medical School, Hanover, NH 03755 **[181]**

Nicholas Bruchovsky, Department of Cancer Endocrinology, Cancer Control Agency of British Columbia, Vancouver, British Columbia, Canada **[247]**

Ricardo S. Calandra, Laboratorio de Esteroides, Instituto de Biología y Medicina Experimental, Buenos Aires, Argentina **[xiii, 97]**

Françoise Capony, Unit 148, Institut National de la Santé et de la Recherche Médicale (INSERM), 60, Rue de Navacelles, Montpellier 34100, France **[37]**

Jan Carlstedt-Duke, Department of Medical Nutrition, Karolinska Institute, Huddinge University Hospital, Huddinge, Sweden **[207]**

Maria-Grazia Catelli, CNRS ER 125 and INSERM Unit 33, Lab Hormones, 94270 Bicêtre, France **[167]**

Dany Chalbos, Unit 148, Institut National de la Santé et de la Recherche Médicale (INSERM), 60, Rue de Navacelles, Montpellier 34100, France **[37]**

Eduardo H. Charreau, Laboratorio de Esteroides, Instituto de Biología y Medicina Experimental, Buenos Aires, Argentina **[97]**

C.J. Conti, Institute for Cancer Research, University of Texas at Austin, Austin, TX 78712 **[119]**

Erik Dahlberg, Department of Medical Nutrition, Karolinska Institute, Huddinge University Hospital F69, Huddinge, Sweden **[261]**

Marie-Anne de Larminat, Laboratorio de Esteroides, Instituto de Biología y Medicina Experimental, Buenos Aires, Argentina **[247]**

J.R. Depaoli, Instituto de Cardiologia, Academia Nacional de Medicina, Buenos Aires, Argentina **[119]**

Giulio De Rossi, Hematology Department, State University, Rome, Italy **[235]**

The number in brackets following each affiliation indicates the opening page of that author's article.

Eugene R. DeSombre, Ben May Laboratory for Cancer Research, The University of Chicago, Chicago, IL 60637 **[1]**

Ejnar Eriksson, Department of Surgery, Section of Trauma, Karolinska Hospital, Stockholm, Sweden **[261]**

Guidalberto Fabris, Istituto di Anatomia e Istologia Patologica, Università di Ferrara, Ferrara 44100, Italy **[109]**

Honorée Fleming, Department of Obstetrics, Gynecology, and Reproductive Science, Mount Sinai School of Medicine, New York, NY 10029 **[145]**

Marcel Garcia, Unit 148, Institut National de la Santé et de la Recherche Médicale (INSERM), 60, Rue de Navacelles, Montpellier 34100, France **[37]**

Martine George, Institut Gustave Roussy, 94800 Villejuif, France **[167]**

L.E. Gerschenson, Department of Pathology, University of Colorado Health Sciences Center, Denver, CO 80262 **[119]**

Patricia Glikman, División de Endocrinología, Hospital Ramos Mejía, Buenos Aires, Argentina **[133]**

Achille Gravanis, CNRS ER 125 and INSERM Unit 33, Lab Hormones, 94270 Bicêtre, France **[167]**

Geoffrey L. Greene, Ben May Laboratory for Cancer Research, The University of Chicago, Chicago, IL 60637 **[1]**

Erlio Gurpide, Department of Obstetrics, Gynecology, and Reproductive Science, Mount Sinai School of Medicine, New York, NY 10029 **[xiii, 145]**

Jan-Åke Gustafsson, Department of Medical Nutrition, Karolinska Institute, Huddinge University Hospital F69, Huddinge, Sweden **[207,261]**

Paul M. Guyre, Department of Physiology, Dartmouth Medical School, Hanover, NH 03755 **[181]**

Tom Häggmark, Department of Surgery, Section of Trauma, Karolinska Hospital, Stockholm, Sweden **[261]**

Nikki J. Holbrook, Department of Physiology, Dartmouth Medical School, Hanover, NH 03755 **[195]**

Stefano Iacobelli, Laboratorio di Endocrinologia Molecolare, Catholic University S. Cuore, Rome, Italy **[53, 235]**

Elwood V. Jensen, Ben May Laboratory for Cancer Research, The University of Chicago, Chicago, IL 60637 **[1]**

William J. King, Ben May Laboratory for Cancer Research, The University of Chicago, Chicago, IL 60637 **[1]**

Jerzy Kulski, National Institute of Arthritis, Diabetes, and Digestive and Kidney Diseases, National Institutes of Health, Bethesda, MD 20205 **[63]**

Claude Laval, Centre René Huguenin, 92211 Saint Cloud, France **[167]**

Carlos Levy, División de Endocrinología, Hospital Ramos Mejía, Buenos Aires, Argentina **[xiii, 133]**

R. Lieberman, Department of Pathology, University of Colorado Health Sciences Center, Denver, CO 80262 **[119]**

M. Lynch, Department of Pathology, University of Colorado Health Sciences Center, Denver, CO 80262 **[119]**

Franco Mandelli, Hematology Department, State University, Rome, Italy **[235]**

Elisabetta Marchetti, Istituto di Anatomia e Istologia Patologica, Università di Ferrara, Ferrara 44100, Italy **[109]**

Paolo Marchetti, Department of Obstetrics and Gynecology, Catholic University S. Cuore, Rome, Italy **[235]**

Geoffrey Mendelsohn, Department of Pathology, The Johns Hopkins Hospital, Baltimore, MD 21205 **[291]**

Jan Mester, Unité 33, INSERM, Lab Hormones, 94270 Bicêtre, France **[133]**

Allan U. Munck, Department of Physiology, Dartmouth Medical School, Hanover, NH 03755 **[181, 195, 223]**

Vittoria Natoli, Laboratorio di Endocrinologia Molecolare, Universita Cattolica S. Cuore, 00168 Rome, Italy **[53]**

Italo Nenci, Istituto di Anatomia e Istologia Patologica, Università di Ferrara, Ferrara 44100, Italy **[23, 109]**

Kevin R. Nicholas, National Institute of Arthritis, Diabetes, and Digestive and Kidney Diseases, National Institutes of Health, Bethesda, MD 20205 [63]

Sam Okret, Department of Medical Nutrition, Karolinska Institute, Huddinge University Hospital, Huddinge, Sweden [207]

D. Orlicky, Department of Pathology, University of Colorado Health Sciences Center, Denver, CO 80262 [119]

Patrizia Querzoli, Istituto di Anatomia e Istologia Patologica, Università di Ferrara, Ferrara 44100, Italy [109]

Paul S. Rennie, Department of Cancer Endocrinology, Cancer Control Agency of British Columbia, Vancouver, British Columbia, Canada [247]

Anna Paola Rimondi, Istituto di Anatomia e Istologia Patologica, Università di Ferrara, Ferrara 44100, Italy [109]

A. Rivas-Berrios, Department of Pathology, University of Colorado Health Sciences Center, Denver, CO 80262 [119]

Paul Robel, CNRS ER 125 and INSERM Unit 33, Lab Hormones, 94270 Bicêtre, France [167]

Henri Rochefort, Unité d'Endocrinologie Cellulaire et Moléculaire, Unit 148, Institut National de la Santé et de la Recherche Médicale (INSERM), 60, Rue de Navacelles, Montpellier 34100, France [37, 79]

Lydie Roger-Jallais, Centre René Huguenin, 92211 Saint Cloud, France [167]

Monique Royer de Giaroli, Laboratorio de Esteroides, Instituto de Biología y Medicina Experimental, Buenos Aires, Argentina [97]

Tönu Saartok, Department of Medical Nutrition, Karolinska Institute, Huddinge University Hospital F69, Huddinge, and Department of Surgery, Section of Trauma, Karolinska Hospital, Stockholm, Sweden [261]

Lakshmanan Sankaran, National Institute of Arthritis, Diabetes, and Digestive and Kidney Diseases, National Institutes of Health, Bethesda, MD 20205 [63]

Giovanni Scambia, Laboratorio di Endocrinologia Molecolare, Università Cattolica S. Cuore, 00168 Rome, Italy [53]

Carlos Scorticati, Servicio de Urología, Instituto Oncología Angel Roffo, U.B.A., Buenos Aires, Argentina [247]

Kendall A. Smith, The Immunology Program, Norris Cotton Cancer Center, Dartmouth Medical School, Hanover, NH 03755 [223]

Marek Snochowski, Department of Medical Nutrition, Karolinska Institute, Huddinge University Hospital F69, Huddinge, Sweden, and Institute of Animal Physiology and Nutrition, Polish Academy of Sciences, Jablonna-near-Warsaw, Poland [261]

Roberto J. Soto, Fundación Argentina de Endocrinología, Buenos Aires, Argentina [xiii, 133]

Yale J. Topper, National Institute of Arthritis, Diabetes, and Digestive and Kidney Diseases, National Institutes of Health, Bethesda, MD 20205 [63]

Irene Vegh, División de Endocrinología, Hospital Ramos Mejía, Buenos Aires, Argentina [133]

Frédéric Veith, Unit 148, Institut National de la Santé et de la Recherche Médicale (INSERM), 60, Rue de Navacelles, Montpellier 34100, France [37]

Françoise Vignon, Unit 148, Institut National de la Santé et de la Recherche Médicale (INSERM), 60, Rue de Navacelles, Montpellier 34100, France [37]

Bruce Westley, Unit 148, Institut National de la Santé et de la Recherche Médicale (INSERM), 60, Rue de Navacelles, Montpellier 34100, France [37]

Örjan Wrange, Department of Medical Nutrition, Karolinska Institute, Huddinge University Hospital, Huddinge, Sweden [207]

Sponsors

The editors would like to thank the following sponsors for helping to make possible the International Symposium on Hormones and Cancer, held in Buenos Aires, May 1983:

Sra. Amalia Lacroze de Fortabat
Alfanuclear SAI y C
Banco de la Nación Argentina
Bayer Argentina Division Farma
Bentley Sorin Biomedica
Laboratorio Elea SACIF y A
Laboratorio Massone
Laboratorio Roussel Lutetia
Montedison Farmaceutica SA
Serono Argentina SA
Shell Compañía Argentina de Petroleo SA

Preface

One of the main objectives of Fundación Argentina de Endocrinología (FAE) is to encourage the progress of basic and clinical endocrinology in Argentina. To this end FAE has already sponsored seven International Symposia to foster interactions between our local scientists and endocrinologists with foremost authority in selected areas of endocrinology.

This volume contains the Proceedings of the Seventh International Symposium organized and sponsored by FAE in Buenos Aires, and devoted to the topic HORMONES AND CANCER.

It deals with the influence that hormones have on the development, maintenance, growth, and evolution of hormone-sensitive tumors—one of the most interesting fields of cancer research.

The activity of hormones as inducers, co-inducers or modifiers of neoplastic processes has to be examined in light of molecular mechanisms of hormone action. It is at this level that the understanding of the intimate relation of a hormone with its receptor, and the resulting modification of genetic expression of the cell, become the key for a better diagnosis and treatment of hormone-dependent tumors.

Recent advances in the knowledge of mechanisms of action of steroid and peptide hormones have changed the classical approach to clinical oncology; studies on the control of endocrine responsive neoplasms now involve multidisciplinary efforts.

This book contains the contributions of several widely known experts working in biochemistry, molecular biology, endocrinology, pathology, and medical oncology. The topics presented include descriptions of methods used to determine hormone receptor levels, mechanisms of action of hormones and antihormones, tests for the prediction of tumor responsiveness to hormones, clinical use of biological tumor markers, and treatment of hormone-dependent cancer.

We wish to thank all who participated in this Symposium and particularly the speakers for their contribution to this important volume. We also wish to express our recognition to Alan R. Liss, Inc., New York, for their assistance in this publication.

Erlio Gurpide
Ricardo Calandra
Carlos Levy
Roberto J. Soto

xiii

Hormones and Cancer, pages 1–21

ESTROGEN RECEPTORS, ANTIBODIES AND HORMONE DEPENDENT CANCER

Eugene R. DeSombre, Geoffrey L. Greene,
William J. King and Elwood V. Jensen

The Ben May Laboratory for Cancer Research
The University of Chicago
Chicago, Ill. 60637

INTRODUCTION

Experiments conducted in many laboratories throughout the world have led to a recognition that steroid hormones in general effect their biologic responses in target tissues through the mediation of high affinity, specific binding proteins, called receptors, which are present in unique amounts in such responsive tissues. The large body of knowledge about steroid hormone mechanism of action has been derived almost entirely from studies in which a radiolabeled steroid hormone has been used as the marker to elucidate the details of the interaction of hormone with responsive cells. Initial studies in vivo (Glascock and Hoekstra, 1959, Jensen and Jacobson, 1960) demonstrated that target tissues for the hormone could take up and retain physiologic amounts of radiolabeled estrogens against a concentration gradient with the blood and that, at least in the immature animal, this uptake occurred without requiring metabolism of the active estrogen. Subsequent studies indicated that while most of the estrogen taken up by target tissues in vivo, or at physiological temperatures in vitro, was associated with the nucleus, smaller but still significant amounts of estrogen were in low salt extracts, and were believed to be extranuclear (Jensen et al, 1968). However after the introduction by Toft and Gorski (1966) of sedimentation analytical methods for the study of receptors, it was found that upon homogenization of the uterus of untreated immature rats with hypotonic Tris–EDTA pH 7.4 buffer almost all of the tissue content of the estrogen receptor protein was obtained in the high speed supernatant or cytosolic

fraction. When such cytosolic estrogen receptor was
incubated with estrogen it underwent an estrogen and
temperature–dependent change (Gorski et al, 1968; Jensen et
al, 1968), which could be recognized by a change in its
sedimentation character from 4S to 5S in 0.4 M KCl. The
transformed estrogen receptor complex was indistinguishable
from the receptor complex extracted by KCl from nuclei of
uteri of estrogen–treated immature rats. Hence a general
pathway for the interaction of estrogen with a target cell,
Fig. 1, evolved in which the steroid entering the cell,

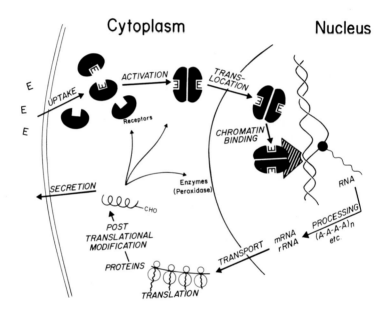

Fig. 1. Schematic diagram of the estrogen interaction
pathway and biochemical response in target cells.

probably by passive diffusion, rapidly binds to its receptor
protein, believed to be present in excess amounts as free
receptor in the extranuclear region of the cell. The
association of estrogen with its receptor leads to a complex
which undergoes activation, possibly involving a
dimerization (Notides et al, 1975), to a form which is

translocated to the nucleus and associates with some yet-to-be definitively characterized acceptors. It appears that this estrogen receptor interaction gives rise to the subsequent initiation of new nucleic acid synthesis leading to the protein, growth and cellular responses that are characteristic of the overall hormone response.

HORMONE DEPENDENCY OF BREAST CANCER

It has been known for some time that some cancers are hormone-dependent. Already in 1896 Beatson reported that several premenopausal breast cancer patients obtained dramatic remission of metastatic disease following removal of their ovaries. However the general acceptance of endocrine ablative surgery for hormone-dependent cancers followed the introduction of orchiectomy for the treatment of prostatic cancer (Huggins and Hodges, 1941), and the use of adrenalectomy (Huggins and Bergenstal, 1952) and hypophysectomy (Luft and Olivecrona, 1953; Pearson et al, 1956) for the treatment of metastatic breast cancer in postmenopausal women.

Thus by the early 1960s when studies in animals were beginning to clarify the nature of differences between the interactions of steroids with target and non-target tissues, it became especially important to apply this emerging basic knowledge to help clinicians properly diagnose and treat breast cancer patients. While the use of endocrine ablation for advanced breast cancer had by this time become a preferred treatment, only 25-35% of all patients obtained benefit. Early studies using tritiated estrogen in vivo in women about to undergo adrenalectomy (Folca et al, 1961) suggested that, as had been found in target tissues of experimental animals, the hormone-dependent lesions, that is cancers of patients who subsequently benefitted from ablative surgery, appeared to show preferential uptake of radioactive estrogen.

While such an in vivo study helped demonstrate an important difference between responsive and non-responsive breast cancers, it did not provide a practical approach to routine diagnosis of the endocrine responsiveness of a lesion. We applied an in vitro assay, developed for animal tissues, in which slices of the breast cancer were incubated with physiologic concentrations of tritiated estradiol

(Jensen et al, 1967) in the absence and presence of an inhibitor of specific uptake. This procedure, while requiring fresh tissue, did provide the first in vitro assay which showed a good correlation with patient response to endocrine ablative therapy (Jensen, 1970). When it became apparent that the basis for the specific uptake of radioactive estradiol in the hormone-responsive cancers was the specific cellular receptors, more convenient and specific assays for the estrogen receptor protein were used. The results (Jensen et al, 1971) indicated that patients whose breast cancers lacked estrogen receptors seldom responded to endocrine therapy while most, but not all, patients with receptor-containing lesions benefitted from such treatment. These findings were soon confirmed and extended by others (Maass et al, 1972, Engelsman et al, 1973, Leung et al, 1973, Savlov et al, 1974) and it became apparent that knowledge of the estrogen receptor status of human breast cancer was an important indicator for proper treatment (McGuire et al, 1975).

As receptor assays were refined and became more sensitive, laboratories began to report that a greater proportion of breast cancers contained detectable estrogen receptor (LeClercq et al, 1975). If assay laboratories found a greater proportion of cancers with estrogen receptors but still only 25-30% of unselected patients responded to endocrine therapies, the assay results would be less accurate for prediction of endocrine responses. One possible solution to this dilemma was that not only the presence of estrogen receptor but also the amount of receptor was of importance for response. When we assessed the quantity of the estrogen receptor present in the cancer, related to the endocrine response of the patient (Fig. 2) it appeared that the patients whose lesions contained low concentrations of receptor, as well as those with no receptor, seldom responded to endocrine therapy (Jensen et al, 1975). When response rates were related to the tumor estrogen receptor content, Figure 3, the low response rate of the patients with tumors having lower estrogen receptor content was apparent. Thus rather than receptor positive and negative lesions, it seemed more appropriate to characterize the cancers as receptor-rich and -poor, with the classification based upon the clinical response rates (Jensen et al, 1976). As can also be seen in Figure 3, there appears to be an increasing response rate with increasing receptor content of the tumor as well (DeSombre

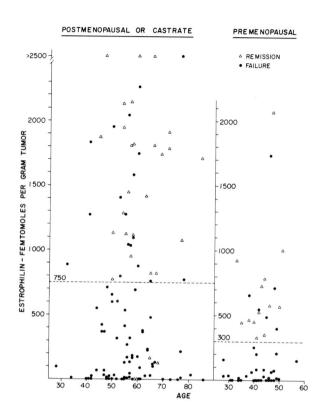

Fig. 2. Correlation of breast cancer cytosol estrogen receptor content with response to endocrine therapy of patients with metastatic breast cancer. Estrogen receptor content was determined by sedimentation analysis of tumor cytosols using 0.5 nM tritiated estradiol (a subsaturating concentration) as described elsewhere (DeSombre et al, 1978).

and Jensen, 1980). This relationship has also been observed by others (Paridaens et al; 1980, Dao and Nemoto; 1980, Lippman and Allegra; 1980, Osborne et al, 1980).

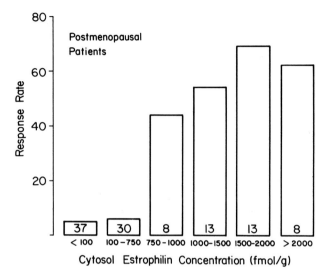

Fig. 3. Relationship between response rates of postmenopausal metastatic breast cancer patients to endocrine therapy and the tumor cytosol estrogen receptor concentration (subsaturating assay as in Figure 2). The number in each bar indicates the number of patients in the group designated by the estrogen receptor concentration given under the bar.

Using the quantitative information from the estrogen receptor assays thus appears to improve the predictability of endocrine responses. In our series of 117 patients treated by endocrine ablative therapy, using the classification of receptor—rich and receptor—poor indicated earlier (Fig. 2), we find that about 71% of the patients in our study who have receptor—rich cancers respond, Table 1. The overall accuracy of prediction of response in fact approaches 90% (i.e. 29 + 74 of 117 = 88%), even though the overall response rate (29 + 2⁄117 = 26.5%) is similar to what is expected for an unselected population. Nonetheless, as is evident from both Figures 2 and 3, there are some patients whose breast cancers contain high concentrations of

Table 1. Objective Remissions to Endocrine Ablation

Treatment	Tumor Classification	
	Receptor-rich	Receptor-poor
Adrenalectomy	4-6[a]	0-20[a]
Adrenalectomy plus oophorectomy	14-19	1-17
Hypophysectomy	2-4	0-9
Oophorectomy	9-12	1-30
Totals (117)	29-41 (71%)	2-76 (3%)

[a]Objective remissions-total cases

estrogen receptor and do not respond. Furthermore, while knowledge of the progestin-receptor content of the cancer, as originally suggested by Horwitz et al, 1975, like quantitation of the estrogen receptor, improves the predictability of endocrine responses, neither is unfailing. Based on the results presented at the Consensus Meeting on Steroid Receptors in Breast Cancer held at the National Cancer Institute in 1979 (DeSombre et al, 1979) the clinical correlations from 10 institutions and over 500 patients indicated a 78% probability of objective response for patients whose lesion has both estrogen and progestin receptor, but also a 33% response rate when only one of the two receptors were present (DeSombre, 1982). Thus, while conventional receptor assays can be of considerable usefulness in predicting endocrine responses, and probably also provide prognostic information (see review in DeSombre, 1982) there is a need to improve the accuracy of such predictions and clearly a need to improve the response rates of patients whose cancers contain receptor proteins. One may hope that the latter goal might be accomplished as we gain more knowledge about the specific molecular details of the regulation of growth by hormones.

RECEPTOR ANTIBODIES AND RECEPTOR ASSAYS

Until very recently all our information about the estrogen-receptor interaction, the subcellular distribution of receptor and quantitative assays for estrogen receptor in both normal and neoplastic tisues were based on the binding of radioactively labeled steroid. Culminating a long effort in the purification of estrogen receptor from calf uterus was the production of polyclonal antibodies to the receptor protein, first obtained in a rabbit (Greene et al, 1977) and subsequently in a goat (Greene et al, 1979). These antibodies were found to react with both cytosolic and nuclear estrogen receptor complexes from calf uterus, as well as estrogen receptors from every receptor containing tissue of each species tested, including even hen oviduct. Nonetheless, these antibodies retain specificity for estrogen receptor and do not react with non-specific, estrogen-binding proteins or with receptor proteins for androgens or progestins. Since the antibodies are non-precipitating, sedimentation analysis has proved to be a convenient, as well as informative, technique for characterization of the association of receptor complex with the antibodies. Both the rabbit and goat antibodies have been shown to bind to the receptor complex and also to the naked receptor protein. While neither the rabbit nor the goat antibodies seem to cause the dissociation of estradiol from the receptor complex, if goat antibodies are allowed to react with the naked receptor protein prior to incubation with estradiol they appear to decrease the affinity of the receptor for estradiol (Greene et al, 1979). Interestingly, while these antibodies will also recognize the estrogen receptor associated with antiestrogen (Garcia et al, 1982), the incubation of goat antibodies with the receptor prior to its incubation with the antiestrogen, hydroxytamoxifen, does not effect any change in the affinity of the receptor for this antiestrogen (Tate et al, 1983). This would suggest that there is a subtle difference in the preferred configuration of the receptor complexed with estradiol and hydroxytamoxifen even though in the absence of antibody the apparent affinity of these 2 ligands for the estrogen receptor is similar.

While the goat and rabbit antibodies to the estrogen receptor are very useful reagents, the heterogeneity of the preparations, which, as polyclonal antibodies, include numerous other immunoglobulins, limits their use in the development of certain new immunochemical assays for estrogen receptor. Therefore monoclonal antibodies were prepared, first using purified estrogen receptor from calf uterus (Greene et al, 1980a). Since the initial monoclonal antibodies against calf uterine receptor did not cross react with estrogen receptors from the human, antibodies were subsequently prepared against the estrogen receptor purified from the human breast cancer cell line, MCF7 (Greene et al, 1980b). The two IgG clonal lines obtained, designated D547 and D75, clearly react with separate and non–overlapping antigenic sites on the receptor protein. As seen in Figure 4, addition of antibody D547 to a cytosol prepared from

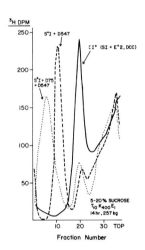

Fig. 4. Independent interaction of two monoclonal antibodies with cytosol estrogen receptor from human endometrium. Particulate free cytosol was prepared from a 10 mM Tris, 1 mM EDTA pH 7.4 homogenate of human endometrium made 400 mM in KCl and, after incubation with tritiated estradiol, aliquots were incubated with 10 ug⁄ml antibody D547 alone or along with 10 ug⁄ml of antibody D75. Following this the samples were layered on 5–20% sucrose gradients in 10 mM Tris, 400 M KCl, 1 mM EDTA, pH 7.4 buffer and centrifuged 14 hours at 257,000 x g. av. After bottom puncture the gradients were collected by displacement and counted for tritium in a scintillation counter.

human endometrium increased the rate of sedimentation of the receptor complex from its usual 4S coefficient, observed in 0.4 M KCl, to the 8S region, characteristic of a ternary complex of antibody-receptor-estrogen. When antibody D75 is also added, the receptor complex sediments even further down the gradient, compatible with the increased size of the receptor complex simultaneously associated with both antibodies.

With 2 monoclonal antibodies which react with independent antigenic sites on the receptor molecule, such that they can both associate with the receptor simultaneously, it becomes possible to develop an immunoradiometric (IRMA) or enzyme immunoassay for receptor (EIA), Figure 5. One of the specific antibodies (Ab1) is

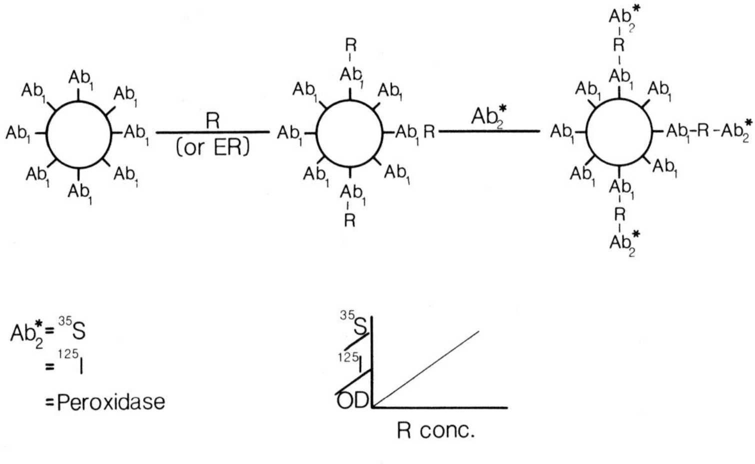

Fig. 5. Schematic for immunoassay for receptor (R) or receptor complex (ER), using two independent monoclonal anti-receptor antibodies (Ab1, and Ab*2) the first of which is associated with a polystyrene bead. The second antibody contains a label or assayable tag, as indicated by *.

attached to a bead which is then incubated with a tissue extract to be assayed for its estrogen receptor content. The receptor (complex or naked receptor as both bind equally well to the antibodies) is retained by the bead, which is washed and then incubated with the second monoclonal antibody containing an assayable tag. After additional washing, the amount of the tagged 2nd monoclonal antibody retained by the bead by virtue of its association with bead-bound receptor is quantified on the basis of the assayable tag. If the tag is a radioactive label (i.e. radioactive iodine by iodination of the antibody, or radioactive sulfur if the antibody is produced from hybridoma cells grown in the presence of methionine labeled with radioactive sulfur) the assay would constitute an IRMA and the amount of receptor present would be assayed by gamma or scintillation counting. If the tag is an enzyme, such as peroxidase, the amount of receptor would be determined by a spectrophotometric assay of the amount of enzyme retained by the incubated beads in an EIA. The initial use of this new type of receptor assay with 18 human breast cancer cytosols using an IRMA and iodine-labeled monoclonal antiestrogen receptor antibody gave an excellent correlation of the receptor content compared with the results of standard sucrose gradient assays for estrogen receptor (Greene et al, 1981; Jensen et al, 1983).

There are several reasons why one might want to change from current biochemical assays for receptor, which are based on the binding of a radiolabeled estrogen to the receptor protein. The most important reasons relate to quality control, receptor lability and assay simplicity. Both sedimentation analysis and titration assays using dextran-coated charcoal, usually with Scatchard plots of the data, are complicated assays which are not only expensive but also are only carried out in major research hospitals and commercial laboratories. Furthermore, while there have been quite a number of serious attempts at quality assurance, none have reached the uniform level of interlaboratory reproducibility that is needed for meaningful use of quantitative receptor results in a multi-institution or collaborative group study of cancer. Certainly part of the reason for the difficulty in reproducing quantitative results across many laboratories relates to the substantial lability of the receptor to partial or complete loss of its ability to bind estrogens under very mild conditions. There is reason to believe that the antigenic sites of the receptor may be more stable to degradation than is the steroid-binding activity. In fact it is clear that these antibodies retain the ability to recognize the receptor which has been denatured in SDS detergent, conditions under which the receptor no longer binds steroid. In addition, while a significant proportion of estrogen receptor titration assays using Scatchard plot analysis are curvilinear, the limited results thus far with the bead type immunoassay for estrogen receptor have not shown such complicating anomalies. Bead assays, like the type under development for estrogen receptor, have been used for other biologically important proteins, such as CEA, and have been found to be very readily quality controlled, by inclusion of internal controls that have a good shelf life even stored at room temperature. It appears that similar quality control materials can also be developed for estrogen receptor for the bead type immunoassay.

While there are a number of attractions to such an antibody-based assay for estrogen receptor, such a new assay will have to be thoroughly tested in a number of laboratories to determine how well the quantitative results of the new assay compare with results of conventional assays before they can be used routinely for breast cancer estrogen receptor assays. Furthermore, if there are any differences between immunoassays and standard assays, it will be important to assess the clinical significance of the differences. Accepting these caveats, it is clear that the potential exists with an immunobead assay to provide simpler, more dependable and more widely available quantitative receptor assays for breast cancers.

One of the limitations of current receptor assays that would not be overcome by an immunobead assay is the inability to assess tissue heterogeneity. There are ample examples of the lack of quantitative agreement even among assays carried out on different portions of the same breast cancer. The inability to characterize the histopathology on the actual assay sample, rather than on an adjacent piece of tissue, has also been worrisome. Indeed, the literature abounds with documentation on histopathologic heterogeneity of many specimens of breast cancer. As a result there have been numerous attempts to use various histologic methods to identify the presence of estrogen receptors in individual cells in frozen or fixed sections of breast cancers. While most of these methods demonstrate apparent heterogeneity of staining of breast cancer sections, in general the details of the techniques used are inconsistent with the detection of receptor (Chamness et al, 1980, DeSombre, 1982;1983). However with the availability of specific monoclonal antibodies prepared against human breast cancer estrogen receptor, specific and also very sensitive methods for immunocytochemical assay of receptor became feasible. Using a sandwich technique, Figure 6, both amplification and

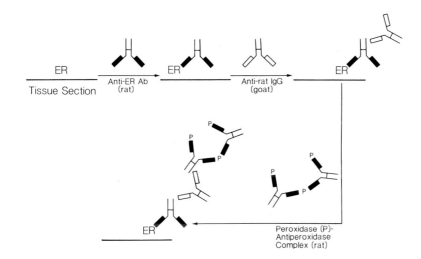

Fig. 6. Immunocytochemical procedure for detection of estrogen receptors in frozen sections of tissue. Lightly fixed frozen sections were incubated with a solution of specific antiestrogen receptor antibody (Anti-ER Ab) followed by bridging antibody (Anti-rat IgG) and peroxidase-antiperoxidase complex (PAP), with appropriate washes between incubations. The localization of the peroxidase is detected following incubation with the substrate, diaminobenzidine (DAB), and hydrogen peroxide.

detection of specific sites are due to the attachment of a rat peroxidase–antiperoxidase complex through a bridging antibody (goat anti–rat IgG) to the specific monoclonal antibodies bound to estrogen receptor present in tissue sections. The method which has been developed in our laboratory uses lightly fixed, frozen sections of tissue, King et al, 1982. As seen in Figure 7, in an estrophilin-rich breast cancer the intense staining of the nuclei of the cancer cells due to receptor antibody (Figure 7A) is not evident when normal rat immunoglobulin is substituted for the specific rat monoclonal antibody against estrogen receptor (Figure 7B). In numerous studies of various normal and neoplastic tissues with several species the only specific staining observed has been nuclear. No significant

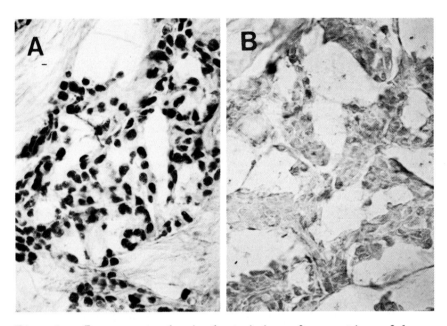

Fig. 7. Immunocytochemical staining of a section of human breast cancer for estrogen receptor. Frozen sections, 8 um thick, lightly fixed with ethanol, of an estrogen receptor rich breast cancer from a postmenopausal patient were incubated with 20 ug/ml antibody H226 (left-7A) or normal rat IgG (right-7B), followed by bridging antibody, PAP complex, and visualized with diaminobenzidine and hydrogen peroxide as indicated in Figure 6. Photomicrograph at 400X magnification.

specific staining in the extranuclear region of estrogen-receptor positive cells have been seen with 5 different monoclonal antibodies, each reacting with different antigenic sites on the receptor, while all these antibodies showed specific nuclear staining (King et al, 1984). Interestingly, all the antibodies demonstrating the exclusive nuclear staining were raised against purified

estrogen receptor from cytosolic extracts of MCF-7 cells
(Greene et al, 1980b). Although in solution the antibodies
react with receptor complexes from cytosolic and nuclear
extracts of target cells, in tissue sections the specific
staining is only nuclear. These results are not only found
with human breast cancers, where one might expect a
reasonable proportion of estrogen receptor to be present in
nuclei, but also with pituitary, ovary and uteri from even
untreated immature rabbits where the classic model would
predict predominantly cytosolic receptor localization.
Results of numerous studies with 5 unique monoclonal
antibodies against the estrogen receptor and various normal
and neoplastic tissues from several species studied under a
variety of different experimental conditions, all indicate
that the specific immunocytochemical staining associated
with receptor antibody is nuclear. Because of these
extensive studies all showing a nuclear localization for the
antibody we believe that there is a good probability that
both forms of receptor, i.e. those referred to previously as
'cytosolic' and 'nuclear', may indeed be located in the
nucleus, Figure 8. While this requires a change in the
model for the subcellular localization of receptor, the new
model can still easily incorporate all the important
phenomena which have been associated with the interaction of
estrogen with a target cell. By this scheme, Figure 8, the
estrogen entering the cell initially associates with low
affinity binders, including type II binders, in the
cytoplasm and then enters the nucleus by virtue of the high
affinity receptors in the nucleus. In this model the low
salt extractible 'native' or 8S form of the receptor, which
appears in 'cytosolic' extracts would, like some mammalian
RNA polymerase molecules, be readily extracted from the
nucleus with such hypotonic media. After association with
estrogen the receptor complex undergoes the steroid-
dependent activation to a more-tightly bound nuclear form, a
process taking place in the nucleus and leading to the
higher affinity association of receptor complex with nuclei.
This latter form of receptor requires a higher salt
concentration for extraction from the nuclei. This model is
in fact more consistent with the model derived from recent
autoradiographic studies on the intracellular localization
of estrogen receptor using tritiated estradiol (Martin and
Sheridan, 1982) in which the naked receptor is believed to
have free access to the nucleus.

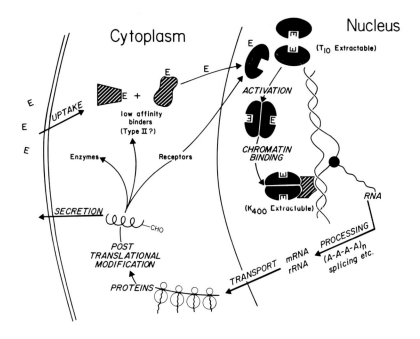

Fig. 8. New schematic diagram of the estrogen interaction pathway and biochemical response in target cells.

With the availability of specific antibodies to the estrogen receptor protein it becomes feasible to study the intranuclear localization of receptor by extending the immunocytochemical approach to the electronmicroscopic level. Results from such studies have the potential to identify the genomic binding site for receptor and also to show any significant changes in the intranuclear localization of receptor which occurs on receptor activation, thereby clarifying details which are important to an understanding of how estrogens act.

Knowledge of the mechanism of estrogen action has clearly improved the ability to predict which cancers are likely to respond to hormone therapies. The development of antibodies to the estrogen receptor promise simpler, more dependable and possibly more meaningful information about receptor content, distribution or activity in cancers. As these new reagents lead to a better understanding of the molecular details of hormone dependency one can hope that more effective treatments can be designed for the one-third of breast cancer patients who have hormone dependent cancers. However, an equally important challenge is to find a way to use the presence of receptor in the nearly equal numbers of breast cancers which have estrogen receptors but do not appear to respond to conventional hormone-based therapies. It may be that identification of the proportion of receptor positive cells by immunocytochemical methods and the synthesis of effective cytolytic estrogen derivatives which can destroy any receptor-containing cell, whether or not it is dependent on estrogen for growth, will enable the design of effective, hormone-based therapies for the nearly 80% of breast cancer patients whose lesions have receptor. With new knowledge and new reagents one can hope that this goal will be realized before too long.

ACKNOWLEDGEMENTS

Investigations in our laboratory were supported by the American Cancer Society (BC-86), Abbott Laboratories, Mead Johnson Pharmaceutical Division and the National Institutes of Health (CA 02897, CA 14599, CA 27476, CB 43969, CB 14358, HD 15513, HD 17103) and by the Womens' Board of the University of Chicago Cancer Research Foundation.

REFERENCES

Beatson GT (1896). On the treatment of inoperable cases of carcinoma of the mamma. Suggestions for a new method of treatment with illustrative cases. Lancet ii:104.

Dao TL, Nemoto T (1980). Steroid receptors and response to endocrine ablations in women with metastatic cancer of the breast. Cancer 46:2779.

DeSombre ER (1982). Breast cancer: hormone receptors, prognosis and therapy. Clinics in Oncol 1:191.

DeSombre ER (1983). Steroid receptors in breast cancer. In McDivitt RW, Oberman H, Ozello L (eds): 'The Breast,' Baltimore: Williams and Wilkens, in press.

DeSombre ER, Jensen EV (1980). Estrophilin assays in breast cancer: quantitative features and application to the mastectomy specimen. Cancer 46:2783.

DeSombre ER, Greene GL, Jensen EV (1978). Estrophilin and endocrine responsiveness of breast cancer. In McGuire WL (ed): 'Hormones, Receptors, and Breast Cancer,' New York: Raven Press, p 1.

DeSombre ER, Carbone PP, Jensen EV, McGuire WL, Wells SA, Wittliff JL, Lipsett MB (1979). Special report: steroid receptors in breast cancer. New Engl J Med 301:1011.

Engelsman E, Persijn JP, Korsten CB, Cleton FJ (1973). Oestrogen receptors in human breast cancer tissue and response to endocrine therapy. Brit Med J 2:750.

Folca PJ, Glascock RF, Irving WT (1961). Studies with tritium labelled hexestrol in advanced breast cancer. Lancet ii:796.

Garcia M, Greene G, Rochefort H, Jensen EV (1982). Effect of antibodies to estrogen receptor on the binding of [3H] antiestrogens and androstanediol in uterus. Endocrinology 110:1355.

Glascock RF, Hoekstra WG (1959). Selective accumulation of tritium-labelled hexoestrol in the reproductive organs of immature female goats and sheep. Biochem J 72:673.

Gorski J, Toft D, Shyamala G, Smith D, Notides A (1968). Hormone receptors: studies on the interaction of estrogen with the uterus. Recent Progr Hormone Res 24:45.

Greene GL, Jensen EV (1981). An immunoradiometric assay for estrogen receptor in breast cancer. Abstr. Endocrine Society p124.

Greene GL, Closs LE, Fleming H, DeSombre ER, Jensen EV (1977). Antibodies to estrogen receptor: immunochemical similarity of estrophilin from various mammalian species. Proc Natl Acad Sci USA 74:3681.

Greene GL, Closs LE, DeSombre ER, Jensen EV (1979). Antibodies to estrophilin: comparison between rabbit and goat antisera. J Steroid Biochem 11:333.

Green GL, Fitch FW, Jensen EV (1980a). Monoclonal antibodies to estrophilin: probes for the study of estrogen receptors. Proc Natl Acad Sci USA 77:157.

Greene GL, Nolan C, Engler JP, Jensen EV (1980b). Monoclonal antibodies to human estrogen receptors. Proc Natl Acad Sci USA 77:5115.

Horwitz KB, McGuire WL, Pearson OH, Segaloff A (1975). Predicting response to endocrine therapy in human breast cancer: an hypothesis. Science 189:726.

Huggins C, Hodges CV (1941). Studies on prostatic cancer. I. The effect of castration, of estrogen and androgen injection on serum phosphatases in metastatic carcinoma of the prostate. Cancer Res 1:293.

Huggins C, Bergenstal DM (1952). Inhibition of human mammary and prostatic cancers by adrenalectomy. Cancer Res 12:134.

Jensen EV (1970). The pattern of hormone-receptor interactions. In Griffiths K, Pierrepoint CG (eds): 'Some Aspects of the Aetiology and Biochemistry of Prostatic Cancer,' Cardiff: Alpha Omega Alpha, p 151.

Jensen EV, Jacobson HI (1960). Fate of steroid estrogens in target tissues. In Pincus G, Vollmer EP (eds): 'Biological Activities of Steroids in Relation to Cancer,' New York: Academic Press, p 161.

Jensen EV, DeSombre ER, Jungblut PW (1967). Estrogen receptors in hormone-responsive tissues and tumors. In Wissler RW, Dao TL, Wood S (eds): 'Endogenous Factors Influencing Host-Tumor Balance,' Chicago: Univ of Chicago Press, p 15.

Jensen EV, Suzuki T, Kawashima T, Stumpf WE, Jungblut, PW, DeSombre ER (1968). A two step mechanism for the interaction of estradiol with rat uterus. Proc Natl Acad Sci USA 59:632.

Jensen EV, Block GE, Smith S, Kyser K, DeSombre ER (1971). Estrogen receptors and breast cancer response to adrenalectomy. Natl Cancer Inst Monogr 34:55.

Jensen EV, Polley TZ, Smith S, Block G, Ferguson DJ, DeSombre ER (1975). Prediction of hormone dependency in human breast cancer. In McGuire WL, Carbone PP, Vollmer EP (eds): 'Estrogen Receptors in Human Breast Cancer,' New York: Raven Press, p 37.

Jensen EV, Smith S, DeSombre ER (1976). Hormone dependency in breast cancer. J Steroid Biochem 7:905.

Jensen EV, Greene GL, Closs LE, DeSombre ER, Nadji M (1982). Receptors reconsidered: a 20-year perspective. Rec Prog Hormone Res 38:1.

King WJ, Jensen EV, Miller L, Greene GL (1982). Immunocytochemical detection of estrogen receptor in frozen sections of human breast tumors with monoclonal anti-receptor antibodies. Abstr Endocrine Soc, p 258.

King WJ, DeSombre ER, Greene GL (1984). Comparison of immunocytochemical and steroid-binding assays for estrogen receptor in human breast cancer. Submitted.

Leclercq G, Heuson JC, Deboel MC, Mattheiem WH (1975). Oestrogen receptors in breast cancer: a changing concept. Brit Med J i:185.

Leung BS, Fletcher WS, Lindell TD, Krippaehne WW (1973). Predictability of response to endocrine ablation in advanced breast carcinoma. Arch Surg 106:515.

Lippman ME, Allegra JC (1980). Quantitative estrogen receptor analyses: the response to endocrine and cytotoxic chemotherapy in human breast cancer and the disease free interval. Cancer 46:2829.

Luft R, Olivecrona H (1953). Experiences with hypophysectomy in man. J Neurosurg 10:301.

Maass H, Engel B, Hohmeister H, Lehmann F, Trans G (1972). Estrogen receptors in human breast cancer tissue. Am J Obstet Gynecol 113:377.

Martin PM, Sheridan PJ (1982). Towards a new model for the mechanism of action of steroids. J Steroid Biochem 16:215.

McGuire WL, Carbone PP, Vollmer EP (eds) (1975). 'Receptors in Human Breast Cancer,' New York: Raven Press.

Notides A, Hamilton DE, Auer HE. A kinetic analysis of the estrogen receptor transformation. J Biol Chem 250:3945.

Osborne CK, Yochmowitz MG, Knight WA III, McGuire WL (1980). The value of estrogen and progesterone receptors in the treatment of breast cancer. Cancer 46:2884.

Paridaens R, Sylvester RJ, Ferrazzi E, Legros N, Leclercq G, Heuson JC (1980). Clinical significance of the quantitative assessment of estrogen receptors in advanced breast cancer. Cancer 46:2889.

Pearson OH, Ray BS, Harrold CC (1956). Hypophysectomy in treatment of advanced cancer,. J Am Med Assoc 161:17.

Savlov ED, Wittliff JL, Hilf R, Hall TC (1974). Correlations between certain biochemical properties of breast cancer and response to therapy: a preliminary report. Cancer 33:303.

Tate AC, DeSombre ER, Greene GL, Jensen EV, Jordan VC (1983). A comparative study of the interaction of monoclonal antibodies with either [3H] estradiol- or [3H] monohydroxytamoxifen-estrogen receptor complexes from human tumor cytosol. Br Ca Res Treat, in press.

Toft D, Gorski J (1966). A receptor molecule for estrogens: Isolation from the rat uterus and preliminary characterization. Proc Natl Acad Sci USA 55:1574.

Hormones and Cancer, pages 23–36
© **1984 Alan R. Liss, Inc., 150 Fifth Avenue, New York, NY 10011**

CHARTING STEROID-CELL INTERACTIONS
IN NORMAL AND NEOPLASTIC TISSUES
Update 1983

ITALO NENCI

Istituto di Anatomia e Istologia Patologica
Universita' di Ferrara, 44100 FERRARA, Italy

The recent period will be remembered in the history
of cell control by steroid hormones as that of the great
breakthrough. As with many scientific advances, new tools,
and new thoughts, rendered possible the massive invasion of
this subcellular world that was launched at that time.
Revolutionary as these developments were, they would,
nevertheless, not have sufficed in themselves for the
construction of an integrated cell biology. Biochemistry
of steroid receptors was expanding rapidly and it seemed
quite natural to try to link biochemistry and physiology
with structural information. What was needed, in addition,
was a bridge between morphology and biochemistry, a junction
between the essentially parallel advances opened by these
two disciplines, a hybrid methodology whereby the visible
and the measurable could be correlated into a unified
picture of the living cell. Cytochemistry provided this
indispensable bridge.

BASIC STEROID RECEPTOR CYTOCHEMISTRY

In effect, during recent years cytochemistry has
become a most valuable methodology for revealing the
distribution in situ of hormone binding sites. Its
application to research problems may provide much information, if care is taken to avoid uncritical appreciation
of the potential and pitfalls of the technology. Before
discussing some of the subjects recently investigated by
these techniques, it seems worthy to summarize the major
trends in steroid receptor cytochemistry over the past few
years.
Until quite recently, the basic methods for the
direct visual study of hormone-cell interaction were

similar to those used in other binding techniques. They
require means to localize the hormone, such as specific
antibodies or appropriately labelled hormones, a suitable
cell or tissue preparation, and plain techniques to distinguish for the hormone bound to specific binding sites from
the hormone interacting with non-specific binders. The
ancestor approach to demonstrate steroid uptake of tissue
section was the autoradiographic technique (Fig. 1). But

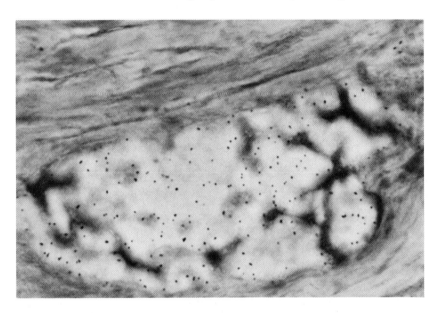

Fig.1. Autoradiography of tritiated estradiol bound to
estrogen receptors of a frozen section from human breast
cancer. The positivity – black spots – is restricted to
neoplastic epithelial cells. The demonstration of estrogen
receptors is very specific – note the unmarked surrounding
stroma – but the structural resolution is very poor.

more suitable and less time consuming means were required
for the precise localization of steroid receptors in human
tissues and at the subcellar level, given the poor, though
specific, resolution achievable by this technique.
     The first generation of cytochemical methods belong
to HORMONE IMMUNOCYTOCHEMISTRY, which has reached such a
sensitive potential of investigation that the opportunity

is given now of detecting hormones at both their site
of production and action. These techniques involve a
specific antisteroid antibody which traces the bound
hormone at the cell level and which is in turn traced by
means of fluorescent or enzymatic tracers at ultraviolet,
light and electron microscopy. These techniques are very
sensitive but need a very complex check-list.

The second generation techniques, that is AFFINITY
CYTOCHEMISTRY, exploit steroid hormones coupled to a
macromolecular protein carrier, for instance estradiol
linked to bovine serum albumin in a molecule highly substituted with either fluorescein or peroxidase labels (Fig. 2).

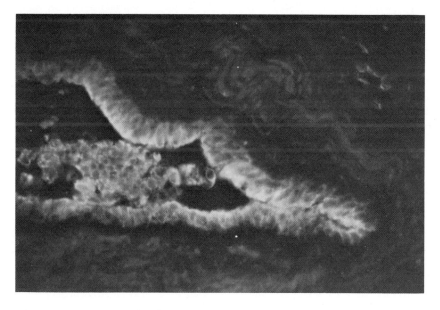

Fig.2. Estrogen binding sites are displayed by macromolecular fluorescent estradiol analog: cytoplasmic unoccupied
estrogen receptors of epithelial normal cells are brightly
demonstrated in breast tissue.

Some of these steroid derivatives retain enough affinity
for specific receptors, but they are prevented by their
size from getting through the plasmamembrane of intact
cells (Fig.3), so that they may be utilized only on tissue
sections for displaying intracellular binding sites.

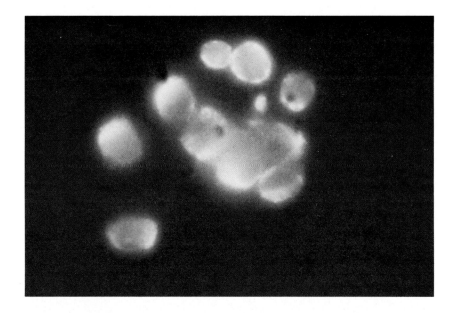

Fig.3. Specific binding sites for estrogens are traced on
the plasmamembrane of isolated cells from human breast
cancer. The incubation with fluorescent estrogen was
carried out at room temperature for 30 min: note that some
cells display the bound estrogen concentrated into polar
caps.

The third generation of techniques could be named
MOLECULAR CYTOCHEMISTRY since exploits steroid molecules
directly labelled with a fluorescent tracer, like estradiol
linked to fluorescein at the seventeen position. These
smaller derivatives have been shown to bind specifically
and with high affinity to cytosolic estrogen receptors and
to interact with intact target cells both in vivo and
in vitro in a way like the native hormone. Therefore these
fluorescent hormonal probes can yield information on the
overall intracellular kinetics of hormone-receptor complexes
in vital cells under appropriate experimental conditions.

VALIDATION OF CYTOCHEMICAL TECHNIQUES

Generally, the success of a given method in achieving its purpose - for instance, the effective detection of specific steroid receptors - may be judged by two main factors, that is its practicability and its reliability. As to PRACTICABILITY a glance at the recent literature leaves no doubt that a sufficient variety of cytochemical methods for hormone receptors is available today to suit almost every purpose. Criteria for RELIABILITY of this particular application of cytochemistry do not differ in essential lines from those defined for other methods of detection exploiting labelled ligands, either hormones or antibodies; they are efficiency, specificity, sensitivity, precision and accuracy. In evaluating the performance of steroid receptor cytochemistry, these classical reliability parameters correspond the accepted criteria for steroid receptors (saturability, high affinity, steroid and tisue specificity, correlation with biological response). When these criteria are appropriately investigated, it can be concluded that in careful hands cytochemical techniques visualize steroid bindig sites which share the same proper-ties with the specific biochemical receptors. In this respect, it has been suggested that at least a part of the cytochemical positivity could be due to the type II sites recently described. These type II sites are known to be present only in target tissues and to be strictly correlated to the type I receptor sites, even if in larger amounts and with a lower affinity constant than receptor sites. They are full-title specific estrogen binding proteins, but their physiological meaning is presently uncertain, even if it has been suggested that they are directly correlated with the effect of estradiol on the control of tissue growth. It has been also suggested that the type II sites could be a form of inactive receptor or of reserve immature receptor.

Above all, the receptor nature of the localizations obtained by the cytochemical ligand techniqeus is now being validated by the results issuing from the last genera-tion of specific cytochemistry, that is RECEPTOR IMMUNOCYTO-CHEMISTRY: polyclonal and chiefly monoclonal antibodies against receptor proteins are now available. This hybridoma technology which allows for the production of monospecific immunoglobulins has revolutionized also this area of the cell biology since these tools may provide information fundamental for fully understanding the complex events of receptor mechanism of action.

When coupled with a high sensitivity display system such as the bridged avidin biotin technique or the peroxidase

antiperoxidase technique monoclonal antibodies prove to be
ideally suited for the immunoenzyme localizatio of estrogen
receptors in tissue and cell preparations. Now, the preliminary results by monoclonal antibody are confirming the
previous basic and applied data obtained with the cytochemical
techniques exploiting the binding properties of the same
receptor molecule of which the antibody traces the antigenic
sites. It seems worth stressing that the antibody recognizes
all the receptor molecules, both occupied and unoccupied by
the hormone, while previous ligand techniques were able to
trace only free receptor sites.

STEROID-CELL INTERACTION. BASIC ASPECTS.

Main events in the steroid-cell interaction may be
traced today thanks to cytochemical methods.

PLASMAMEMBRANE. While the major evidence is unques-
tionably in support of the prominence of the intracellular
receptor mechanism, evidence has been provided for the
occurrence of specific binding sites for steroid hormones in
the plasmamembrane of steroid-target cells. Affinity
binding approaches on intact cell system appear to be
ideally suited for binding studies to the cell surface more
than disrupting procedures. Such an approach using protein
linked fluorescent estrogen and steroid derivatized agarose
beads have demonstrated that estrogen target cells are
equipped with a structural component fully integrated in the
fluid mosaic of the plasmamembrane, which represents a level
of steroid-cell interaction additional to the classical
cytoplasmic receptor.

STEROID RECEPTOR MECHANISM. A prevalent cytoplasmic
localization of the receptor protein in the absence of the
hormone is well documented by all cytochemical techniques.
Electron microscopy resolves the cytoplasmic positivity
into a main localization at the level of microsomal profiles.
Though the soluble phase of cell homogenates is widely
considered as the major subcellular localization of steroid
receptors, recent studies have shown that the structure
(like membrane, microsomal and cytoskeletal components) -
associated receptor represents a major, if not the entire,
receptor population in the cell. On the contrary, in the
presence of steroid hormones, like the normal in vivo
situation, the receptor is traced predominantly in the cell
nucleus. The most vital element in the steroid action chain

is the translocation of steroid-receptor complexes from the cytoplasm to the nucleus within target cells. The shift of the steroid receptor subcellular distribution in favor of the nucleus upon warming is a reproducible step in whole cell systems. It is worth noting that the translocation step seems to be subserved, at least in part, by a vesicular shuttle system ("transferosome") providing a particulate channel for the intracellular steroid information flow, like the "receptosome" and "diacytosome" transport systems recently described for polypeptide hormones. Such a particulate channel implies that the nuclear entry has to employ a non-diffusional mechanism at the nuclear membrane level. In the electron microscopic pictures it appears as though, getting into touch with the nuclear membrane, the shuttle particles may adhere to and incorporate into the membrane then dissolving in the nuclear interior. Moreover, it appears that the shifting of receptors from the cytoplasm to the nucleus may be brought about in intact cells by hyper-termic treatment through some presently unknown induced change in the receptor molecule, in the absence of the specific hormone, too (Fig.4).

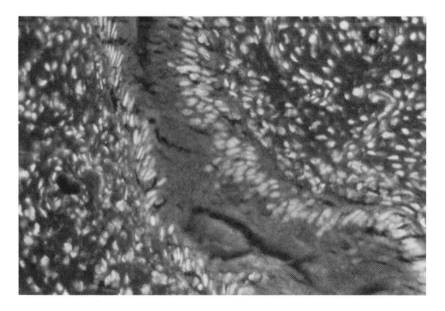

Fig.4. Estrogen receptors are traced at the nuclear level of both epithelial and stromal cells of a spayed rat uterus preheated at 39°C for 30 min: the nuclear translocation of free receptors has been induced by the hyperthermic treatment.

STEROID ACTION MECHANISM. APPLIED ASPECTS.

The opportunity of interfacing biochemical findings
with biological processes allowed by steroid receptor
cytochemistry appears chiefly appreciable when dealing with
the hormonal control of heterogeneous tissues such as cancer
tissues.

BREAST CANCER. One of the most significant outcomes
of estrogen receptor cytochemistry in human breast cancer
has been the very apparent heterogeneity in hormone receptivity of tumor cells. Most of the investigated breast
tumors have proved to be composed of mixed receptor-positive
and receptor-negative cell populations in a variable proportion. Tumors displaying homogeneous cell types - all cells
exhibiting estrogen receptors or not - are seen rarely (Fig. 5).

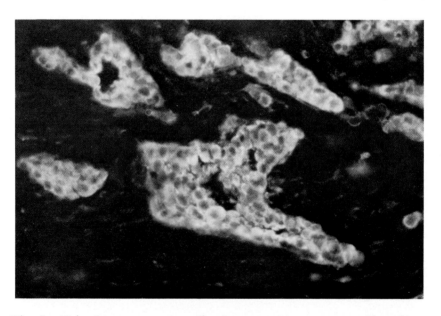

Fig.5. This breast cancer displays an homogeneous distribution of cytoplasmic free estrogen receptors among neoplastic
cells.

Moreover, positive tumor cells frequently express different
amounts of receptors; it may be that this varying positivity

is related to some extent to the cell cycle.

This very apparent heterogeneity may explain the fact that the probability of tumor regression after endocrine therapy correlates better with a quantitative than a simply qualitative assessment of estrogen receptors.

Besides, the dynamic monitoring of the receptor mechanism has shown that many tumors contain a varying number of cells that fail to translocate the bound estradiol into the nucleus in spite of a normal cytoplasmic receptor uptake, so that many cells do not display any nuclear estradiol incorporation at permissive temperature. It is also worthy of note that in some tumours there are a number of cells that lack the prolonged nuclear retention of the translocated complexes. Such a failure of translocation or binding of estrogen receptor complexes into nuclei of receptor-positive breast tumours, demonstrated at first by cytochemical techniques, has been later confirmed by in vitro tissue slice technique combined with a biochemical assay. These defects in the receptor pathway distal to the initial estrogen binding may be considered to involve the insensitivity of receptor-positive cells to hormonal effects. So that it has been suggested that the assessment of either the nuclear bound receptors or a final product of the hormone receptor mechanism may provide a better indicator of hormone responsiveness that just the assay of cytoplasmic receptors.

Finally, uncharged nuclear receptors have sometimes been demonstrated in histochemical preparations: a predominant nuclear estrogen receptor pattern has been seen in a limited number of cases (Fig. 6); more often a significant combination of nuclear and cytoplasmic positivity was observed (Fig. 7). These observations are in keeping with the recent demonstration that breast tumours may contain uncharged nuclear estrogen receptors also in the absence of cytosolic receptors, chiefly in the central part of the tumor mass. It may be that in central districts of the tumour some metabolic event happens which brings about the nuclear receptor translocation in a way like that obtained by the experimental tissue heating.

This cell heterogeneity in cytoplasmic uptake, nuclear translocation and binding is very apparent with all of the cytochemical techniques and it seems so constitutive of breast cancer that it stands out as a biological constant of this tumor (Fig.8).

It seems also worthy of mention that it seems to be sufficient the positivity of 20% of the cell pupulation to give a positive result by biochemical assays. This in turn signifies that in tumors considered as positive by biochemical receptor assays, the hormone responsiveness could be actually restricted to one fifth of their cell population, a thing to

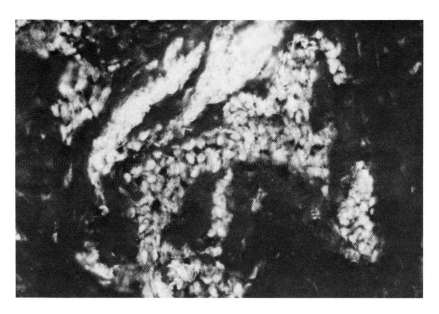

Fig.6. Uncharged nuclear estrogen receptors are shown in the central area of the same tumor presented in Fig.4; the two diffused flourescent areas on top of the figure represent yellow autofluorescence of elastosis.

keep in mind when dealing with the clinical management.

These observations concerning cell heterogeneity are clinically relevant, in that the demarcation line between hormone responsiveness and refractoriness not only splits different tumors - that is at the clinical level - but it runs through each tumor at the biological level. Generally, this cell heterogeneity is not reflected by distinctive morphological features, which offer little clue as to the scope of hormone sensitivity; nevertheless, in some instances a relationship between the presence of estrogen receptors and the cell differentiation can be recognized at the cytological level. As a general rule, it could be said that when differentiated features are present in breast cancer cells, they couple with the presence of estradiol receptors; while the contrary is not mandatory.

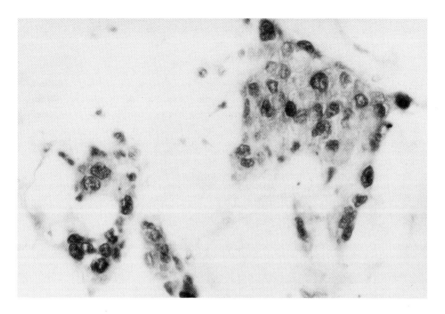

Fig.7. Monoclonal antibody against estrogen receptor traces both cytoplasmic and nuclear, filled and unfilled, receptor molecules in breast cancer cells.

Clearly, it is not possible at present to say because and when in neoplastic transformation this cell heterogeneity arises. However, cytochemical data suggest that breast cancer is a very complex entity from its first detectable expression: at the cellular level a heterogeneous cell the hormone receptivity is already present in the incipient esent tumor and appears to be a trait of breast cancer from its inception.

The logic of almost all existing strategies for cancer therapy can be summarized in these terms: "malignant cells resemble each other and differ from normal cells: identify and exploit the difference". A fundamental weakness of this notion is that it neglects variation within a given tumor cell population. This is true also for receptor distribution and hormone responsiveness. The evolution of diversity among the progeny of tumor cells is clearly a major factor

in cancer progression and it is probably the fundamental
reason for the shortcomings of current therapy, included

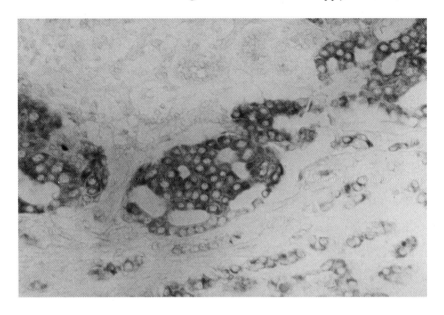

Fig.8. Cell heterogeneity in estrogen receptor levels is
very apparent in breast cancer: positive and negative cells
by monoclonal receptor antibody are irregularly intermingled.

endocrine therapy. At the same time, heightened awareness
of the fact that tumour cells are heterogeneous may offer
scope for alternative strategies.

ACKNOWLEDGEMENT. The experimental work was supported in
part by the National Research Council, Special Project
"Control of Neoplastic Growth" (grants n.81.01361.96 and
82.00301.96) and by the Ministero della Pubblica Istruzione,
Italy.

REFERENCES
Only the relevant personal references are cited.

STEROID RECEPTOR CYTOCHEMISTRY

-Nenci I, Beccati MD, Piffanelli A, Lanza G (1976). Detection

and dynamic localisation of estradiol receptor complexes in intact target cells by immunofluorescene technique. J Steroid Biochem 7:505.
-Nenci I (1979). Estrogen receptor immunocytochemistry. J Histochem Cytochem 27:1053.
-Nenci I, Dandliker WB, Meyers CY, Marzola A, Marchetti E, Fabris G (1980). Estrogen receptor cytochemistry by fluorescent estrogen. J Histochem Cytochem 28:1081.
-Nenci I, Fabris G, Marzola A, Marchetti E (1980). Hormone receptor cytochemistry in human breast cancer.
In Iacobelli S, King RJB, Lindner HR, Lippman ME (eds): "Hormones and Cancer", New York: Raven Press, p 227.
-Nenci I, Marchetti E (1982). Evaluating the performance of steroid receptor cytochemistry. In Kaiser E, Gabl F, Muller MM, Bayer M (eds): "XI International Congress of Clinical Chemistry", Berlin: Walter de Gruyter & Co., p 487.

STEROID-CELL INTERACTIONS

PLASMAMEMBRANE
-Nenci I, Fabris G, Marchetti E, Marzola A (1980). Cytochemical evidence for steroid binding sites in the plasmamembrane of target cells. In Bresciani F (ed): "Perspectives in Steroid Receptor Research", New York: Raven Press, p 61.
-Nenci I, Marchetti E, Marzola A, Fabris G (1981). Affinity cytochemistry visualizes specific estrogen binding sites on the plasma membrane of breast cancer cells. J Steroid Biochem 14:1139.
-Nenci I, Fabris G, Marzola A, Marchetti E (1981). The plasma membrane as an additional level of steroid-cell interaction. J Steroid Biochem 15:231.
-Nenci I (1983). Specific cell adhesion to estradiol-derivatized agarose beads. J Steroid Biochem 17:in press.

RECEPTOR MECHANISM
-Nenci I, Piffanelli A, Beccati MD, Lanza G (1976). In vivo and in vitro immunofluorescent approach to the pathophysiology of estradiol kinetics in target cells. J Steroid Biochem 7:883.
-Nenci I, Beccati MD, Piffanelli A, Lanza G (1977). Dynamic immunofluorescence tracing of estradiol interaction with cytoplasmic and nuclear constitutents in target cells. Res Steroids 7:137.
-Nenci I, Fabris G, Marzola A, Marchetti E (1980). Steroid-

cell interactions revealed by immunological probes and electron microscopy. In Genazzani E, DiCarlo F, Mainwaring WIP (eds): "Pharmacological Modulation of Steroid Action", New York: Raven Press, p 99.
-Nenci I, Fabris G, Marchetti E, Marzola A (1980). Intra-cellular flow of particulate steroid-receptor complexes in steroid target cells. Virchows Arch B Cell Pathol 32:139.
-Nenci I, Fabris G, Marzola A, Bagni A, Poli G, Marchetti E (1983). Charting steroid-cell interaction by visual means. In McKerns KW (ed): "Regulation of Target Cell Responsiveness", New York: Plenum Press (in press).

BREAST CANCER
-Nenci I (1978). Receptor and centriole pathways of steroid action in normal and neoplastic cells. Cancer Res 38:4204.
-Nenci I (1981). Estrogen receptor cytochemistry in human breast cancer. Status and prospects. Cancer 48:2674.
-Nenci I, Marchetti E, Marzola A, Fabris G, Rotola A (1982). Bases et applications de la cytochemie des recepteurs steroidiens. Int J Breast Mammary Pathol 1:15.

Hormones and Cancer, pages 37–51
© 1984 Alan R. Liss, Inc., 150 Fifth Avenue, New York, NY 10011

EFFECT OF ESTROGEN IN BREAST CANCER CELLS IN CULTURE :
RELEASED PROTEINS AND CONTROL OF CELL PROLIFERATION *

Henri Rochefort, Dany Chalbos, Françoise Capony,
Marcel Garcia, Frédéric Veith, Françoise Vignon
and Bruce Westley

Unité d'Endocrinologie Cellulaire et Moléculaire
U 148 I.N.S.E.R.M.
60, Rue de Navacelles - 34100 Montpellier France

1. INTRODUCTION

Estrogens stimulate both gene expression and cell
proliferation in breast cancer cells. Specific intracellular estrogen receptors are required to mediate these
effects but not sufficient, since 50 % of human breast
cancers containing estrogen receptor (RE+) will not
respond to endocrine therapy (McGuire, 1975). In order to
evaluate the estrogen responsiveness, McGuire and
colleagues (Osborne, McGuire, 1979 ; Horwitz et al, 1978)
have proposed that the progesterone receptor (RP) is
assayed in addition to the RE as the RP is known to be
stimulated by estrogen. However, there are many examples
of discrepancy between the effect of estrogens on RP
induction and the stimulation of breast cancer growth
(Koenders et al, 1977 ; Ip et al, 1979 ; Rochefort et al,
1980 b). Besides, antiestrogens prevent cell growth while
they induce the RP (Horwitz et al, 1978). Moreover, there
are still 20 % of RP (–) patients who respond to endocrine
therapy and 20 % of RP (+) who do not respond (Osborne,
McGuire, 1979). In order to find better marker than the RP
to predict the responsiveness of tumor to estrogens, it is
useful to understand better the mechanism by which
estrogens stimulate cell proliferation. For this purpose,
we have choosen to use the in vitro cell culture approach
which present many advantages over the in vivo approach as
far as it is able to reproduce the effect of hormones
observed in vivo. We have therefore investigated the
effect of estrogen in vitro on the cell proliferation and
the synthesis of specific proteins in MCF_7 and $T_{47}D$ human

---

* Presented at the International Symposium on "Hormones and
Cancer", Buenos Aires, 9-13 May 1983.

breast cancer cell lines both of which were established from metastatic pleural effusions.

We will successively discuss : 1°. The effect of estradiol on the growth of these cells. 2°. The effect of estrogens on protein synthesis with the evidence for an increased production in the medium of a 52 K glycoprotein. 3°. The possible relationship between the estrogen regulated released proteins and the control of cell proliferation including the negative effect of antiestrogens on these responses. 4°. The evidence that the 52 K protein is present and released in primary culture by estrogen receptor positive metastatic breast cancer and the potential clinical applications of this protein in breast cancer.

2. IN VITRO EFFECT OF ESTRADIOL ON CELL PROLIFERATION

It is generally agreed that estrogens in vivo stimulate the growth of some hormone dependent tumors (Banbury Report, 1981). The extent of their direct effect on breast cancer cell lines in vitro, however, has varied considerably according to the investigators and the cells being studied. Many laboratories have failed to show an in vitro effect of estrogens (Sonnenschein, Soto, 1980 ; Shafie, 1980) and one popular hypothesis is that estrogens act indirectly via the liberation of growth factors (estromedins) released from other tissues (Sirbasku, Benson, 1979).

To demonstrate a mitogenic effect of estrogens in cells containing estrogen receptor, the cell culture conditions and the withdrawal of cells from endogenous estrogens (Vignon et al, 1980) are critical. One laboratory has previously shown that estradiol (E_2) is able to stimulate directly the growth of MCF_7 (Aitken, Lippman, 1980) and ZR_{75-1} (Allegra, Lippman, 1978) cells. In order to confirm and extend this finding, we have studied the regulation of the growth of two cloned sublines derived from the $T_{47}D$ metastatic human breast cancer cells (Keydar et al, 1979). Cell proliferation was evaluated by DNA assay, cell counts and thymidine incorporation. In clone 11 which contains estrogen and progesterone receptors, estradiol (1 pM to 1 nM) stimulated cell proliferation 2 to 5 fold after a lag period of 6 days (Fig. 1). Maximal stimulation by estradiol was observed in the presence of 1 or 3 % fetal calf serum and without added insulin. The effect of estradiol was biphasic since the growth rate was stimulated at E_2 concentrations 10 nM and then progressively inhibited at higher concentrations. Dexamethasone, Dihydrotestosterone, Progesterone and R_{5020} (at 1 nM or 1 μM) did not modify cell growth.

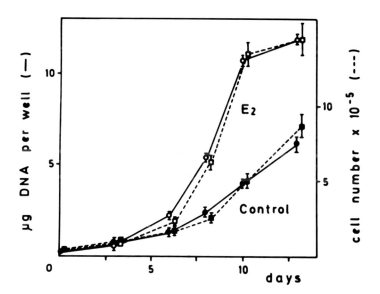

Figure 1. Effect of estradiol on the growth of $T_{47}D$ cells in function of time. On day -2, cells were plated in medium containing 3 % FCS/DCC and without added insulin. They were then incubated from day 0 with (o,□) or without (●,■) 1 nM E_2. The amount of DNA (●,o,——) was evaluated by the diaminobenzoic acid fluorescence assay in triplicate wells and represented as the mean ± SD of 3 determinations. Cell numbers (■,□,---) were counted in 3 other wells, using a hemocytometer and represented as the mean ±SD of 6 determinations.

(From Chalbos et al, 1982, by permission).

By contrast, in clone 8 which contains low concentrations of estrogen and progesterone receptors, estradiol was ineffective on cell growth. Recently, we have also confirmed that estradiol stimulates the growth rate of MCF$_7$ cells, while for all estrogen receptor positive cell lines, Tamoxifen and hydroxytamoxifen drastically decrease this growth rate below the control level (Keydar et al, 1979 ; Chalbos et al, 1982 ; Coezy et al, 1982). Contrary to the absolute requirement of estrogens for growth observed in vivo with MCF$_7$ cells, in vitro these cells were however able to grow in the absence of estrogens, suggesting either some synergic effect of extra ovarian and extra tumoral factor, or the artefactual stimulation of growth in the culture medium (Shafie, 1980 ; Sirbasku, Benson, 1979 ; Leung, Shiu, 1981). However other laboratories (Darbre et al, 1983 ; Page et al, 1983) have now reported that estrogens can stimulate the growth of breast cancer cells in culture and it is likely that the failure to demonstrate such an effect was due to different experimental conditions or to the use of cells having lost their estrogen responsiveness for growth. Other general responses are also observed in addition to the stimulation of cell proliferation. These are a general increase of RNA and protein synthesis and morphological modifications of the cells, as observed by transmission and scanning electron microscopy (Vic et al, 1982). The major modifications concern the surface of the cell membrane where estradiol provokes a large increase in the number and the length of microvillae within 2 days of treatment followed by the occurrence of secretory like granules at the cell surface. Moreover, the cells become more rounded after E$_2$ treatment and have a greater tendency to become detached from the substrate (Vic et al, 1982). Similar modifications are observed in the androgen responsive Shionogi 115 cell line (Yates, King, 1981).

3. EVIDENCE FOR ESTROGEN INDUCED PROTEINS IN MCF$_7$ - THE 52 K PROTEIN

Several proteins induced by estrogen in breast cancer cell lines have been described (Butler et al, 1979 ; Edwards et al, 1980 ; Mairesse et al, 1980 ; Bronzert et al, 1981). We actually found several estradiol stimulated proteins by using ^{35}S-methionine labelling of proteins and two dimensional gel analysis (Westley, Rochefort, 1980 ; Kaye et al, 1981). Some of these cellular proteins have potential interests, however they can only be assayed in tumor samples collected during surgery. This is why we have searched for estrogen induced proteins which would be secreted by the cells in an attempt to find potential circulating marker(s) of hormone dependency in breast cancer.

We have therefore analysed the proteins released into the medium by several continuous breast cancer cell lines which are either hormone responsive (MCF_7, ZR_{75-1} and $T_{47}D$) or hormone unresponsive (BT_{20}, HBL_{100} - clone 8 of $T_{47}D$).

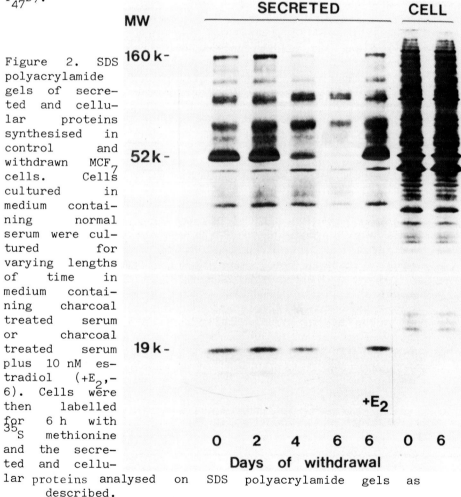

Figure 2. SDS polyacrylamide gels of secreted and cellular proteins synthesised in control and withdrawn MCF_7 cells. Cells cultured in medium containing normal serum were cultured for varying lengths of time in medium containing charcoal treated serum or charcoal treated serum plus 10 nM estradiol ($+E_2$,-6). Cells were then labelled for 6 h with ^{35}S methionine and the secreted and cellular proteins analysed on SDS polyacrylamide gels as described.

(From Westley and Rochefort, 1980, by permission).

Using protein labelling by ^{35}S-methionine followed by SDS polyacrylamide gel electrophoresis and fluorography, we found that estrogens stimulated the production of proteins which were released into the medium (Westley, Rochefort, 1980). Some of them were more particularly induced, a 160 K protein and a major one, representing 20 to 40 % of these secretory proteins[*1] which had a molecular weight of 52,000 daltons in denaturating conditions (Fig. 2). The increased production of this protein was specific for physiological concentrations of estrogens. Progesterone and Dexamethasone were inactive. Any steroid able to activate the RE after binding was also able to induce this protein which therefore gave a very convenient in vitro test to assess the estrogenic activity of ligands (Rochefort et al, 1980 b). For instance, the 52 K protein was also induced by the estrogen 3 sulfate but not the 17 sulfate in MCF$_7$ cells. This finding was surprising since estrogen sulfates have no or only a low affinity for RE. However, we found that MCF$_7$ cells are able to hydrolyse the sulfate$_3$ ester bond of ^{3}H estrone 3 sulfate thus liberating ^{3}H estrone which was recovered, bound to the nuclear RE (Vignon et al, 1980). Androgens were also able to stimulate this protein but only when their concentrations and affinities for RE were sufficient to occupy the RE sites (Rochefort et al, 1980). Thus, pharmacological concentrations of DHT (0.5μM) behave as estrogen agonist. This effect of androgens on the induction of the 52 K protein was inhibited by antiestrogen. Adrenal androgens such as 5-androstenediol and DHEA were also able to induce in vitro the 52 K protein at physiological concentrations (Adams et al, 1981), suggesting that they could behave directly as estrogens. These results indicate that these steroids, chemically defined as androgens, are also biologically active estrogens and that the plasma concentration of adrenal androgens mostly in post-menopausal or ovariectomised women, may play a role in stimulating the growth of hormone dependent cancer. Other hormones (Prolactin, Insulin) or growth factors (charcoal treated fetal calf serum and EGF), were found inactive in stimulating the production of the 52 K protein suggesting that this protein was not triggered by these mitogenic agent (Vignon, unpublished) (Table 1).

*1. The molecular weight was first found to be 46,000 daltons when using 15 % polyacrylamide gels. It seems to be closer to 52,000 daltons in 10 % polyacrylamide gels and using the NEN protein markers.

PRODUCTION OF THE 52 K PROTEIN IN MCF7 : HORMONE SPECIFICITY

STIMULATION		NO EFFECT	
Estradiol	0.1 nM	Progesterone	up to 1 μM
Diethylstilboestrol	0.1 nM	Dexamethasone	
Estrone	1 nM	Estradiol 17β SO_4	
Estriol	1 nM	T_3, up to 0.1 μM	
DHT	0.5 μM	Prolactin, up to 20 nM	
Estradiol 3 SO_4	1 nM	Insulin, up to 0.1 μM	
Estrone 3 SO_4	10 nM	EGF, from 16 pM to 16 nM	
		Charcoal treated FCS up to 10%	

Table 1. Hormonal specificity for the increased production by MCF_7 cells of the 52 K glycoprotein in the medium. The 52 K glycoprotein was evaluated in percent of total released protein as described in Fig. 1. Results from Westley and Rochefort (1980), Vignon et al (1980) and Vignon (unpublished experiments) are summarized. Only ligands able to activate the RE were efficient to stimulate the production of the 52 K protein showing that it is strictly an estrogen specific response. Hormones which also increase cell proliferation of MCF_7 cells such as Insulin or EGF were inefficient in the range of concentration tested.

The 52 K protein has been characterized and antibodies have been developped (Capony et al, 1982). This is a glycoprotein as shown by its micro heterogeneity in 2D gel electrophoresis, its sensitivity to neuraminidase and tunicamycin, its labelling by ^3H fucose and other sugar, and its selective retention on Con A Sepharose. A regulation at the transcriptional level is likely as suggested by the effect of Actinomycin D and α Amanitin (M. Garcia et al, in preparation). Whether the protein is secreted by exocytosis or shedded from plasma membranes cannot be presently specified since electron microscopic studies indicate that estrogens both stimulate the secretory activity of MCF_7 cells and modify markedly the plasma membrane surface (Vic et al, 1982).

The identity and function of this 52 K protein is presently unknown. We can however exclude that it is a major milk protein such as the human casein and α lactalbumin, which have different MW and do not seem to be present or estrogen induced in MCF_7 cells.

4. POSSIBLE RELATIONSHIP BETWEEN THE ESTROGEN REGULATED RELEASED PROTEINS AND CONTROL OF CELL PROLIFERATION

Several evidences support the hypothesis that the regulation of the proteins released into the medium is correlated to, if not responsible for, the regulation by estrogens and antiestrogens of cell growth (Rochefort et al, 1980 a).

The effects of estrogens and of several antiestrogens on the production of the 52 K (or related) secretory protein and on the control of cell proliferation appear to be parallel.

a. Estrogens Stimulate both Responses

Estrogens stimulate <u>in vitro</u> the growth of RE positive breast cancer cells (MCF_7, ZR_{75-1}, $T_{47}D$) and the production of the 52 K (or 60 K) protein at the same physiological concentrations (Table 2).

MARKERS OF RESPONSES TO ESTROGEN IN HUMAN BREAST CELL LINES

	MCF_7	ZR_{75-1}	$T_{47}D$ CL. 11	BT_{20}	$T_{47}D$ CL. 8	HBL_{100}
R_E	+	+	+	−	−	−
R_P	+	+	++	−	--	−
52 K $-E_2$	−	−	− (60 K)	+	−	−
52 K $+E_2$	+	+	+	+	−	−
E_2 ON CELL PROLIFERATION	+	+	+	ND	−	ND

Table 2. Results obtained from three estrogen responsive metastatic breast cancer cell lines (MCF_7, ZR_{75-1} and $T_{47}D$ cells clone 11) contrast with results obtained in three unresponsive human mammary cell lines. BT20 = primary breast cancer, $T_{47}D$ cl. 8 = pleural metastasis, HBL100 = "normal" mammary cells (milk). Receptors for estrogen (RE) and progesterone (RP) were determined by charcoal assay. The presence and inducibility of the 52 K protein was determined after ^{35}S methionine labelling by SDS PAGE and effect of estradiol on cell proliferation by DNA assay. ND = not determined.

On the basis of its molecular weight, Concanavalin A reactivity, inducibility by estrogens and antigenic reactivity with polyclonal antibodies to the 52 K protein, we could identify this glycoprotein in both the MCF_7 and ZR_{75-1} cell lines. By contrast, it was not detected in the $T_{47}D$ cell line where another group of released proteins (60 K) was stimulated by estradiol (Capony et al, 1982). Another breast cancer cell line (BT20) which is unresponsive to estrogen, appears to produce constitutively the 52 K protein in the medium (Capony et al, in preparation). In the estrogen responsive cell lines, the induction of these proteins (52 K and 60 K) by E_2 clearly anticipates (2 days-lag) the stimulation of cell growth.

When the culture media are changed less often, the effect of E_2 on cell growth, compared to the control, is much greater suggesting that the medium is conditioned by factors released by the cells.

b. Several Antiestrogens (Progestins and non Steroidal) Inhibit both Responses for the same Concentrations

In MCF_7 cells, tamoxifen is totally inactive in inducing the 52 K protein but prevents E_2 action in a molar ratio of $\simeq 10^3$. Monohydroxy tamoxifen, a metabolite of tamoxifen which binds RE with a high affinity, is 100 fold more potent than tamoxifen itself for blocking the cell growth (Coezy et al, 1982) and the induction of the 52 K secreted protein by E_2 (Westley, Rochefort, 1980).

By contrast in the R_{27} cells, an antiestrogen resistant clone of MCF_7 cells established by Nawata et al (1981), tamoxifen does not inhibit cell growth but stimulates markedly the biosynthesis of the 52 K protein (Vignon et al, submitted).

Progestins such as R5020 are able to inhibit successively and at the same concentrations the production of estrogen induced released protein and the estrogen stimulated cell proliferation (Vignon et al, 1983 b ; Chalbos et al, submitted, see also in this Book Rochefort, 1983).

c. More Direct Evidence

Recent experiments indicate that conditioned medium from cells treated by estrogens stimulate the growth of MCF_7 cells to a larger extent than the conditioned medium from cells which had not been treated (Vignon et al, 1983 a). This conditioned medium has no growth stimulatory activity after its passage through a Concanavalin A Sepharose column which retains glycoproteins including the estrogen stimulated protein 52 K. The E_2 conditioned medium also induces the appearance of numerous microvillae on the cell surface.

These results suggest that glycoproteins present in the medium, might act as growth factors, mediating, as 2nd extracellular messengers, the mitogenic effect of estrogen on mammary cells. The 52 K protein is a good candidate for being such a growth factor since it is the major estrogen regulated protein of the medium. However, this conditioned medium also contains other minor estrogen regulated proteins. Moreover in the $T_{47}D$ cell line, estradiol stimulates the cell proliferation and the production of 60 K protein(s) and not of the 52 K protein. Therefore the 52 K protein does not seem to be required in these cells and may be replaced by other estrogen induced growth factors. The availibility of specific antibodies against the 52 K protein might allow us to prove whether or not the 52 K protein is a growth factor responsible for the stimulatory activity of media conditioned in the presence of estrogens (Garcia et al, in preparation). Other function of this protein are currently not excluded such as protease, spreading, attachment or angiogenic factors, protein kinase, etc...

5. PRESENCE OF THE 52 K PROTEIN IN HUMAN BREAST CANCER AND POSSIBLE CLINICAL APPLICATIONS

In addition to their basic interest for understanding the mechanism of modulation of breast cancer by hormones, the E_2 induced proteins have potential clinical applications. The evidence that the 52 K protein might be a better marker of estrogen responsiveness than the RP is presently mostly circumstancial. It is certain that this protein is a very specific criterion of estrogen responsiveness. Without estrogen its level is near negligible and it is very specifically regulated by estrogens. Its assay also requires less cells (5×10^4 cells) than the assay of the RP (5×10^7 cells). As already mentioned, it is likely that this protein is more closely related to cell growth that the RP. Finally, the 52 K protein being released into the medium, could be secreted into the blood and serve as a usefull circulating marker of hormone dependency in human breast cancer. The 52 K protein appears therefore to be a potentially interesting marker for estrogen responsiveness of breast cancers.

However, before suggesting any clinical application, it was most important to demonstrate that this protein is actually made and secreted by breast cancer tissue and not only by continuous cell lines.

We have recently demonstrated its presence in patients bearing breast cancer by using two different approaches to assess its hormonal regulation. In the first approach, biopsies were taken in patients having cutaneous metastasis, before and after Tamoxifen treatment. This work performed in collaboration with the Centre de Lutte contre le Cancer of Montpellier (Prs Pujol and Pourquier) allowed us to show that in some patients the pattern of secretory proteins was different before and after Tamoxifen treatment (Veith et al, 1981). In most cases, a majoritary protein located in the 40-60 K region was markedly decreased after antiestrogen. The second approach was to study the in vitro effect of estrogens on protein synthesis in primary culture of pleural metastasis of human breast cancer. A 52 K glycoprotein induced by E_2 was demonstrated in most of the E_2 responsive pleural effusions. It displayed the same characteristics (hormone regulation, Con A reactivity, mol. weight, pHi and antigenicity) as the protein described in MCF_7 cells (Veith et al, 1983). These results indicate that the 52 K protein is not restricted to continuous cell line but is also made in the human breast cancer and that the MCF_7 cell line is a good model to study metastatic breast cancer.

6. CONCLUSIONS

Estrogen responsive breast cancer cell lines (MCF_7, $T_{47}D$) provide an excellent in vitro experimental system to study the mechanism by which estrogen stimulate the growth of epithelial breast cancer cells. We have described a 52 K glycoprotein released by cell lines and primary culture of metastatic breast cancer which is specifically increased by estrogen. This protein is a potential circulating marker of estrogen responsiveness of breast cancer. We propose that this (or other) estrogen induced protein(s) is (are) acting on the same breast cancer cells to autostimulate their growth as has been described for transforming growth factors (DeLarco, Todaro, 1978). Such transforming growth factors could be produced constitutively in hormone independent cancer or under hormonal control in hormone responsive cancer.

However, further work is required to specify the mechanism of the regulation by estrogens of these proteins, to determine their biological function and tissue specificity. The purification of the 52 K protein, the preparation of monoclonal antibodies and the purification of the cDNA and genomic sequence coding for this protein would help to reach these aims. The possible role of these proteins in earlier estrogen regulated step(s) of mammary cancerogenesis might also stimulate further experiments.

This study was supported by the "Institut National de la Santé et de la Recherche Médicale", the NCI-INSERM cooperation on "Hormones and Cancer" and the "Fondation pour la Recherche Médicale Française". We thank Mrs D. Derocq, Mr C. Rougeot and Mrs J. Vanbiervliet for their excellent technical assistance and Miss E. Barrié for her skilfull preparation of the manuscript. We are grateful to Drs M. Lippman, M. Rich, I. Keydar, and the Mason Research Institute, for their gifts of mammary cell lines.

REFERENCES

Adams J, Garcia M, Rochefort H (1981). Estrogenic effects of physiological concentrations of 5-Androstene-3 ,17 - diol and its metabolism in MCF7 human breast cancer cells. Cancer Res 41:4720.

Aitken SC, Lippman ME (1980). Hormonal regulation of net DNA synthesis in human breast cancer cells in tissue culture. In De Asua J et al. (eds): "Control Mechanisms in Animal Cells", New York: Raven Press, p 133.

Allegra JC, Lippman ME (1978). Growth of a human breast cancer cell line in serum-free hormone supplemented medium. Cancer Res 38:3823.

Banbury Report 8 (1981). "Hormones and Breast Cancer". Pike MC, Siiteri PK, Welsch CW (eds) Cold Spring Harbor Laboratory.

Bronzert DA, Monaco ME, Pinkus L, Aitken S, Lippman ME (1981). Purification and properties of estrogen-responsive cytoplasmic thymidine kinase from human breast cancer. Cancer Res 41:604.

Butler WB, Kirkland WL, Jorgensen TL (1979). Induction of plasminogen activator by estrogen in a human breast cancer cell line (MCF7). Biochem Biophys Res Commun 90:1328.

Capony F, Garcia M, Veith F, Rochefort H (1982).
Antibodies to the estrogen induced 52 K protein
released by human breast cancer cells. Biochem Biophys
Res Commun 108:8.

Chalbos D, Vignon F, Keydar I, Rochefort H (1982)
Estrogens stimulate cell proliferation and induce
secretory proteins in a human breast cancer cell line
(T47D). J Clin Endocrin Metab 55:276.

Chalbos D, Rochefort H. Dual effects of the progestin
R5020 on proteins released by the T47D human breast
cancer cells. Submitted for Publication.

Coezy E, Borgna JL, Rochefort H (1982). Tamoxifen and
metabolites in MCF7 cells : Correlation between binding
to estrogen receptor and inhibition of cell growth.
Cancer Res 42:317.

Darbre P, Yates J, Curtis S, King RJB (1983). Effect of
estradiol on human breast cancer cells in culture.
Cancer Res 43:349.

DeLarco JE, Todaro GJ (1978). Growth factors from murine
sarcoma virus-transformed cells. Proc Natl Acad Sci
USA 75:4001.

Edwards DP, Adams DJ, Savage N, McGuire WL (1980).
Estrogen-induced synthesis of specific proteins in
human breast cancer cells. Biochem Biophys Res Commun
93:804.

Horwitz KB, Kosedi Y, McGuire WL (1978). Estrogen control
of progesterone receptor in human breast cancer : Role
of estradiol and antiestrogen. Endocrinology 103:1742.

Ip M, Milholland RJ, Rosen F, Kim U (1979). Mammary
cancer : Selective action of the estrogen receptor
complex. Science 203:361.

Kaye AM, Reiss N, Shaer A, Sluyser M, Iacobelli S,
Amroch D, Soffer Y (1981). Estrogen responsive
creatine kinase in normal and neoplastic cells.
J Steroid Biochem 15:69.

Keydar I, Chen L, Karby S, Weiss FR, Delarea H, Radu M
(1979). Establishment and characterization of a cell
line of human breast carcinoma origin. Eur J Cancer
15:659.

Koenders AJM, Geurts-Moespot A, Zolinger SJ, Benraad TJ
(1977). Progesterone receptors in normal and neoplastic
tissues. New York: Raven Press, p 71.

Leung CKH, Shiu RPC (1981). Required presence of both
estrogen and pituitary factors for the growth of human
breast cancer cells in athymic nude mice. Cancer Res
41:546.

Mairesse N, Deuleeschonuer N, Leclerq G, Galand P (1980).
Estrogen-induced protein in the human breast cancer
cell line MCF7. Biochem Biophys Res Commun 97:1251.

McGuire WL, Carbonne PP, Vollmer EP (1975). Estrogen
receptors in human breast cancer. New York: Raven Press

Nawata H, Bronzert D, Lippman M (1981). Isolation and
characterization of a tamoxifen-resistant cell line
derived from MCF7 human breast cancer cells. J Biol
Chem 256:5016.

Osborne CK, McGuire WL (1979). The use of steroid hormone
receptors in the treatment of human breast cancer :
a review. Bulletin du Cancer 66:203.

Page MJ, Field JK, Everett NP, Green CD (1983). Serum
regulation of the estrogen responsiveness of the human
breast cancer cell line MCF-7. Cancer Res 43:1244.

Rochefort H, Coezy E, Joly E, Westley B, Vignon F
(1980 a). Hormonal control of breast cancer in cell
culture. In Iacobelli S, King R, Lindner H, Lippman M
(eds): "Progress in Cancer Research and Therapy,
Hormones and Cancer", New York: Raven Press, Vol 14,
p 21.

Rochefort H, Garcia M, Vignon F, Westley B (1980 b).
Proteins induced by the estrogen receptor in uterus
and breast cancer cells. In Beato M (ed): "Steroid
Induced Uterine Proteins", Amsterdam, New York, Oxford:
Elsevier/North-Holland Biomedical Press, p 171.

Shafie M (1980). Estrogen and the growth of breast
cancer new evidence suggests indirect action. Science
209:701.

Sirbasku DA, Benson RH (1979). Estrogen-inducible growth
factors that may act as mediators (estromedins) of
estrogen-promoted tumor cell growth. In Sato JH, Ross R
(eds): "Hormones and Cell Culture", Cold Spring Harbor
Conferences on Cell Proliferation, Cold Spring Harbor
Laboratory, Vol 6, p 477.

Sonnenschein C, Soto AM (1980). But... are estrogens
perse growth-promoting hormones ? J Natl Cancer Inst
64:211.

Veith F, Rochefort H, Saussol J, Bressot N, Pourquier H,
Pujol H (1981). Proteins secreted by human breast
cancer : Effect of tamoxifen. In "Reviews on Endocrine-
Related Cancer", Proceedings of International Symposium
on Anti-hormones and Breast Cancer, Nice, 26-27 Sept
1980, ICI, Suppl 9, p 229.

Veith F, Capony F, Garcia M, Chantelard J, Pujol H,
    Veith F, Zajdela A, Rochefort H (1983). Release of
    estrogen-induced glycoprotein with a molecular weight
    of 52,000 by breast cancer cells in primary culture.
    Cancer Res 43:

Vic P, Vignon F, Derocq D, Rochefort H (1982). Effect
    of estradiol on the ultrastructure of the MCF7 human
    breast cancer cells in culture. Cancer Res 42:667.

Vignon F, Terqui M, Westley B, Derocq D, Rochefort H
    (1980). Effects of plasma estrogen sulfates in mammary
    cancer cells. Endocrinology 106:1079.

Vignon F, Derocq D, Chambon M, Rochefort H (1983 a).
    Endocrinologie. Les protéines oestrogéno-induites
    sécrétées par les cellules mammaires cancéreuses
    humaines MCF7 stimulent leur prolifération. C R Acad
    Sci Paris 296:151.

Vignon F, Bardon S, Chalbos D, Rochefort H (1983 b).
    Antiestrogenic effect of R5020, a synthetic progestin
    in human breast cancer cells in culture. J Clin Endocr
    Metab (June).

Vignon F, Derocq D, Lippman M, Rochefort H. Antiestrogens
    induce two estrogen-responsive proteins in a tamoxifen
    resistant R27 clone of MCF7 cells. Submitted for
    publication.

Westley B, Rochefort H (1980). A secreted glycoprotein
    induced by estrogen in human breast cancer cell lines.
    Cell 20:353.

Yates J, King RJB (1981). Correlation of growth
    properties and morphology with hormone responsiveness
    of mammary tumor cells in culture. Cancer Res 41:258.

Hormones and Cancer, pages 53–62
© 1984 Alan R. Liss, Inc., 150 Fifth Avenue, New York, NY 10011

ESTROGEN-INDUCED PROTEINS IN ESTROGEN-SENSITIVE CELLS

Stefano Iacobelli, MD, Vittoria Natoli and Giovanni Scambia

Laboratorio di Endocrinologia Molecolare
Università Cattolica S. Cuore
00168 Roma - Italia

INTRODUCTION

Estrogen receptors are present in approximately 60% of primary human breast cancers. Only about half of these tumors respond to endocrine manipulations (Lippman, Allegra 1978). In patients with tumors having high levels of estrogen receptors the response rate to endocrine therapy is about 75% (Lippman, Allegra 1978; Horwitz, McGuire 1977). Some patients with estrogen receptors respond to endocrine therapy (McGuire et al. 1978). Conversely, some patients with tumors lacking receptors respond to hormones (McGuire et al. 1977). Thus, the presence of estrogen receptors does not necessarily indicate that a patient will respond to endocrine therapy.

The discrepancy between the presence of estrogen receptors and the absence of clinical response to endocrine therapy has led investigators to search for alternative indicators of estrogen action in breast cancer. The ideal indicator would be one which closely correlated with estrogen-dependent stimulation of cell proliferation under all assay conditions. Progesterone receptor might be one such marker. In fact, progesterone receptor has been shown to be induced by estrogen in breast cancer cells in vitro (Horwitz, McGuire 1978) as well as in vivo (Namer et al. 1980) and the presence of progesterone receptor in breast cancer tissue does increase the likelihood of the patient's response to endocrine manipulations. However this relationship is not fixed. Moreover, there are human breast cancer cell lines, such as MCF-7 and CG-5, in which progesterone receptor is present in the absence of estrogens. Also, antiestrogenic compounds such as tamoxifen prevent proliferation of MCF-7 cells and yet induce progesterone receptor (Horwitz et al. 1978), indicating that in breast cancer cells there may be a dissociation between the two responses (proliferation and induction of a specific protein).

In the past few years, we have focused on biological markers of hormone action which would more consistently correlate with estrogen-dependent stimulation of cell proliferation. The final goal would be to relate these markers to the in vivo response of breast cancer to endocrine therapy. In 1981, two years after the original discovery by a research group in Montpellier (France) of a 46,000 dalton glycoprotein which is induced in breast cancer cells in tissue culture (Westley, Rochefort 1979), we found a protein with similar physicochemical properties in freshly obtained primary human breast cancer (Iacobelli et al. 1981). This was the first evidence that estrogen regulates specific protein synthesis in human breast cancer cells in vitro. For reasons that will be described below, we thought that this protein (now referred to as 52K following a more precise evaluation of its molecular weight, Capony et al. 1982) may prove to be an interesting molecule to study in relation to hormone-dependency in breast cancer.

Effect of Estrogen and Antiestrogen on 52K Labelling and Cell Proliferation

As mentioned above, the perfect indicator of estrogen dependency in breast cancer would have characteristics such as (i) specific stimulation by physiological doses of estrogen (ii) a close relationship to hormone-stimulated cell proliferation and (iii) ease of detection in tumor extracts or biological fluids. Most if not all of these requirements are met by the 52K protein.

Fig.1 illustrates that the addition of physiological concentrations of either estradiol, estrone or the synthetic steroid diethylstilbestrol to CG-5 cells – an estrogen-supersensitive variant of the MCF-7 cell line (Natoli et al. 1983) – results in a dramatic stimulation of a secreted 52K protein band evidenced by sodium dodecylsulfate gel electrophoresis. Maximal stimulation was obtained with 1 nM estradiol and diethylstilbestrol had an analogous effect, whereas estrone was approximately ten times less effective.

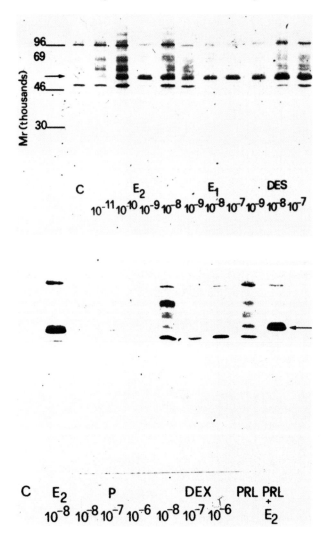

Fig. 1. Effect of different steroids on 52K protein synthesis in human breast cancer cell cultures. Samples were subjected to sodium dodecylsulfate-polyacrylamide gel electrophoresis followed by fluorography. C, Medium derived from control cells; E_2, 17β-estradiol; E_1, estrone; DES, diethylstilbestrol; P, progesterone; DEX, dexamethasone; PRL, prolactin. Full details are given in Iacobelli et al. (in press)

Other steroids tested were completely ineffective in the
induction of the synthesis of the 52K protein at
concentrations up to 1 µM (Fig. 1, lower panel). Prolactin has
no effect when added either alone or in combination with
estradiol. This suggests that only those steroids which
act on the estrogen receptors are capable of modifying the
synthesis of the 52K.

Interestingly enough, hydroxy tamoxifen, a tamoxifen
derivative which is more potent than tamoxifen itself in
occupying estrogen receptors (Jordan et al. 1977), while
incapable of inducing the 52K at every concentration used,
antagonized the effect of estradiol when used at a molar ratio
greater than 100 (Fig. 2).

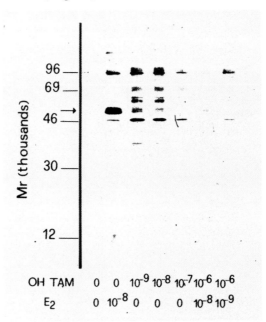

Fig. 2. Effect of different concentrations of mono-hydroxytamoxifen (OH TAM) and 17β-estradiol (E$_2$) on 52K protein
synthesis. Full details are given in Iacobelli et al.(in press)

Given that estrogen specifically stimulates the label
ling of the 52K before any effect on cell proliferation is

seen (the earliest time of appearance of 52K after estrogen exposure of the cells is 8 h) and the evidence that in clones deriving from the T47D human breast cancer cell line estrogen affects in a parallel way the labelling of a group of secretory proteins and cell proliferation (Chalbos et al. in press), we attempted to correlate the presence of 52K with proliferation of CG-5 cells. As shown in Fig. 3, extremely low concentrations - i.e., 0.01 nM of estradiol - already increased both the labelling of 52K and cell proliferation. The decreased effect on 52K labelling but not on cell proliferation seen at higher hormone concentrations - i.e. greater than 1 nM - is still not clearly understood. A suggestive hypothesis in keeping with that of other authors (Westley, Rochefort 1980) is that the 52K is a "growth factor" for the cells and that the decrease in this protein seen at high hormone concentrations may reflect the still unexplained growth inhibitory effects at high doses of estrogen seen in vivo in patients with breast cancer.

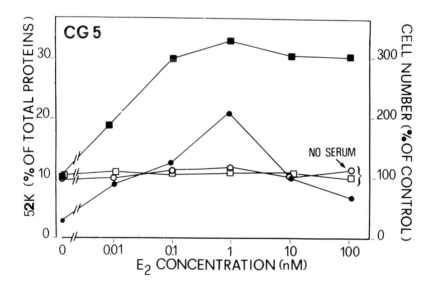

Fig. 3. Effects of estradiol on proliferation and 52K labelling in CG-5 cells. Full details are given in Iacobelli et al. (in press)

Finally, Fig. 4 shows that all concentrations of 4-hydroxytamoxifen used are similarly effective in preventing estrogen-stimulated cell proliferation and 52K labelling.

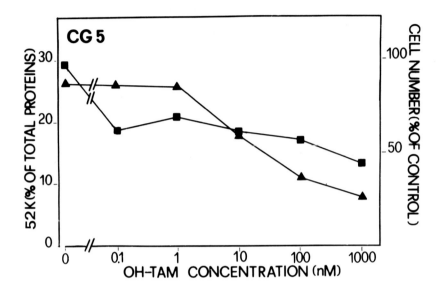

Fig. 4. Effects of mono-hydroxytamoxifen (OH TAM) on proliferation and 52K labelling in CG-5 cells. Full details are given in Iacobelli et al. (in press)

While the above data indicate that the 52K may be a specific and sensitive marker of estrogen action - probably in relation to hormone-stimulated cell proliferation - no information is yet available concerning the physiological role of this protein. Nor is it known whether estrogen simply increases its rate of synthesis or also accelerates its appearance in the culture medium. In trying to answer these questions, we have first focused on 52K purification. Prior purification is essential to the development of an immune assay of the 52K and an evaluation of its effectiveness as a marker for clinical breast cancer.

Purification of 52K

As outlined above, the 52K is primarily found in the culture medium of human breast cancer cells where it amounts to 20 to 40% of all extracellular labelled proteins.

However, a rough calculation in terms of protein concentration proved that the 52K was present in trace amounts, in the order of a few hundred picograms per ml of medium, thus making it quite uneconomical to use the medium as starting material for purification. Therefore, we decided that the most convenient source of material for 52K purification was human breast cancer cells.

The sequence of steps in the preparation of purified 52K is outlined in Fig. 5. Typically, starting material consisted of 5 to 10 x 10^9 CG-5 cells, which yielded 2 to 4 mg of purified 52K. The main step is purification by polyacrylamide gel electrophoresis under denaturing conditions. The fractions richest in 52K, i.e., M1 (corresponding to light membranes) and P2 (corresponding to crude nuclei) were pooled for electrophoresis. Several gels were processed at once; gels were then stained and destained and the protein band corresponding to the labelled 52K from the culture medium (evaluated from parallel electrophoreses in which a small amount of ^{35}S-methionine-labelled 52K was added to cold cellular proteins to permit fluorographic visualization) cut out by means of a scalpel. Several hundred gel fragments were extracted with sodium dodecylsulfate containing buffer and the extracted protein precipitated with trichoroacetic acid. The purification protocol outlined in Fig. 5 gave a 52K preparation that was approximately 60% pure as judged by protein staining after electrophoresis.

The 52K purified by the procedures described here should provide an appropriate antigen for the development of a specific antibody. Capony et al. 1982 recently described a rabbit antibody to a crude nuclear pellet of MCF-7 cells which recognized the radioactive 52K released into the culture medium. However, the antibody prepared in this manner was not monospecific and, in addition to the 52K, it precipitated many cellular proteins. Very recently, an antiserum against the cellular 52K produced in mice has been obtained in our laboratory and work is in progress to prepare hybrids secreting monoclonal antibodies (Iacobelli et al. in preparation).

PURIFICATION OF 52K

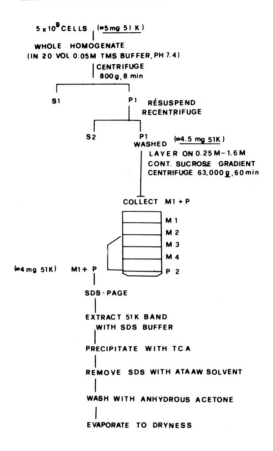

Fig. 5. Purification protocol of 52K from CG-5 cells.

Interestingly enough, the antiserum gave an intense membrane fluorescence when tested against intact CG-5 cells, suggesting that at least some antigenic determinants of the 52K are localised at the cell surface. Once it has been confirmed that the presence of 52K is restricted to malignant cells (Westley, Rochefort 1980), this antibody will be of specific interest from the clinical standpoint since it will allow the production of cytotoxic drug or toxin-antibody conjugate for a selective drug targetting to breast cancer cells.

Conclusion and perspectives

Among the various estrogen-induced proteins reported in the literature, we have focused our attention on the 52K as a potential marker for hormone-dependent human breast cancer. This for several reasons. First, the 52K is not confined to or acquired by cells in long-term tissue culture but is even produced in breast cancer tissue (Iacobelli et al. 1981; Natoli et al. 1981) as well as in breast cancer cells in early stages of culturing (S. Iacobelli, unpublished data), which suggests that its synthesis actually occurs in vivo. Second, as 52K is released into the medium of cultured cells, it might be secreted into the blood and provide a circulating indicator of hormone-dependency. If this were so, precise information could be obtained on the clinical outcome of spreading disease as well as the onset. Last but not least, the already mentioned possibility of building up of monoclonal antibodies carrying toxic agents or toxins with a high degree of selectivity for breast cancer cells.

Capony F., Garcia M., Veith F., Rochefort H. (1982). Antibodies to the estrogen induced 52K protein released by human breast cancer cells. Biochem. Biophys. Res. Comm. 108:8.

Chalbos D., Vignon F., Keydar I., Rochefort H. Estrogens stimulate cell proliferation and induce secretory proteins in a human breast cancer cell line (T47D). J. Clin. Endocrin. Metab. (in press).

Horwitz K.B., McGuire W.L. (1977). Estrogen and progesterone: Their relationship in hormone-dependent breast cancer. In McGuire W.L., Raynaud J.P., Baulieu E.E. (eds.) "Progesterone Receptors in Normal and Neoplastic Tissue". New York: Raven Press, p. 103.

Horwitz K.B., Koseki Y., McGuire W.L. (1978). Estrogen control of progesterone receptor in human breast cancer: role of estradiol and antiestrogen. Endocrinology 103:1742.

Horwitz K.B., McGuire W.L. (1978). Estrogen control of progesterone receptor in human breast cancer. J. Biol. Chem. 253:2223.

Iacobelli S., Marchetti P., Bartoccioni E., Natoli V.,

Scambia G., Kaye A.M. (1981). Steroid-induced proteins in human endometrium. Cell Molec. Endocrinol. 23:321.

Iacobelli S., Natoli V., Natoli C., Scambia G., Kaye A.M. (1981). Proceedings Second Innsbruck Winter Conference on Biochemistry in Clinical Medicine: Hormone-Cell Interactions in Reproductive Tissues, Igls 1981, Masson Publ. Inc. USA (in press).

Iacobelli S., Scambia G., Natoli V., Natoli C., Sica G. Estrogen stimulates cell proliferation and the increase of a 52,000 dalton glycoprotein in human breast cancer cells. J. Steroid Biochem. (in press).

Jordan V.C., Collins M.M., Rowsby L., Prestwhich R. (1977). A monohydroxylated metabolite of tamoxifen with potent antiestrogenic activity. J. Endocrinol. 75:305.

Lippman M.E., Allegra J.C. (1978). Receptors in breast cancer. N. Engl. J. Med. 299:930.

McGuire W.L., Horwitz K.B., Pearson O.H., Segaloff A. (1977). Current status of estrogen and progesterone receptors in breast cancer. Cancer 39:2934.

McGuire W.L., Horwitz K.B., Zava D.T., Garola R.E., Chamness G.C. (1978). Hormones in breast cancer: update 1978. Metabolism 27:487.

Namer M., Lalanne C., Baulieu E.E. (1980). Increase of progesterone receptor by tamoxifen as a hormonal challenge test in breast cancer. Cancer Res. 40:1750.

Natoli C., Sica G., Natoli V., Serra A., Iacobelli S. (1983). Two new estrogen-supersensitive variants of the MCF-7 human breast cancer cell line. Breast Cancer Res. Treat. 3:23.

Natoli V., Marchetti P., Natoli C., Sica G., Iacobelli S. (1981). Estrogen and antiestrogen effects on protein synthesis in human breast cancer cells. Current Chemotherapy & Immunology, Proceedings 12th Internat'l Congr. of Chemotherapy Florence, p. 1465.

Westley B., Rochefort H. (1979). Estradiol induced proteins in the MCF-7 human breast cancer cell line. Biochem. Biophys. Res. Commun. 90:410.

Westley B., Rochefort H. (1980). A secreted glycoprotein induced by estrogen in human breast cancer cell lines. Cell 20:353.

Hormones and Cancer, pages 63–77
© **1984 Alan R. Liss, Inc., 150 Fifth Avenue, New York, NY 10011**

INSULIN AS A DEVELOPMENTAL HORMONE

Yale J. Topper, Kevin R. Nicholas, Lakshmanan
Sankaran and Jerzy Kulski
National Institute of Arthritis, Diabetes, and
Digestive and Kidney Diseases, National Institutes
of Health, Bethesda, Maryland   20205

I.   INTRODUCTION

This is an account of some of our studies on the relationship between insulin and the terminal differentiation of
mammary epithelium. Organogenesis includes two major types
of developmental change: 1) Morphogenetic, i.e., the multiplication of the various cellular elements and their characteristic juxtaposition in relation to one another. 2) Terminal differentiation, i.e., the phenotypic expression of the
cellular components of the tissue, elicited by a number of
kinds of stimuli, including hormones. This report is not
concerned with the control of morphogenesis. Rather, it is
restricted to a discussion of aspects of the terminal differentiation of the epithelial cells in the mammary gland
under the influence of hormones. The emphasis here is on
insulin.

The mammary epithelial cell is one of the few cell
types which is not yet in a mature functional state in the
adult, non-pregnant animal. Maturity is attained only during pregnancy and lactation. After weaning of the suckling
young, the cells revert to a condition resembling that in
the mature virgin. Two markers of the fully-developed
mammary epithelial cell are the caseins and α-lactalbumin.
Caseins comprise a group of phosphoproteins; α-lactalbumin
is one of the two protein components of the lactose syn-
thetase system. The present report deals primarily with
these two markers. Most of the studies to be described concern the determination of the minimal hormone requirements
for the premature expression of the casein and α-lactalbumin

genes in mouse and rat mammary epithelial cells. Of the
several hormones required, insulin is the major point of emphasis.

The experimental system used was first described by
Elias (1957). Small mammary explants are supported at the
surface of Medium 199 containing various combinations of
several hormones, and the system is incubated for some days
at 37°. Usually, no macromolecules other than the hormones
are added. Tissue from both virgin and pregnant animals has
been employed. After incubation, the premature presence of
casein and α-lactalbumin in the tissue and media and the
premature accumulation of the corresponding mRNAs in the tissue, are determined.

The premature phenotypic expression of the casein genes
in isolated mouse and rat mammary tissue requires insulin,
glucocorticoid, prolactin and estrogen. Before beginning a
detailed discussion of insulin in this system it is of interest to provide a brief account of the other hormones
needed for this aspect of mammary development. Using tissue
from intact immature mice (Voytovich and Topper 1967) and
mice in mid-pregnancy (Turkington et al., 1965) it was demonstrated that all 4 caseins can be induced in the presence
of exogenous insulin, glucocorticoid and prolactin. No incomplete complement of these 3 hormones is effective (Juergens et al., 1965). Furthermore, the coordinate pattern of
induction of the 4 mouse caseins which occurs in vitro is
similar to that which takes place throughout mammary gland
development in vivo (Lockwood et al., 1966). In the in
vitro conditions described, the need for estrogen is not apparent. However, an estrogen requirement can be demonstrated
using tissue from ovariectomized mice (Bolander and Topper,
1980) and rats (Sankaran and Topper unpub.). This tissue
does not synthesize casein in vitro in response to insulin,
glucocorticoid and prolactin. Also, it does not accumulate
casein mRNA in these conditions (Bolander and Topper, 1981).
While addition of estrogen during culture does not correct
the problem, estrogen replacement therapy in vivo does re-
store the responsiveness of the tissue as tested in vitro.
Apparently, mammary tissue isolated from intact animals can
retain endogenous estrogen, or its effects, for an extended
period, thus making it appear that the tissue is independent
of the steroid. Long-term retention of estrogen by a mammary cell line has been demonstrated directly (Strobl and
Lippman, 1979).

It is clear that prolactin is required not only for the formation of caseins, but is also essential for premature accumulation of the corresponding mRNAs (Guyette et al., 1979) in rat mammary tissue. Similar observations have been reported (Ganguly et al., 1980; Nagaiah et al., 1981) in regard to the relationship between glucocorticoid and isolated mouse tissue. However, other reports (Hobbs et al., 1982) have suggested that glucocorticoid is not essential, but is merely potentiative for the accumulation of casein mRNAs in rat mammary explants. This is incorrect, at least in terms of certain rat casein mRNAs. Depletion of endogenous glucocorticoids by adrenalectomy of virgin rats 2 weeks prior to isolation of the tissue renders the tissue completely dependent on exogenous glucocorticoid for accumulation of certain casein mRNA species (Kulski, et al., unpub.). Tissue survival in vitro is not compromised by absence of the steroid. Long-term retention of glucocorticoid by the rat tissue has been demonstrated directly (Bolander et al., 1979).

These observations on the relationships of estrogen and glucocorticoid to mammary tissue re-emphasize an important general consideration. Isolated tissue may not be devoid of the humoral factors to which it has been exposed in vivo.

It was stated above that a minimum of 4 hormones, insulin, glucocorticoid, prolactin and estrogen, is essential for phenotypic expression of casein genes in mouse and rat mammary tissue in vitro. The essential hormonal determinants for the premature induction of α-lactalbumin in this tissue in vitro are less rigid. Under some circumstances, particularly when the prolactin concentration is high, glucocorticoid may not be essential. Mammary cells from rats also appear to possess a prolactin-independent pathway leading to α-lactalbumin synthesis (Nicholas and Topper, 1980). However, no conditions are known in which the induction of α-lactalbumin in murine cells in vitro can occur in the absence of insulin and estrogen. In this respect, the hormonal requirements for casein and α-lactalbumin are the same.

II. INSULIN IN RELATION TO TERMINAL DIFFERENTIATION OF
     THE MURINE MAMMARY EPITHELIAL CELL

Most studies on insulin have been concerned with acute metabolic effects, such as glucose tolerance. This aspect

of insulin biology is of great clinical importance in relation to diabetes. Insulin, of course, exerts other acute
effects on its target tissues. In addition, insulin is
known to elicit growth responses, and to evoke other "late"
or long-term biological effects. For example, insulin treatment of 3T3-L1 fatty fibroblasts increases the activity of
lipoprotein lipase maximally after 2-4 days, but is without
effect during the first 4 hours (Spooner et al., 1979).
Such late effects have occasionally been termed "chronic
metabolic" responses to insulin (Van Obberghen et al., 1979).
Other instances of such "late" effects will be presented
later. Here we wish to suggest that it might be useful to
regard at least some so-called chronic metabolic responses
to insulin as developmental effects of the hormone. More
particularly, that insulin may be essential for selective
gene expression in certain cells at particular stages of
ontogeny. Regardless of whether or not such functions of
insulin are critical in relation to diabetes, they are probably significant in terms of general developmental biology.
In this section the role of insulin as an essential developmental agent for the terminal differentiation of murine mammary epithelial cells will be discussed. This system may
serve as a prototype for similar studies on other systems.

A. Physiological Levels of Insulin Suffice For Milk Protein
Gene Expression In Murine Mammary Epithelium In Vitro

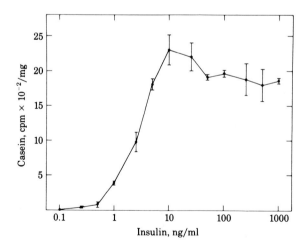

Fig. 1. Insulin dose-response relationship for casein synthesis in mammary gland explants from midpregnant mice. Explants were cultured for 44 hr in medium 199 containing cortisol (1 µg/ml), prolactin (1 µg/ml), and insulin and then pulsed for 4 hr with $^{33}P_i$ (10 µCi/ml). Casein was determined by immunoprecipitation; results (radioactivity per mg of tissue) are mean ± SEM of three pools of tissue.

    It was stated earlier that glucocorticoid and prolactin, in the absence of insulin, do not support the induction of casein or α-lactalbumin in murine mammary tissue <u>in-vitro</u>. Supporting evidence is provided in figure 1. However, a physiological level of insulin, in the presence of cortisol and prolactin, does support the induction of casein synthesis by mouse mammary explants (Fig. 1) (Bolander et al., 1981) and does promote the induction of α-lactalbumin activity in cultured rat mammary tissue (data not shown). These effects of insulin do not require the presence of glucose in the medium; similar responses are observed when the Medium 199 contains fructose, instead.

B.   Specificity of Insulin For Milk Protein Synthesis and mRNA$_{csn}$ Accumulation

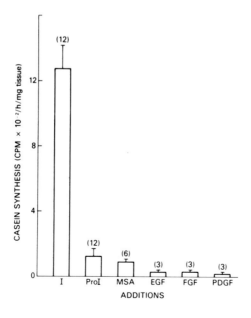

Fig. 2. Comparison of insulin, proinsulin and several growth factors for their ability to induce casein synthesis in pregnant rat mammary gland explants. Explants from 14 day pregnant rats were cultured for 72 h in medium containing hydrocortisone and prolactin each at 1 µg/ml, and either insulin(I), proinsulin(proI) or the growth factors, each at 0.25 µg/ml. The explants were pulsed with 20 µCi/ml of [^{3}H]-L-amino acid mixture during the last 16 h of incubation and the amount of casein formed was measured by immunoprecipitation using sheep anti-rat casein serum. Values are mean ± SEM for the number of rats shown, each analyzed separately.

In an effort to determine whether insulin is unique in its ability to support milk protein induction, other factors have been tested in the culture system containing cortisol and prolactin. In the experiment depicted in Fig. 2, relating to rat casein synthesis, each factor was tested at 0.25 µg/ml, a concentration considerably above their physiological level (Cohen and Savage 1974; Antoniades and Scher 1977; Jaffe and Behrman 1979; Wilde and Kuhn 1979; Moses et al., 1980); the blood level of FGF has not been reported. In addition, both MSA and EGF were tested at a concentration of 1 µg/ml, with similar results (data not shown). Appreciable induction occurs only in the presence of insulin. Proinsulin and multiplication stimulating activity are less than 10% as active as insulin. Similar results were obtained in terms of α-lactalbumin; in this case, nerve growth factor was also tested, and had virtually no activity (data not shown).

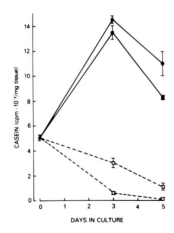

Fig. 3.   Capacity of insulin and ARS to induce casein in
pregnant mouse mammary gland explants.   All media contained
F(1 μg/ml), P(1 μg/ml) and BSA (1 mg/ml).   Tissue was cultured for the times indicated with these 2 hormones only ( )
or together with either I (0, 20 ng/ml) ARS ( ) or CS ( )
[serum was added at a 1:50 dilution].   Explants were pulsed
with ^{3}H-amino acid mixture (35 μCi/ml) at 0-6h, 66-72h and
114-120h of culture, and casein formed was measured in tissue
extracts by immunoprecipitation with sheep anti-mouse casein.
Mammary glands from six mice were pooled and casein determined in tissue from triplicate culture dishes.   Each value
represents mean ± SEM.

Actually, the only substance found capable of substitu-
ting for insulin in the induction of murine milk protein is
anti-insulin receptor antibody.   Its effect on the induction
of mouse casein synthesis is depicted in Fig. 3 (Nicholas
and Topper, 1983).   The implications of such a "late" effect
in terms of insulin biology have been discussed by Van Obberghen et al., (1979).

TABLE 1.   Effect of growth factors on mRNA$_{csn}$ accumulation
and RER formation

Addition	mRNA$_{csn}$ %	RNA in RER μg/100 mg
None (t_o)	0.099 ± 0.011	2.2 ± 0.2
None (cultured)	0.020 ± 0.004	2.0 ± 0.4
Insulin	1.39 ± 0.16	9.9 ± 0.5
Epidermal growth factor	0.093 ± 0.008	8.8 ± 0.5
Somatomedin C	0.103 ± 0.011	9.1 ± 0.3

Mammary gland explants from midpregnant mice were
either assayed immediately (t_o) or cultured for 48 hr in
medium 199 containing growth factor (50 ng/ml) and cortisol (1 μg/ml).   When mRNA$_{csn}$ was to be assayed, prolactin
(1 μg/ml) was also present.   mRNA$_{csn}$ was determined by RNA
excess hybridization (Nagaiah et al. 1981) and RNA in RER
was measured in an epithelial cell-enriched fraction (Oka
and Topper, 1971).   Results are mean ± SEM of three pools
of tissue, except for somatomedin C which, because of
limited supplies, was assayed twice and is average ± range.

Insulin is not only specifically required for the formation of the milk proteins, but is also essential for the
accumulation of mRNA$_{csn}$.   Culture for 48 hours in the pres-

ence of cortisol and prolactin alone results in an 80% loss of the mRNA$_{csn}$ present in the freshly isolated mouse tissue (Table 1) (Bolander et al., 1981). Addition of epidermal growth factor or somatomedin C maintains the initial level of the messenger, but does not enhance its level. By contrast, insulin evokes a 14-fold increase in the accumulation of mRNA$_{csn}$.

The accumulation of rat casein mRNA also appears to have a specific requirement for insulin. As can be seen in Fig. 4, during incubation in the presence of FCS, F and P the level of 42 K mRNA falls below that in the freshly isolated tissue. Subsequent addition of either MSA or EGF does not result in an increment of the 42 K mRNA. By contrast, addition of insulin does lead to an elevated level of the messenger. Similar results were obtained with the 25 K mRNA (data not shown).

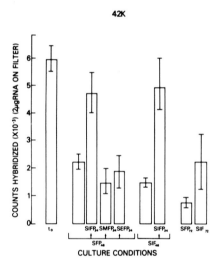

Fig. 4. Effect of insulin or prolactin on the accumulation of 42 K casein mRNA. Mammary explants from pregnant rats were cultured with 20% fetal calf serum (S), hydrocortisone (F) and prolactin (P) for 48 h, and then for another 24 h with insulin (I), multiplication stimulating activity (M) or epidermal growth factor (E), in addition; or with S, I and F for 48 hr, and then with P, in addition. The concentrations of I, E, M, F and P were 10, 100, 100, 50 and 1000 ng/ml; respectively. RNA (1 or 2 ng) was bound to DBM paper for the hybridization assay. Each value represents mean ± SEM for 3 groups of rats with 2 animals per group.

C. Cell Maintenance

Barnawell (1965) reported that the epithelial cells in rat mammary explants lose viability during culture in the absence of exogenous insulin. The observation (Table 1) that much of the mRNA$_{csn}$ present in freshly isolated mouse mammary tissue is lost during culture in the absence of insulin is consistent with this conclusion. A critical question, then, is whether the unique ability of insulin to promote milk protein gene expression reflects a unique ability of the hormone to maintain the cells, or whether, in addition to its cell maintenance function, it also participates more directly in casein and α-lactalbumin gene expression. An approach to this question is to determine whether any of the factors found to be ineffective in such gene expression can, nevertheless, maintain the cells.

Table 1 (Bolander et al., 1981) demonstrates that cortisol alone does not produce an increment in the rough endoplasmic reticulum (RER) of cultured mouse mammary epithelium. When insulin is also present a 4-5 fold increase in RER accumulation occurs. Despite the fact that neither EGF nor SmC elicited any increase in the accumulation of mRNA$_{csn}$, they were as effective as insulin in promoting enhanced accumulation of the RER. Epidermal growth factor is also as effective as insulin in maintaining general cellular responsiveness to prolactin (Bolander et al., 1981). The results suggest that although both EGF and SmC can maintain the cells as well as insulin, only insulin has the additional capacity to participate in milk protein gene expression.

TABLE 2. Capacity of insulin, MSA and EGF to maintain NADH-cytochrome C reductase activity in pregnant rat mammary gland explants

Culture Conditions	NADH-Cytochrome C Reductase (ΔA_{550nm}/min/g tissue)	
Uncultured	0.377 ± 0.08	(2)
Hydrocortisone	0.119 ± 0.01	(5)
Insulin + Hydrocortisone	0.400 ± 0.07	(4)
MSA + Hydrocortisone	0.373 ± 0.03	(5)
EGF + Hydrocortisone	0.344 ± 0.02	(2)

Tissue was cultured for 96 h in media containing hydrocortisone (0.05 µg/ml) alone, or a combination of hydrocortisone and either insulin, MSA or EGF (each at a concen-

tration of 0.25 µg/ml). NADH-cytochrome C reductase was
measured (Oka and Topper, 1971) in epithelial cell enriched
fractions following collagenase digestion of the explants
(Freeman and Topper, 1978). Values represent mean ± SEM or
mean ± range with the number of observations shown in paren-
thesis.

Similarly, Table 2 shows that hydrocortisone alone does
not maintain the initial level of rat mammary epithelial
NADH-cytochrome C reductase activity in culture. Addition
of insulin, MSA or EGF does result in maintenance of the initial enzyme activity, which denotes maintenance of cellular
responsiveness to hydrocortisone (Oka and Topper, 1971). A-
gain, it appears that while MSA and EGF can sustain the cells
as well as insulin, only insulin can function in the production of the milk proteins.

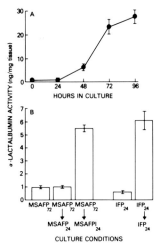

Fig. 5. Capacity of MSA to maintain hormone-responsive mammary epithelial cells. (A) Explants from pregnant rat mammary glands were cultured in media containing insulin (0.25
µg/ml), hydrocortisone (0.05 µg/ml) and prolactin (1 µg/ml),
and the α-lactalbumin activity in tissue extracts determined
at daily intervals. Each value represents mean ± SEM for 3
groups of rats (2 rats/group). (B) Explants were cultured
in media containing hydrocortisone (F, 0.05 µg/ml), prolactin
(P, 1 µg/ml) and MSA (0.25 µg/ml) for 72 h, and then the
media were changed to fresh MSAFP medium, or MSAFPI medium
(I = 0.25 µg/ml); culture was continued for an additional
24 h. α-Lactalbumin activity was determined in tissue ex-

tracts. The values shown for the IFP system correspond to those shown in (A). Each value represents mean ± SEM for 3 groups of rats (2 rats/group).

Although the type of evidence presented above is consistent with the possibility that other factors can sustain murine mammary epithelial cells as well as insulin, it might be argued that the particular activities selected do not adequately represent cell maintenance as required for the complex processes involved in the induction of the milk proteins. A more direct experimental approach to this issue is presented in Figure 5. Here it is apparent that although MSA in the presence of glucocorticoid and prolactin, has little ability to promote the induction of α-lactalbumin activity, it does maintain, during 3 days of culture, the cells' potential for prompt response to the delayed addition of insulin. More specifically, the presence of insulin for 1 day following 3 days with MSA, glucocorticoid and prolactin resulted in approximately as much induction as that which occurred during a 1 day period in a system containing insulin from the start.

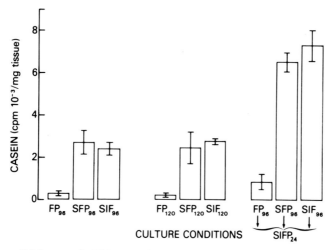

Fig. 6. Effect of FCS on the maintenance of mammary epithelial cells and the synthesis of casein. Mammary explants were cultured with F and P; S, F and P; or S, I and F for 96 h. Then the media contained S, I, F and P for an additional 24 h. After pulsing with ^{3}H-amino acids (30 μCi/ml) during the last 4 h, casein was assayed by immunoprecipitation.

The concentration of S was 20%, and those of I, F and P were 25, 50 and 1000 ng/ml, respectively. Each value represents mean ± SEM for 3 groups of Day 13 pregnant rats, with 2 animals per group.

A similar approach, using FCS instead of MSA as a maintenance agent is shown in Fig. 6. It is clear that after 4 days in the presence of only F and P the tissue does lose viability, i.e. it loses the ability to respond to the delayed addition of insulin. However, FCS maintains the tissue so that it can respond to the delayed addition of insulin. the tissue did not respond to MSA or EGF.

It is clear that while insulin is not unique in terms of cell maintenance, it does appear to have an essential and unique role in the phenotypic expression of the murine mammary epithelial cell.

E. Conclusions Concerning Insulin As A Developmental
    Hormone In The Mammary System

The explant system used in these studies has made it possible to demonstrate a unique role of insulin in the phenotypic expression of murine mammary epithelial cells unrelated to its function in cell maintenance. The biological events involved in this role are virtually completely dependent on insulin. By contrast, the events related to the acute metabolic functions of the hormone, such as transport of substrates, general protein synthesis, etc., generally do not show such total dependency.

F. Other Systems In Which Insulin May Function As A
    Developmental Hormone

There have been sporadic reports in the literature which suggest that insulin may play a role in selective gene expression in other cell types also. Some of these studies were carried out in the whole animal, non-diabetic and diabetic, with the usual attendant difficulties of interpretation. Others demonstate a direct effect of insulin on isolated tissues or cells, but the specificity of the hormone has not been established.

Administration of insulin to adrenalectomized rats increases the accumulation of mRNA for tyrosine aminotrans-

ferase in the liver (Hill et al., 1981). This may not be a
unique response to insulin, since glucocorticoid can induce
the corresponding enzyme in isolated rat hepatoma cells (Tomkins et al., 1966). The pancreas of diabetic rats manifests
a selective reduction in the level of mRNA for amylase (Korc
et al., 1981), and the livers of mildly diabetic rats show
a selective reduction in the level of mRNA for α_{2u} globulin
(Roy et al., 1980). It is not clear, however, whether the
defects are the result of deprivation of insulin per se, or
of the systemic derangements of diabetes.

Insulin can induce δ-crystallin mRNA in cultures of
chicken lens epithelial cells (Milstone and Piatiogorsky,
1977). Serum is also effective in this system, but the active component of serum has not been identified. Lipoprotein lipase activity in 3T3-L1 fibroblasts is stimulated
to maximum levels after 4 days of culture in the presence
of insulin (Spooner et al., 1979), as mentioned earlier,
and insulin can effect the determination of pre-adipocytes
(Sager and Kovac, 1981).

We suggest that such effects, variously termed "late",
"long-term" and "chronic metabolic," and which we have referred to as developmental effects , probably represent a
category of biological activity distinct from the more commonly studied acute effects of the hormone. More particularly, they may represent important influences of insulin
at the level of gene expression, and warrant greater attention than they have received heretofore. It will be of
great interest to determine whether the isolated systems
cited above are similar to the mammary system, i.e., whether
they too, have a unique requirement for insulin unrelated
to its efficacy in cell maintenance.

Antoniades HN, Scher, CD (1977). Radioimmunoassay of a
human serum growth factor for Balb/c-3T3 cells: derivation from platelets. Proc Natl Acad Sci USA 74:1973
Barnawell EB (1965). A comparative study of the responses
of mammary tissues from several mammalian species to hormones in vitro. J Exp Zool 160:189.
Bolander FF, Jr., Nicholas KR, Topper YJ (1979). Retention
of glucocorticoid by isolated mammary tissue may complicate
interpretation of results from in vitro experiments. Biochem Biophys Res Comm 91:247.
Bolander FF, Jr., Topper YJ (1980). Loss of differentiative

potential of the mammary gland in ovariectomized mice:
prevention and reversibility of the defect. Endocrinology
107:1281.

Bolander FF, Jr., Nicholas KR, Van Wyk JJ, Topper YJ (1981),
Insulin is essential for accumulation of casein mRNA in
mouse mammary epithelial cells. Proc Natl Acad Sci USA
78:5862.

Bolander FF, Jr., Topper YJ (1981). Loss of differentiative
potential of the mammary gland in ovariectomized mice:
Identification of a biochemical lesion. Endocrinology 108:
1649.

Cohen S, Savage CR (1974). Recent studies on the chemistry
and biology of epidermal growth factor. Rec Prog Horm Res
30:551.

Elias JJ (1957). Cultivation of adult mouse mammary gland
in hormone-enriched synthetic medium. Science 126:842.

Ganguly R, Ganguly N, Mehta NM, Banerjee MR (1980). Absolute
requirement of glucocorticoid for expression of the casein
gene in the presence of prolactin. Proc Natl Aca Sci USA
77:6003.

Guyette WA, Matusik RJ, Rosen JM (1979). Prolactin-mediated
transcriptional and post-transcriptional control of casein
gene expression. Cell 17:1013.

Hill RE, Lee LL, Kenney FT (1981). Effects of insulin on
messenger RNA activities in rat liver. J Biol Chem 256:
1510.

Hobbs AA, Richards DA, Kessler DJ, Rosen JM (1982). Complex
hormonal regulation of rat casein gene expression. J Biol
Chem 257:3598.

Jaffe BM, Behrman HR (1979). Methods of Hormone Radioimmunoassay Acad. Press NY Appendix 3:1005.

Juergens, WG, Stockdale FE, Topper YJ, Elias JJ (1965). Hormone-dependent differentiation of mammary gland in vitro.
Proc Natl Acad Sci USA 54:629.

Korc M, Owerbach D, Quinto C, Rutter WJ (1981). Pancreatic
islet-acinar cell interaction: amylase messenger RNA
levels are determined by insulin. Science 213:351.

Lockwood DH, Turkington RW, Topper YJ (1966). Hormone-
dependent development of milk protein synthesis in mammary gland in vitro. Biochim Biophys Acta 130:493.

Milstone LM, Piatigorsky J (1977). δ-Crystallin gene expression in embryonic chick lens epithelia cultured in
the presence of insulin. Exp Cell Res 105:9

Moses AC, Nissley SP, Short PA, Rechler MM, White RM, Knight
AB, High OZ (1980). Increased levels of multiplication-
stimulating activity, an insulin-like growth factor, in

fetal rat serum. Proc Natl Acad Sci USA 77:3649.

Nagaiah K, Bolander FF, Jr., Nicholas KR, Takemoto T, Topper YJ (1981). Prolactin-induced accumulation of casein mRNA in mouse mammary explants: A selective role of glucocorticoid. Biochem Biophys Res Comm 98:380.

Nicholas KR, Topper YJ (1980). Enhancement of α-lactalbumin-like activity in mammary explants from pregnant rats in the absence of exogenous prolactin. Biochem Biophys Res Comm 94:1424

Nicholas KR, Topper YJ (1983). Anti-insulin receptor serum mimics the developmental role of insulin in mouse mammary explants. Biochem Biophys Res Comm 111:988.

Oka T, Topper YJ (1971). Hormone-dependent accumulation of rough endoplasmic reticulum in mouse mammary epithelial cells in vitro. J Biol Chem 246:7701

Roy AK, Chatterjee B, Prasad MSK, Unaker NJ (1980). Role of insulin in the regulation of the hepatic messenger RNA for α_{2u}-globulin in diabetic rats. J Biol Chem 255:11614.

Sager R, Kovac P (1981). Pre-adipocyte determination either by insulin or by 5-azacytidine. Proc Natl Acad Sci USA 79:480.

Spooner PM, Chernick SS, Garrison MM, Scow RO (1979). Development of lipoprotein lipase activity and accumulation of triacylglycerol in differentiating 3T3-L1 adipocytes. J Biol Chem 254:1305.

Strobl JS, Lippman ME (1979). Prolonged retention of estradiol by human breast cancer cells in tissue culture. Cancer Res 39:3319.

Tomkins GM, Thompson EB, Hayashi S, Gelehrter T, Granner D, Peterkofsky B (1966). Tyrosine transaminase induction in mammalian cells in tissue culture. Cold Spring Harbor Symp Quant Biol 31:349.

Turkington RW, Juergens WG, Topper YJ (1965). Hormone-dependent synthesis of casein in vitro. Biochim Biophys Acta 111:573.

Van Obbergen E, Spooner PM, Kahn CR, Chernick SS, Garrison, MM, Karlsson FA, Grunfeld C (1979). Insulin-receptor antibodies mimic a late insulin effect. Nature 280:500

Voytovich AE, Topper YJ (1967). Hormone-dependent differentiation of immature mouse mammary gland in vitro. Science 158:1326.

Wilde CJ, Kuhn NJ (1979). Lactose synthesis in the rat, and the effects of litter size and malnutrition. Biochem J 182:287.

Hormones and Cancer, pages 79–95
© **1984 Alan R. Liss, Inc., 150 Fifth Avenue, New York, NY 10011**

BIOCHEMICAL BASIS OF BREAST CANCER TREATMENT BY ANDROGENS
AND PROGESTINS *

Henri Rochefort

Unité d'Endocrinologie Cellulaire et Moléculaire
U 148 I.N.S.E.R.M.
60, Rue de Navacelles
34100 MONTPELLIER France
Tél. : (67) 54.13.79 – 54.15.44.

1. INTRODUCTION

Even though other mechanisms are not excluded, the
endocrine treatment of breast cancer is based on the
assumption that estrogens are the major mitogenic hormones
and that it is necessary to suppress their production
(ablative therapies) and their action at the tumor level
(additive therapies). That the predictive value of the
assay of estrogen and progesterone receptors in breast
cancer tissue is similar whether the treatment is made by
non steroidal antiestrogen, androgens or progestins,
support such an assumption. The different endocrine
therapies of breast cancer are indicated in Table 1. We
will consider here only the mechanisms by which hormones
and drugs act at the tumor level, to inhibit estrogen
action and tumor growth. The negative feedback effect of
these steroids on gonadotrophin release, leading to a
decreased ovarian secretion will not be considered even
though this mechanism may obviously be involved in vivo.
An extensive literature is available concerning the mode
of action of non steroidal antiestrogens (Furr et al,
1979 ; Rochefort, 1981 ; Sutherland, Jordan, 1981). These
are currently thought to work by forming a partially
active complex with the estrogen receptor, thus preventing
the binding and the action of estrogens, and explaining
the higher efficiency of this drug on RE positive breast
cancer. By contrast, the mode of action of androgens and
progestins in breast cancer cells has been less studied
and we will limit our contribution to these two mode of

* Presented at the International Symposium on "Hormones and
  Cancer", Buenos Aires, 9-13 May 1983.

endocrine therapy. In a given target cell, it is currently considered that the biological effect of a hormone is related to the concentration of the activated hormone receptor complex. Effect = $f\left(hR\right)$.

ENDOCRINE TREATMENT OF BREAST CANCER

To decrease :

1. Estrogen production
         - ovariectomy, adrenalectomy
         - amino-glutetimide
         - chemotherapy

2. Estrogen action (Antiestrogen)
         - tamoxifen

3. Both estrogen action + production
         - progestins, androgens

Table 1

Since $hR = f\left(h\right) \times \left(R\right) \times KA$, the biological effect of estrogen is a function of the concentration in target cell of estrogens (h) and of the affinity (KA) and concentration of binding sites (R) of the estrogen receptor. Estrogen antagonists can therefore decrease any factor among h, R or KA. The decrease of KA is triggered by non steroidal antiestrogens acting as competitive inhibitors. By contrast, we will see that androgens and progestins are rather decreasing the concentrations of estrogens (h) and/or of the receptor sites (R) in the cell. We will review the literature on the anti proliferative and anti estrogenic effect of androgens and progestins and give results from our laboratory aiming to answer the following questions.

1. Do androgen and progestins act directly as antiestrogens in breast cancer cells ?

2. If no, what are the initial steps and receptors responsible for these antiestrogenic effects ?

3. Estrogens being mitogenic, do androgens and progestins act simply by inhibiting the estrogenic effect, or do they have additional antiproliferative effect(s) by themselves on breast cancer cells ?

4. Finally, what is (are) the final step(s) mechanism(s) by which androgens and progestins inhibit tumor growth ?

2. ANDROGEN THERAPY OF BREAST CANCER

Androgens (Testololactone dromostandone calusterone, halotestin) were used before the advent of tamoxifen for both pre and post menopausal advanced breast cancer (Ulrich, 1939 ; Lacassagne, 1936).

Their mode of action is complex and may be both indirect by blocking pituitary gonado trophin release and subsequently ovarian secretion and direct on breast cancer cells. The mechanism of the direct effect of androgens on estrogen target cells has mainly been investigated in the uterus and mammary tumors. Androgens have been shown to display both an estrogenic effect and an antiestrogenic effect according to the nature of the receptor that they predominantly activate.

A. Estrogenic Effect of Androgens Mediated by the Estrogen Receptor

Several pieces of evidence support the idea that androgens behave as full estrogens when they bind to the estrogen receptor (Rochefort, Garcia, 1983). This was first demonstrated with DHT which was shown to translocate the RE to the nucleus (Rochefort et al, 1972) and to subsequently induce estrogen-specific responses such as the rat uterine induced protein, the progesterone receptor (RP) and the 52 K protein in MCF_7 cell. At very high concentrations, DHT also stimulate the growth of DMBA-induced rat mammary tumors (Garcia, Rochefort, 1978). Some androgens, like the 5-androstene 3 β 17β diol metabolite of the adrenal DHEA, and 5α androstane 3β 17β diol which have a high affinity for the estrogen receptor (Garcia, Rochefort, 1979), are estrogenic at near physiological concentrations and might therefore stimulate the growth of hormone dependent mammary cells. The use of androgen in breast cancer therapy is obviously not based on this estrogenic activity which is only observed for higher concentrations that those used in therapy.

B. Evidence for the Antiestrogenic Activity of Androgens
in vivo

Regression of rat mammary tumors has been obtained mainly by daily administration of moderate doses of androgens (0.2 to 4 mg/rat) for 10 to 30 days. In the uterus, the demonstration of an antiestrogenic effect of androgens has been shown by the inhibition of the estrogen induced increase in progesterone receptor content (Li, Li, 1978 ; Ip et al, 1982). The antiestrogenic effects of androgen are obtained only with concentrations lower than those which translocate the estrogen receptor to the nucleus and require at least 5 daily injections. Androgens therefore appear much less efficient than synthetic antiestrogens to inhibit estrogen-induced uterotrophy (Rochefort et al, 1979 b). Moreover, from these in vivo data, an indirect effect of androgens, perhaps mediated by a feedback mechanism, was not excluded.

C. Evidence for a Direct Antiestrogenic Effect of Androgens

McIndoe and Etre (1981) have studied the effects of androgens on the estrogen-dependent accumulation of progesterone receptor in MCF_7 human breast cancer cell line. A complete inhibition of the estradiol induced increase of progesterone receptor level was obtained by 10 nM concentration of testosterone or DHT. We also studied the effects of androgen in MCF_7 cells on the estrogen-induced 52 K glycoprotein secreted into the medium (Westley, Rochefort, 1980). Androgens for 2 days treatment did not modify the levels of the estradiol-induced 52 K glycoprotein. When DHT (10 to 100 nM) was administered for 5 to 19 days, a two-fold inhibition of the 52 K estrogen induced protein was observed. However, this inhibition was not specific for the 52 K protein since other secreted proteins were also inhibited. A significant inhibition by 100 nM DHT of the estradiol-increased growth of MCF_7 cells was observed in parallel (Garcia, Rochefort, unpublished). These results taken together suggest a general inhibition of secretion and of cell proliferation by DHT (10 to 100 nM) and a more specific inhibition of the progesterone receptor induction than for the 52 K protein.

D. Mechanisms of the Antiestrogenic Activity of Androgens

The possible nature of the receptor responsible for this antagonism has been studied recently. In any target cells for example, hormone dependent breast cancer cells, androgens bind to the androgen receptor at low physiological concentrations, and also to the progesterone receptor and the estrogen receptor at higher concentrations (Fig. 1). Since high doses of androgen can interact with the 3 classes of steroid receptors, each has been proposed to trigger the antiestrogenic activity of androgen.

a. <u>Antiestrogenic effect via the estrogen receptor ?</u> This first hypothesis was strengthened by the observation that androgens, as well as classical non steroidal antiestrogens, interact with the RE with a low affinity and a similar rapid dissociation rate (Rochefort et al a, 1979). However, long-term treatment by androgen was necessary to obtain an antiestrogenic effect, while the synthetic antiestrogens inhibit estrogen action more rapidly (within 2 days). Moreover, there was no general correlation between the binding affinity of a ligand for the RE and its antiestrogenic activity (Rochefort et al b, 1979) since high affinity ligands such as 4-hydroxytamoxifen (Borgna, Rochefort, 1980) or the Ci 628 metabolites (Katzenellenbogen et al, 1981) were full antiestrogens, while low affinity ligands such as DHT can behave as full estrogens. Adrenal androgens having a high affinity for the RE could therefore be considered as potential estrogens rather than antiestrogens.

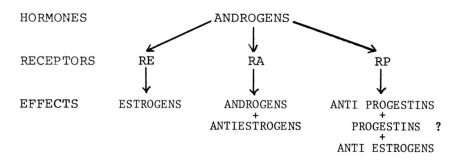

Figure 1. Androgens in mammary cancer cells may trigger different biological or pharmacological responses according to the nature of the sex steroid receptors on which they interact. While the consequences of their interaction with the estrogen receptor (RE) and the androgen receptor (RA) are well documented, the effects of their binding to the progesterone receptor (RP) are less understood.

b. Antiestrogenic effect via the progesterone receptor ? Androgens which also bind to the progesterone receptor could also behave as antiestrogens by the same mechanism as progestins. However, DHT appears unable both to translocate the progesterone receptor into the nucleus in vivo (Rochefort, Garcia, 1983) and to induce progestin specific responses in the MCF_7 or $T_{47}D$ cell lines (Chalbos, Rochefort, 1983). It is therefore unlikely that DHT is antiestrogenic as a result of its interaction with the progesterone receptor.

c. Antiestrogenic effect via the androgen receptor. Two lines of evidence indicate that the antiestrogenic effects of androgens are mediated by the androgen receptor. The doses of androgens which antagonize estrogen action are lower than those which are required for an interaction with, and nuclear translocation of the estrogen receptor, but are in the range required to occupy the androgen receptor (Garcia, Rochefort, 1979 ; Zava, McGuire, 1978). Antiandrogens inhibit the antiestrogenic effects of androgens. In MTW9 rat mammary tumor (Ip et al, 1982) and in MCF_7 cells (McIndoe, Etre, 1981), the androgen mediated inhibition of the induction of the progesterone receptor by estrogen is reversed by anti-androgens (Flutamide, Cyproterone and SCH-16, 423).

It is therefore suggested that the androgens used in breast cancer therapy have more affinity for the RA than for the RE and act chiefly by displaying an antiestrogenic activity mediated by the RA. Whether this effect is due to regulation of the concentration of estrogen receptor, of its activity or of the concentration of active estrogen, has not been specified.

E. Conclusions

Recent studies on the interactions of androgens with different receptors in estrogen target tissues and their effects on estrogen specific responses have provided some basic information on the mechanism of action of androgens in endocrine related tumors. The mechanism of the estrogenic activity of androgens seems to be fairly well understood. First, androgens can be aromatised into estrogen ; this might be the case for testosterone in the hypothalamus. Second, they might displace free active estrogens from their plasma binding protein such as the Sex Hormone Binding Globulin. Third, some of them such as

5-androstenediol, 3β-adiol and DHEA might act as full estrogens via an efficient interaction with the estrogen receptor. From the estrogenic effects triggered by RE-androgen complexes, one can therefore conclude that the specificity of the hormonal response depends more upon the nature of the receptor translocated to the nucleus than upon that of the hormone. This indicate that the tissue protein which is being characterized and defined as a putative receptor is actually responsible for triggering the action of an hormone, rather than a cellular binding protein which simply carries the hormone into the chromatin (Rochefort, Westley, 1983).

In contrast, the mechanism by which androgens are able to act as antiestrogens is not yet fully understood. In vitro cell culture studies suggest that this effect is possibly mediated by the RA. However, a progestin like effect is not totally excluded and androgens may have a more complex action in vivo. Moreover, the mechanism by which the RA inhibits the effect or the concentration of RE demands further experiments.

A better understanding of the mechanism by which androgens regulate tumor cell proliferation is to be expected from progress which is being made in the assay of the different hormones, metabolites and receptors, and in the study of proteins specifically regulated by androgens or estrogens in target tissues.

3. MECHANISM OF ACTION OF PROGESTIN IN BREAST CANCER CELLS

A. Introduction

17-hydroxy progesterone derivatives (megestrol, medroxy progesterone, acetate (MPA)) and 19-nor testosterone derivatives (lynestrenol, orgametryl) are used in the treatment of both benign and malignant human breast diseases (McGuire, Horwitz, 1977). Their use is based on the assumption that progesterone prevents the mitogenic activity of estrogens in breast cancer cells. While this has been clearly demonstrated in human endometrium (Tseng et al, 1977 ; Gurpide et al, 1979) the antiestrogenic effect of progesterone had not, to our knowledge, been demonstrated in human breast cancer cells (Banbury Report, 1981). The effect of progestins on the growth of mammary adenocarcinoma appears to vary among different species. In rodents, and in Beagle dogs, it is generally agreed that progestins act synergistically with estrogens to promote the growth of mammary tumors (Mühlbock, 1972) and the normal mammary gland (Delouis, 1980). In humans, however, it has been proposed that progestins display an antiestrogenic effect on mammary cancer and that women with unbalanced estrogen and progesterone levels would be more likely to develop breast cancer. This situation could arise in luteal phase defect (Sherman et al, 1981) and during puberty and the premenopausal period when the mammaray cells could be exposed to estrogens with insufficient control by progesterone (Korenman, 1980). The mechanism of action of progestins either directly on the epithelial cancer cells, and/or indirectly via the hypothalamo-pituitary axis is unknown and difficult to determine in vivo. By contrast, the in vitro approach with the MCF_7 and $T_{47}D$ estrogen-responsive cell lines might allow the study of the direct effect of progestin in breast cancer.

In order to look for a direct antiestrogenic activity of progestin on the growth of these cells, we have studied in culture the effects of R5020, a progestin derivative from the 17-hydroxy progesterone (Ojasoo, Raynaud, 1978) on the growth of two cloned variants of $T_{47}D$ and MCF_7 cells in the presence and absence of estradiol.

B. Antiestrogenic Effect of R5020 (Vignon et al, 1983)

R5020 significantly inhibited the growth of both cell lines in the presence of estradiol (1 nM). The effect was most clear cut after 10-12 days of treatment and was dose-dependent, a half maximal inhibition being obtained with 1 nM R5020. R27, a cloned MCF_7 variant resistant to tamoxifen (Nawata et al, 1981), remained responsive to R5020 which prevented the effect of E_2 and inhibited cell growth in the presence of Tamoxifen. This suggests that the 2 antiestrogens are acting through different mechanisms. Dihydrotestosterone and dexamethasone did not reproduce or inhibit the effect of R5020 on cell growth suggesting that R5020 probably acts via RP rather than via the androgen or glucocorticoid receptors. Using SDS-polyacrylamide gel electrophoresis, we found that R5020 specifically decreased the production of the 52 K protein, a major glycoprotein released by MCF_7 cells after E_2 stimulation.

We concluded that R5020 has an antiestrogenic activity on breast cancer cells in culture since it prevents the stimulation of cell growth and protein synthesis by E_2.

C. Direct Progestin Effects of R5020 without added estrogens (Chalbos, Rochefort, submitted, 1983).

These have been studied mostly in the $T_{47}D$ cell line (clone 11) where the RP is known to be present in high concentrations even in the absence of added estrogens (Horwitz et al, 1982).

a. Effect on cell growth. R5020 inhibits the growth of $T_{47}D$ cells in a dose dependent manner. This inhibitory effect was also observed independently by K. Horwitz (personnal communication) and also shown with other synthetic compounds such as the RU38,486, a specific progestin inhibitor (Chalbos, unpublished experiments). The effect was more important with estradiol than without added estrogens (Vignon et al, 1983). Even though it is difficult to totally exclude some estrogen in the control serum and cells, progestins may act not only as anti-estrogens but also independently as cytostatic and/or cytotoxic agents.

b. Effect on proteins released into the culture medium. Before cell growth inhibition, there is a marked decrease of the total amount of proteins released into the medium. This effect occurs with similar concentrations of R5020 (ED50 $\simeq$ 0.1 nM) and appears to be specific to progestins. It is not observed in the RP negative cell line BT20 and is less in MCF_7 than in the $T_{47}D$ cell line. This general inhibitory effect on the production of released protein therefore appears to be mediated by the RP. However, the mechanism of this inhibition (decreased protein synthesis, shedding, or secretion) is unknown.

c. Progestin specific proteins. An earlier effect is observed, (within 2 days) prior to this general inhibition (5 days). The amount and percentage of some proteins labelled by ^{35}S methionine and released into the medium are specifically increased by R5020, medroxy progesterone acetate and progesterone. The production of a 48 K protein which is not seen without added progestins is particularly increased. The stimulation is specifically inhibited by RU38,486, (a progestin inhibitor), is concentration dependent and absent in the RP-negative cell line BT20. Other steroids are totally unable to increase the production of this protein suggesting that it is a useful marker to assess the progestin (and antiprogestin) activity of a hormone or drug.

D. Mechanisms of the Antiestrogenic Effect

The molecular mechanism of the antiestrogenic activity of progestins has been mainly studied in endometrium (Gurpide et al, 1979). Progesterone and progestins may be acting at a different level : a) They might decrease the concentration of active estrogens, such as estradiol, by increasing its rate of metabolism in target tissue. This is due to the induction of 17 hydroxysteroid oxydo reductase by progestins. This induction by progestin was observed in epithelial cells of human endometrium (Tseng et al, 1977) and in fibro-adenoma of mammary glands (Sitruh Ware et al, 1983). However, in other species (rat endometrium) or other tissues (human stromal endometrium), while progestins do not induce the enzyme, they remain antiestrogens. Thus, this mechanism may not be considered as general (King, 1983). b) Progestins also decrease the efficiency of the RE by decreasing the concentration of RE and/or its nuclear translocation. It has been proposed that progestin increases the RE inactivation by a dephosphorylation mediated by acid phosphatases (McDonald et al, 1982).

4. CONCLUDING REMARKS

The studies of androgen and progestin action in breast cancer cell lines provide two series of information which improve our basic understanding of hormone action and the practical treatment of breast cancer.

A. Mode of Action of Estrogen and their Antagonists

Androgens and progestins clearly modulate the growth and protein production of breast cancer cells under in vitro conditions indicating that in vivo they may also act directly on the tumoral cells in addition to their indirect effect on gonatrophin release. In contrast to non steroidal antiestrogen which competitively inhibit estrogen binding, and act relatively rapidly, androgens and progestins are only antiestrogenic after a lag period of several days. This suggests that mechanisms such as protein synthesis or degradation and receptor sites regulation are involved. The concentration of RE has in fact been shown to be decreased by progesterone.

The receptor involved in these antagonistic activities is likely to be the physiological receptor responsible for the agonist activity of the hormone. For instance, the antiestrogenic activity of androgen is prevented by treatment with antiandrogens. There is a correlation between the concentrations of drug able to saturate this receptor and their observed antiestrogenic activity. For instance, for concentrations of androgens which occupy the RE, no antiestrogenic activity is observed but rather a full estrogenic activity (Rochefort and Garcia, 1983). The final steps of the antiproliferative effect of androgens and progestins is not understood. According to an oversimplified diagram, one can discriminate between three series of mechanisms : 1. These steroids might stimulate a pathway inhibiting DNA replication and/or cell division such as the increased production of androgens or progestins induced growth inhibitory factors. 2. They might inhibit an estrogen-induced stimulatory pathway such as the synthesis or release of estrogen-induced proteins behaving as growth factors (Vignon et al, 1983). 3. Finally, they could modulate the effect of any other mitogens besides estrogens, since cell proliferation can be regulated by multiple hormone and factors. All three mechanisms are possible since both androgen-, progestin- and estrogen- specific induced proteins have recently been observed in breast cancer cells in culture (Chalbos, Rochefort, 1983 ; Westley, Rochefort, 1980). These different hypotheses are being tested for progestin. We found a remarkable correlation between the inhibition by R5020 of the production of the released proteins by T47D and MCF_7 cells and the inhibition of E_2-stimulated cell growth (Fig. 2). On the basis of recent results showing a mitogenic effect of conditioned media (Vignon et al, 1983), we favor the second mechanism by why progestins could inhibit the E_2-induced cell proliferation by inhibiting the production of E_2 induced secreted growth factors. As compared to the non-steroidal antiestrogens, progestins appear therefore to act by different initial mechanisms involving different receptors. However, the final steps by which they control tumor growth may be similar since tamoxifen and metabolites have also been shown to specifically decrease the production of estrogen-induced released proteins. Further work is required to prove and to analyse such mechanisms.

Figure 2. Effects of R5020 on the bio-synthesis of relea-sed proteins and cell growth in T47D cells. T47D cells were cultured with 3 % charcoal treated fetal calf serum for 5 days and plated in 96-microwell dishes. Two days later, cells were treated with (a) or without 1 nM estradiol (b) and increasing con-centrations of R5020 for 5 days, media being replaced every 2 days. After ^{35}S methionine labelling of the cells, TCA precipitable counts of the media were measured and the amount of secreted proteins was calcula-

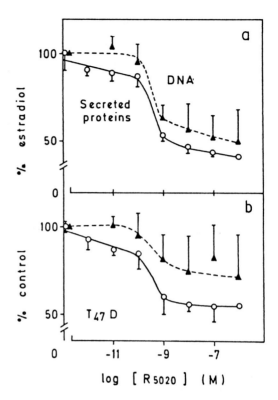

ted as a percentage of the amount of proteins in the estradiol-treated cells (a) or in the control cells (b). DNA values were determined in parallel after 12 days of treatment and expressed as a percentage of control or E_2-treated cells.

From Vignon et al, 1983, by permission.

B. Practical and Clinical Consequences for Therapy

The recent progress in the understanding of the mode of action of additive therapy aimed at inhibiting estrogen action give a rationale for an improved use and new approaches for treating breast cancer.

a. The concentration of estrogen and progesterone receptors should be sufficiently high to allow full effi-ciency of tamoxifen and progestins. It is known (McGuire, Horwitz, 1977) that progestins rapidly and drastically decrease the concentration of its specific receptor. By contrast, estrogen and also antiestrogen increase the RP concentration, and the use of tamoxifen has been proposed for this purpose (Namer et al, 1980). Sequential association of tamoxifen and progestins have therefore been proposed to increase the efficiency of these two compounds. Firstly, tamoxifen acts via RE to inhibit tumor growth and to stimulate the progesterone receptors. Secondly, progestogens can then act, but this reduces the concentration of RP and RE and requires further tamoxifen treatment.

   b. Antiestrogen-resistant tumors may still be responsive to androgens and/or progestins. This has been observed clinically and is beginning to be understood biochemically since the mechanism and the receptor responsible for the action of these hormonal therapy are different, as reported above. Furthermore, recent analysis of an antiestrogen resistant clone (R27) selected from MCF$_7$ cells by its ability to grow with 1 μM tamoxifen (Nawata et al, 1981) has indicated that in this particular case, when cells contained RE, tamoxifen was not inactive but acted as a full estrogen. More precisely it was able to increase the production in the medium of the 52 K glycoprotein while in the antiestrogen sensitive cell it is totally ineffective for this particular effect (Vignon et al, 1983). In the same clone, R5020 a synthetic progestin has been shown to prevent cell growth in vitro indicating that at least in vitro a second type of endocrine therapy could be efficient while classical antiestrogen become inefficient or even dangerous. Before extrapolating the conclusions of these in vitro studies to the in vivo situation, additional experiments are necessary.

   c. Progression to hormone resistance. Unfortunately in metastatic diseases the efficiency of hormone-related therapy decreases with time, due to the progressive selection of hormone-resistant cells which are less differentiated, having lost their RE and RP. Moreover, responsive cells are not always destroyed, but blocked in a G0 (non dividing) stage. They are at rest but they are not always destroyed and can redivide again. Research to develop ways to maintain cells under a differentiated state and to rapidly eliminate the totality of cancer cells before this progression is urgently required.

This work was supported in part by the "Institut National de la Santé et de la Recherche Médicale", the University of Montpellier 1 and the "Fondation pour la Recherche Médicale Française". We are grateful to the skilful assistance of E. Barrié for preparing the manuscript. We thank our colleagues and particularly D. Chalbos, M. Garcia and F. Vignon for their ideas and experimental results.

REFERENCES

Banbury Report (1981). "Hormones and Breast Cancer". Pike MC, Siiteri PK, Welsch CW (eds) Cold Spring Harbor Laboratory.

Borgna JL, Rochefort H (1981). Hydroxylated metabolites of tamoxifen are formed in vivo and bound to estrogen receptor in target tissues. J Biol Chem 256:859.

Chalbos D, Vignon F, Keydar I, Rochefort H (1982). Estrogens stimulate cell proliferation and induce secretory proteins in a human breast cancer cell line (T47D). J Clin Endocrin Metab 55:276.

Chalbos D, Rochefort H. Dual effects of the progestin R5020 on proteins released by the T47D human breast cancer cells. Submitted for publication.

Delouis C (1980). Histopathologie du sein, rôle des hormones dans l'élaboration de la maturation du tissu mammaire. In Martin PM (ed): "Récepteurs Hormonaux et Pathologie Mammaire", Paris: Medsi, Vol 11.

Fournier S, Kuttenn F, De Cicco F, Baudot N, Mallet C, Mauvais-Jarvis P (1982). Estradiol 17 β-hydroxysteroid dehydrogenase activity in human breast fibroadenomas. J Clin Endocrin Metab 55:428.

Furr BJ, Patterson JS, Richardson DN, Slater SR, Wakeling AE (1979). Tamoxifen. In Goldberg ME (ed): "Pharmacological and Biochemical Properties of Drugs Substances" Washington: American Pharmaceutical Association, Vol 2, p 335.

Garcia M, Rochefort H (1978). Androgen effects mediated by estrogen receptor in 7, 12 Dimethylbenz(a)anthracene-induced rat mammary tumors. Cancer Res 38:3922.

Garcia M, Rochefort H (1979). Evidence and characterization of the binding of two ^{3}H androgens to the estrogen receptor. Endocrinology 104:1797.

Gurpide E, Satyaswaroop PG, Fleming H, Bressler RS (1979). Hormonal aspects of carcinoma of the endometrium. In Thatcher N (ed): "Advances in Medical Oncology, Research and Education, Gynecological Cancer", Oxford, New York, Toronto, Sydney, Paris, Frankfurt: Pergamon Press, Vol VIII, p 191.

Horwitz KB, Mockus MB, Lessey BA (1982). Variant T47D human breast cancer cells with high progesterone receptors levels despite estrogen and antiestrogen resistance. Cell 28:633.

Ip M, Milholland RJ, Kim U, Rosen F (1982). Androgen control of cytosol progesterone receptor levels in the MT-W9B transplantable mammary tumor in the rat. J Natl Cancer Inst 69:673.

Katzenellenbogen BS, Pavlik EJ, Robertson DW, Katzenellenbogen JA (1981). Interaction of a high affinity antiestrogen (α- 4-pyrrolidinoethoxy phenyl-4-hydroxy-α'-nitrostilbene, CI628M) with uterine estrogen receptors. J Biol Chem 256:2908.

King RJB (1983). Steroid receptors in normal and abnormal endometrium. 2nd International Meeting on Hormonal Receptors, Barcelona, 14-19 March 1983.

Korenman S (1980). The endocrinology of breast cancer. Cancer 46:874.

Lacassagne A (1936). A comparative study of the carcinogenic action of certain oestrogenic hormones. Am J Cancer 27:217.

Li SA, Li JJ (1978). Estrogeninduced progesterone receptor in the Syrian Hamster Kidney. Modulation by antiestrogens and androgens. Endocrinology 103:2119.

MacDonald RG, Okulicz WC, Leavitt WW (1982). Progesterone induced inactivation of nuclear estrogen receptor in the hamster uterus is mediated by acid phosphatase. Biochem Biophys Res Commun 104:570.

MacIndoe JH, Etre LA (1981). An antiestrogenic action of androgens in human breast cancer cells. J Clin Endocrin Metab 53:836.

McGuire WL, Horwitz KB (1977). A role of progesterone in breast cancer. In Gurpide E (ed): "Biochemical Actions of Progesterone and Progestins", New York: Annals of the New York Academy of Sciences, Vol 286, p 90.

Namer M, Lalanne C, Baulieu EE (1980). Increase of progesterone receptor by tamoxifen as a hormonal challenge test in breast cancer. Cancer Res 40:1750.

Nawata H, Bronzert D, Lippman ME (1981). Isolation and characterization of a tamoxifen-resistant cell line derived from MCF7 human breast cancer cells. J Biol Chem 256:5016.

Ojasoo T, Raynaud JP (1978). Unique steroid congeners for receptor studies. Cancer Res 38:4185.

Rochefort H, Lignon F, Capony F (1972). Formation of estrogen nuclear receptor in uterus : Effect of androgens, estrone and nafoxidine. Biochem Biophys Res Commun 47:662.

Rochefort H, Capony F, Garcia M (1979a). Mechanisms of action of antiestrogens and androgens on the estrogen receptor. J Steroid Biochem 11:1635.

Rochefort H, Garcia M, Borgna JL (1979b). Absence of correlation between antiestrogenic activity and binding affinity for the estrogen receptor. Biochem Biophys Res Commun 88:351.

Rochefort H (1981). Données récentes sur le mécanisme d'action des antioestrogènes de synthèse. Biochimie 64:89.

Rochefort H, Bardon S, Chalbos D, Vignon F (1983). Steroidal and non steroidal antiestrogen in breast cancer cells in culture. J Steroid Biochem, In press.

Rochefort H, Garcia M. The estrogenic and antiestrogenic activities of androgens in female target tissues. In Clark JH, Markaverich B (eds): "Pharmacology of Steroid Hormone Antagonists", International Encyclopedia of Pharmacology and Therapeutics, Submitted for publication (1983).

Rochefort H, Westley B (1983). Role of the estrogen receptors in estrogen responsive mammalian cells. In Litwack G (ed): "Biochemical Actions of Hormones", Academic Press.

Sherman BM, Wallace RB, Korenman SG (1981). Corpus luteum dysfunction and the epidemiology of breast cancer : A reconsideration. Breast Cancer Res Treatment 1:287.

Sitruk-Ware R, Sterkers N, Mowszowicz I, Mauvais-Jarvis P (1977). Inadequate corpus luteal function in women with benign breast diseases. J Clin Endocrin Metab 44:771.

Sutherland RL, Jordan VC (1981). In "NonSteroidal Antiestrogens", Sydney: Harcourt Brace Jovanovitch Group, Academic Press.

Tseng L, Gusberg SB, Gurpide E (1977). Estradiol receptor and 17 -dehydrogenase in normal and abnormal human endometrium. In Gurpide E (ed): "Biochemical Actions of Progesterone and Progestins", New York, Annals of the New York Academy of Sciences, Vol 286, p 190.

Ulrich P (1939). La testostérone (hormone mâle) et son rôle possible dans le traitement de certains cancers du sein. Acta Un Int Cancer 4:377.

Vignon F, Bardon S, Chalbos D, Rochefort H (1983). Antiestrogenic effect of R5020, a synthetic progestin in human breast cancer cells in culture. J Clin Endocrin Metab, June, in press.

Vignon F, Derocq D, Chambon M, Rochefort H (1983). Endocrinologie. Les protéines oestrogéno-induites sécrétées par les cellules mammaires cancéreuses humaines MCF7 stimulent leur prolifération. C R Acad Sci PARIS 296:151.

Vignon F, Lippman M, Nawata H, Derocq D, Rochefort H. Antiestrogens induce two estrogen responsive proteins in a tamoxifen resistant clone, R27, of MCF7 cells. submitted for publication.

Westley B, Rochefort H (1980). A secreted glycoprotein induced by estrogen in human breast cancer cell lines. Cell 20:353.

Zava DT, McGuire WL (1978). Androgen action through estrogen receptor in a human breast cancer cell line. Endocrinology 103:624.

Hormones and Cancer, pages 97–108

INCIDENCE OF ESTROGEN, PROGESTERONE AND PROLACTIN
RECEPTORS IN HUMAN BREAST CANCER

R.S. Calandra, E.H. Charreau, M. Royer de
Giaroli, A. Baldi
Laboratorio de Esteroides, Instituto de Biología y Medicina Experimental, Obligado 2490,
1428 Buenos Aires, Argentina

INTRODUCTION
     The first event on the molecular mechanism of ac-
tion of sex steroid hormones consists in the interaction between these steroids and the macromolecules
within the cells of target organs. Following this inter
action, the sexual steroids bind to the cytoplasmic
receptor and subsequently the hormone-receptor complex
is transfered into the nucleus where it is associated
with the chromatin and stimulates transcription (Baldi,
Charreau 1981).

     In the last decade it has been accepted that estrogen
-receptor (ER) assay predicts the clinical response to
endocrine manipulations in patients with mammary carcino
ma. The response rate to hormone treatments is high in
patients with ER$^+$ tumors (Mc Guire 1978).

     Since in estrogen target tissues, either normal or
neoplastic cells, estrogen administration induces cytoso
lic progesterone receptors (PR), the possibility arises
that its measurement be an excellent biochemical marker
for estrogen action. Therefore, the quantitation of both,
ER and PR, have shown to be a better indicator of human
mammary cancer response to hormone therapy (Osborne et
al.1980) than the determination of ER alone.

     Questions has been raised about the role of prolac
tin (PRL) in the development and maintenance of human
breast carcinoma (Pearson et al., 1978). Some studies
indicated that PRL and estrogens are the two main hormones

implicated in the regulation of mammary gland growth.
No correlation has been shown between serum PRL levels
and sex steroid receptors values in breast cancer (Vihko
et al. 1980). Nevertheless, a recent publication (Ben—Da
vid et al. 1981), reported a higher dependency of breast
cancer on PRL than on steroid receptors, according to
their study on binding sites for PRL (PRL-R).

With the above questions in mind, the aims of the
present study were: 1) to investigate the receptor
status (ER y PR) in primary and metastatic mammary carci
noma; 2) to correlate in some of our cases the existence
of ER/PR with some clinical features; 3) to assess the
interrelationship between ER/PR with PRL-R in some tumors
and 4) to establish the incidence of these receptors in
the local population*, in comparison with what has been
published by other groups (McGuire 1978; Vihko et al.
1980; Wittliff et al. 1978).

MATERIAL AND METHODS

Samples were obtained from a total of 1150 patients.
Patients were grouped as pre or postmenopausal according
to their menstrual history. Breast tumor specimens obtain
ed by biopsy or mastectomy were divided for receptor
assays and histological examination.

Fat—free and nonhemorrhagic specimens were quickly
frozen on dry ice and transported to the laboratory.
Dissected tumors were stored at $-70^{\circ}C$ until receptor
assay was performed and stored for no longer than
three weeks. A group of 5 male with primary breast
tumors were also included. No patient received any
endocrine treatment before operation.

Tissue references were made from prepuberal rat
uterus for ER and similar rats treated with 17β-estra-
diol (12.5 μg/rat/day) for three days for PR. These
internal control tissues were proccessed as the human
specimen and remain stable for at least three months at
$-70^{\circ}C$.

Chemicals:
$[2,4,6,7 -{}^{3}H]$ —Estradiol, 85—106 Ci/mMol; 1,2,4,5,

*Part of this work had been reported previously

6,7 -^{3}H] -Dihydrotestosterone, 100 Ci/mMol; [1,2,6,7-^{3}H]
-Progesterone, 90Ci/mMol; R5020 [6,7-^{3}H] 17,21-dimethyl
-19-nor-4,9-pregnadiene-3,10-dione, 87Ci/mMol and R1881
[6,7-^{3}H]-17α -hydroxy-17α -methyl-4,9,11-estratien-3-
one, 58Ci/mMol, were purchased from New England Nuclear,
U.S.A. Non-labelled steroids (estradiol,diethylstil-
bestrol (DES), cortisol, dihydrotestosterone (DHT),
triamcinolone acetonide); Tris-base, dithiothreitol and
disodium ethylenaminotetra-acetate (EDTA) were obtained
from Sigma Chem.,Co., St.Louis,Mo.,U.S.A. Nafoxidine
was a gift from Upjohn Co.,U.S.A. Norit-A was purchased
from Amend Drug Chem.Co.Inc. and Agar form Behringwerke,
Marburg, W.G. Other chemicals were reagent of analytical
grade.
Human PRL (h-PRL) and ovine PRL (o-PRL) were a kind
gift from the National Pituitary Agency NIAMDD,U.S.A.
(NIH-h-PRL-VLS3 and NIH-oPRL-P-S12 respectively). Ultra
gel ACA-54 was obtained from LKB,Sweden.

Processing of the Tissues:
All procedures were performed at 0-4ºC. The frozen
tissue was thawed, washed with a buffer A (20mM Tris-
HCl, pH 7.4, containing 1.5 mM EDTA, 0.25 mM DTT and
10%, v/v glycerol), an aliquot weighed and minced.
Tissue was homogenized with the same buffer in a ratio
1 to 4, w/v, with a Polytron desintegrator Pt10 (Brink
man Instruments Inc., N.Y.) for three 10-second bursts
with 1 min. cooling intervals on ice. The homogenate
was centrifuged at 800xg for 15 min. to remove large
particles and the supernatant was spun for 60 min. at
105,000xg in an ultracentrifuge (Beckman Inst., model
L2-65B). The soluble supernatant fraction (cytosol) was
used inmediately for steroid receptor assays. When
PRL-R was performed, the postnuclear pellet was washed
twice with buffer PBS (Phosphate buffered saline, pH7.4)
resuspended in the original volume with PBS and procceed
as described below.

Measurement of steroid receptor:
a) Sucrose gradients analysis.
Aliquots of 500 μl of cytosol were incubated
with saturating concentration of [^{3}H]estradiol, [^{3}H]-
progesterone or [^{3}H] -R5020 (5-8nM). Non-specific
binding of the tracer was estimated from tubes contain
ing a 500-fold molar excess of non-radioactive Nafoxidi
ne, estradiol or DES for ER; progesterone plus cortisol

or R5020 plus cortisol for PR. To rule out the influence
of SHBG and CBG on the assay for ER and PR, aliquots
were incubated with DHT or cortisol respectively (200-
fold molar excess). From the incubation mixtures 250 μl
were taken and layered on top of 5-20% linear sucrose
gradient. Samples were centrifuged in a SW56 rotor at
205,000xg for 15 hr (0-4ºC).
Alternatively, before ultracentrifugation, the incubation mixture was adsorbed with dextran-coated charcoal
suspension (0.05-0.5%,w/v respectively) in order to
remove most of free radioactivity (Calandra et al. 1977).
The tubes were centrifuged and bound steroids counted
as published elsewhere (Calandra et al. 1980).
      b) Agar gel electrophoresis.
      Agar gel electrophoresis was performed essential
ly as described by Wagner (Wagner 1972). Cytoplasmic
fractions were incubated as in a) with $[^3H]$-estradiol or
$[^3H]$-DHT for ER and androgen receptor (AR). Aliquots of
50 μl of these tritium labelled cytosols were applied
on agar and run at 130mA, 120 volts, during 90 min. Gel
temperature was mantained at 0-5ºC.
      c) Analysis by charcoal technique.
      This method based on the original described by
Korenman and Dukes (Korenman, Dukes 1970), was recently
adapted (Calandra et al. 1980). Aliquots in duplicate of
200 ul cytosol were incubated with a series of concentra
tions of $[^3H]$ -estradiol (0.2-5nM), $[^3H]$ -progesterone or
$[^3H]$ R5020 (0.2-8nM), with or without 100-fold molar
excess of Nafoxidine or DES (ER), progesterone or R5020
(PR) respectively. The binding of estradiol and progeste
rone/R5020 to SHBG and CBG was eliminated by adding 200-
fold molar excess of DHT and cortisol respectively. In
the few cases of male breast cancer studied for AR, the
tracer $[^3H]$-R1881 was used and an excess of triamcinolone
acetonide was also added to the incubation medium to
prevent binding of radioligand to the PR. Scatchard plots
were used to analyse the data (Scatchard 1949). In many
occassions the assay was carried out by a single saturat
ing dose, due to the limitation on the specimen size.
The tubes were incubated for 4 hr at 0-4ºC, and then 400μl
of Dextran-Charcoal suspension in Buffer A were added.
Tubes were centrifuged at 1000xg for 10 min and aliquots
of supernatant (bound fraction) were counted for radioacti
vity in a Packard Tricarb Model 3320 Scintillation Counter
with an efficiency of 49% (Calandra et al. 1980).
For both ER and PR the results were expressed as fmoles

per mg of cytosol protein.

    d) Prolactin binding assay.

    Iodination of h-PRL was performed using the lactoperoxidase method (Thorell, Johansson, 1971). The iodinated hormone had a specific activity between 20-30 μCi/ug and was weekly purified by Ultragel ACA-54 column chromatography as reported earlier (Charreau et al.1977). The membrane suspension was centrifuged and washed with PBS buffer twice, filtered through a nylon cloth and spun at 12,000xg for 20 min. Pellets were resuspended in PBS in a ratio 1:2 (w/v) and aliquots of 100 μl of the membrane suspension were equilibrated with 50,000 dpm I^{125}-h-PRL for 90 min at 34ºC. Non-specific binding was considered to be that binding occurring in the pre sence of 500 ng exccess of h-PRL (total binding was between 5—10%). Once the non-specific binding was correct ed, the results were expressed as fmoles per mg of mem brane suspension protein.

    e) Miscellaneous methods.

    Yeast alcohol dehydrogenase (ADH, 7.55) and bovi ne serum albumin (BSA, 4.65), were used as internal standards in the sucrose gradients. Protein in the cyto sol and membrane suspension was determined by the method of Lowry et al. (Lowry et al. 1951).

RESULTS AND DISCUSSION

    Cytosol reference made of prepuberal rat uterus (ER) and estradiol treated prepuberal rat uterus (PR), were prepared and run in each assay. Both receptors were stable for at least three months at -70ºC.

    We considered a positive ER (ER$^+$) assay for human breast specimens when the number of binding sites was equal to/or higher than 2 fmol/mg protein and for PR (PR$^+$) level equal to/or higher than 5 fmol/mg protein. The first approach to the study of ER was done using the sucrose gradient method. In our hands, the sedimenta tion profiles of ER fell into four categories for the first 180 human breast carcinomas. From these data it can be seen (Table I) from the ER$^+$ cases that 64.2% of breast tumors containing ER exhibited the 8Sform, almost 25% only the 4S type and 11% contained both the 8S and 4S components, using low ionic strenght gradients. The remaining tumors did not contain any type of binding. These results are interesting in relation to the finding

TABLE I

DISTRIBUTION OF ESTROGEN RECEPTORS (ER) FORMS[*] IN A GROUP OF 180 HUMAN BREAST CARCINOMA.

TOTAL ER+	8S	4.5S	8 +4.5S	TOTAL ER –
109 (60.6 %)	70 (64.2 %)	27 (24.7 %)	12 (11.0 %)	71 (39.4 %)

[*] BY SUCROSE GRADIENT ANALYSIS

reported by Wittliff et al (1978) who initiated a long term study to examine the presence of different binding complexes as a predictive tool of clinical response. It appears from these studies that, the molecular proper- ties of the 8S tumors who exhibiting remissions to endo crine therapy, are different from those unresponsive breast tumors which contained other components.

It is well known that it is more accurate to predict the prognosis and clinical response to endocrine treatment of breast cancer if both, the ER and PR are measured simultaneously (Osborne et al. 1980; Edwards et al.1979). The assumption for this is that estrogens exert its biological effect through the formation of PR.

We have now analysed 970 samples and the mean concentra tions of both receptors in the whole group are shown in Table II. It can also be seen a lower ER levels in premenopausal women in comparison to postmenopausal women (60.8 fmol/mg prot.vs 175.2 fmol/mg prot). On the other hand, there was no difference on the PR levels between both groups of patients.

TABLE II

CONCENTRATIONS OF ESTROGEN AND PROGESTERONE RECEPTORS (ER,PR IN CYTOSOL, f mol/mg prot.) IN THE WHOLE GROUP AND THE COMPARISON BETWEEN PRE AND POSTMENOPAUSAL PATIENTS WITH HUMAN BREAST CARCINOMA.

WHOLE GROUP :	
E R	140.3 ± 11.1[*] (970)[**]
P R	210.2 ± 16.3 (970)
PREMENOPAUSAL :	
E R	60.8 ± 7.3 (168)
P R	190.1 ± 23.1 (168)
POSTMENOPAUSAL :	
E R	175.2 ± 13.2 (802)
P R	205.4 ± 19.6 (802)

[*] MEAN $\pm$ SEM
[**] NUMBER OF PATIENTS INVESTIGATED

These results agree with the findings of another groups and particularly to the higher ER levels in post menopausal patients, which is well interpreted by the lower estradiol levels in this study (Vihko et al.1980; Bird et al. 1981) and is correlated with age.

From the entire group, 776 (80%) were primary and 194 (20%) metastatic lesions. In all samples, ER was present in 77.6% and PR in 61.4%, while both receptors were found simultaneously in 59% (Table III). Negative specimens in the whole group were 20% whereas ER^+ only in 18.6% of the cases, and PR^+ only in approximately 2%.

TABLE III
DISTRIBUTION OF ESTROGEN AND PROGESTERONE RECEPTORS (ER,PR) IN THE WHOLE GROUP AND IN SAMPLES CLASSIFIED ACCORDING TO THE TYPE OF LESION.

DISTRIBUTION	WHOLE GROUP	PRIMARY SPECIMENS	METASTATIC SPECIMENS
ER^+/PR^+	572/970*(59.0%)	450/776 (57.9%)	78/194 (40.2%)
ER^+/PR^-	180/970 (18.6%)	124/776 (15.9%)	49/194 (25.2%)
ER^-/PR^+	24/970 (2.4%)	24/776 (3.0%)	5/194 (2.5%)
ER^-/PR^-	194/970 (20.0%)	180/776 (23.2%)	62/194 (32.1%)

✦ NUMBER OF PATIENTS INVESTIGATED

The present findings are similar to the data previously reported by several other groups (Mc Guire 1978; Osborne et al.1980; Vihko et al. 1980).
In this study we have also compared the receptor distribution between primary and metastatic samples. It is shown in the same table (Table III) that ER was present with less frecuency in secondary than in primary lesions (73.8vs 65.4%) and the differences were even greater for the PR (60.9vs 42.7%). The presence of both steroid receptors are also more frequently seen in the primary lesions as well as the incidence of megative tumors (23.2vs 32.1%). On this basis some authors, postulate that secondary breast carcinoma is less hormone-dependent than primary tumors (Vihko et al 1980). Despite previous and present findings, a long-term follow up study is required in order to give more support to this idea.

According to other clinical features no association was found between the tumor size, location, age of menarche, latency and the presence of ER. Regarding the tumor histology and its ability to bind estradiol, no correlation was found between both parameters. Furthermore,Witt

liff et al. (1978), have given some evidences that there
is relationship between the number of estrogen binding
sites and the proportion of tumor epithelium. In consequence, the differences in binding activity may be relat
ed to the number of binding sites per tumor cell rather
than to the number of tumor cells.
As has been already mentioned, several groups have
demonstrated the presence of cytoplasmic steroid receptors in female breast malignant tumors. However, there
is little information concerning hormone receptor studies
in male breast carcinoma. Less than 1% of breast carcinoma occur in men and therefore few centers have the
opportunity to study a reasonable number of patients. In
most of these studies only ER determined and almost all
cases contain this binding protein.
    We have studied five primary male breast carcinoma
and AR/ER were quantitated simultaneously. It was seen
in our limited group that three out of five specimens
possess only AR whereas the remaining two cases were
ER⁺. These data do not allow to draw any conclusion, but
it is striking that a 45 to 68% (Holleb et al. 1968; Tre
ves 1959) of men with metastatic mammary carcinoma pre—
sent a regression of their secondary tumor following
orchidectomy. The availability of the synthetic radioligand R1881 and specific competitive inhibitors will
allow a more accurate estimation of AR in male breast
carcinoma and its significance.
    The biological response of breast tumors is not
only under the action of steroid sexual hormones. The
effect of peptide hormones, like PRL, has been well
described in experimental models (Kelly et al, 1974;
Costlow et al. 1975). Since early studies it was suggest
ed that PRL is one of the main stimulus for breast tumor
growth and estrogen may be mediating these PRL effects.
In the present study, we have measured PRL binding sites
in a limited number of female breast tumors. The specificity was confirmed by the abscense of displacement
with other peptide hormones like FSH and LH (data not
shown).
    As shown Table IV, the incidence of breast tumors
containing or not PRL-R is equally distributed (48% vs
52%) and there was a lack of correlation between PRL-R
and ER. ER were approximately equally seen in the presence or absence of PRL-R (34% vs 42%). The incidence
of PRL R⁺ tumors in our serie is slightly higher than the
binding sites showed by Holdaway and Friesen (1977) and

Table IV
DISTRIBUTION OF PROLACTIN AND ESTROGEN RECEPTORS (PRL-R,ER)
IN HUMAN BREAST CARCINOMA.

PRL-R⁺ ER⁺	17/50*	34 %
PRL-R⁺ ER⁻	7/50	14 %
PRL-R⁻ ER⁺	21/50	42%
PRL-R⁻ ER⁻	5/50	10 %

* NUMBER OF PATIENTS INVESTIGATED

this may result from some differences in the specific
activity of the labelled hormone as well as to the
minimun specific binding fixed to define a tumor as
positive. In contrast, Ben-David et al. (1981), have
presented some evidences that human breast cancer mantain
binding sites for PRL without correlation with age,
hormonal milieu and stage of the disease. Whether or not
the determination of PRL-R will improve the accuracy of
prediction for hormonal dependence in the breast cancer
needs to be confirmed by a larger group of patients and
the correlations between laboratory data and response
in clinical trials.

SUMMARY

Analysis of estrogen and progesterone cytosolic
receptors (ER, PR) has been studied in human breast
carcinoma. ER were assayed by sucrose density gradients
and dextran coated-charcoal method. In a serie of 109
ER⁺ breast tumors, 64.2% exhibited the 8S form, 25% the
4S and 11% both the 8S and 4S components.

From a total number of 970 specimens, 776 (80%)
were primary and 194 (20%) metastatic lesions. In the
whole group, ER was positive in 77.6% and PR in 61.4%,
while both receptors were found simultaneously in 59%.
The concentration of ER was higher in postmenopausal
women in comparison to premenopausal women. On the other
hand, the levels of PR were rather similar in both groups.
In primary lesions, PR was more frequently seen than in
secondary tumors and the same holds true for the presence
of ER and PR and the frecuency of negative tumors.

Specific prolactin (PRL) binding assay was performed

in a group of 50 breast tumors. Positive and negative distribution was almost equal (48 vs 52%) and there was not correlation between PRL-R and ER.

In addition, a limited group of male breast cancer, showed that three out of five patients possess only androgen receptors, whereas the remaining two cases were exclusively ER+.

In summary, the present results indicate that the local incidence of steroid receptors in female breast carcinoma, are very likely similar to previous reports either in premenopausal and postmenopausal women and in primary and secondary lesions. The importance of PRL-R assay requires a further evaluation.

ACKNOWLEDGEMENTS

The excellent technical assistance of Mrs. Ana Rosa de la Cámara and Diana Bas are greatly appreciated. This work was partially supported by the Consejo Nacional de Investigaciones Científicas y Técnicas de la República Argentina (CONICET) and the Comisión Nacional de Energía Atómica (CNEA).

Human prolactin, FSH, LH and ovine prolactin were kindly supplied by the National Pituitary Agency (NIAMDD, U.S.A.). We are also indebted to Upjohn Co. for providing the Nafoxidine.

REFERENCES

Baldi A, Charreau EH (1981). Effects of estradiol-receptor complexes on the template activity of human breast tumor chromatin. In: Soto RJ, De Nicola A, Blaquier J (eds):"Physiopatology endocrine diseases and mechanisms of hormone action", New York: Alan R Liss, Inc, p 447.

Ben-David M, Dror Y, Biran S (1981). Maintenance of prolactin receptors in human breast cancer. Isr J Med Sci 17: 965.

Bird CE, Houghton B, Westnbrink W, Tenniswood M, Sterns EE, Clark AF (1981). Estradiol receptor levels in human breast carcinomas. Can Med Assoc J 124: 1010.

Calandra RS, Purvis K, Hansson V (1977). Measurement of specific androgen-binding proteins in target tissues. In: Hafez,ESE (ed):"Techniques of Human Andrology", Amsterdam, Elsevier, North Holland, p 287.

Calandra RS, Charreau EH, Royer de Giaroli M, Baldi A,

Calvo JC, Pujato D, Arrighi L (1980). Receptores para esteroides y prolactina en carcinomas mamarios humanos. Medicina 40: 718.

Costlow ME, Buschow RA, Richert NJ, Mc Guire WL (1975). Prolactin and estrogen binding in transpantable hormone-dependent and autonomous rat mammary carcinoma. Cancer Res 35: 970.

Charreau EH, Attramadal A, Torjesen PA, Purvis K, Calandra RS, Hansson V (1977). Prolactin binding in rat testis: specific receptors in interstitial cells. Molec Cell Endocr 6: 303.

Edwards OP, Chamness GC, Mc Guire WL (1979). Estrogen and progesterone receptor protein in breast cancer. Biochem Biophys Acta 560: 457.

Holdaway IM, Friesen HG (1977). Hormone binding by human mammary carcinoma. Cancer Res 37: 1946.

Holleb AI, Freeman HO, Farrow JH (1968). Cancer of the male breast. N.Y. State J Med 68: 544.

Kelly PA, Bradley C, Shiu RPC, Meites J, Friesen HG (1974). Prolactin binding to rat mammary tissues. Proc Soc Exptl Biol Med 146: 816.

Korenman SG, Dukes BA (1970). Specific estrogen binding by the cytoplasm of human breast carcinoma. J Clin Endocr Metab 30: 639.

Lowry OH, Rosebrough NJ, Farr AL, Randall RJ (1951). Protein measurement with the Folin Phenol Reagent. J Biol Chem 193: 265.

Mc Guire WL (1978). "Hormones, receptors and breast cancer. Progress in cancer research and therapy", vol 10, New York, Raven Press.

Osborne CK, Yochmowitz MG, Knight WA, Mc Guire WL (1980). The value of estrogen and progesterone receptors in the treatment of breast cancer. Cancer 46: 2884.

Pearson OH, Manni A, Chambers M, Brodkey J, Marshall JS (1978). Role of pituitary hormones in the growth of human breast cancer. Cancer Res 38: 4323.

Scatchard G (1949). The atractions of proteins for small molecules and ions. Ann N Y Acad Sci 51: 660.

Thorell JI, Johansson BG (1971). Enzymatic iodination of polypeptide with ^{125}I to high specific activity. Biochem Biophys Acta 251: 363.

Treves N (1959). The treatment of cancer, specially in operable cancer of male breast by ablative surgery (orchiectomy, adrenalectomy and hypophysectomy) and hormone therapy (estrogen and corticosteroids). An analysis of 42 patients. Cancer 12: 820.

Vihko R, Jänne O, Kontula K, Syrjälä P (1980). Female
    sex steroid receptor status in primary and metastatic
    breast carcinoma and its relationship to serum steroid
    and peptide hormone levels. Int J Cancer 26: 13.
Wagner RK (1972). Characterization and assay of steroid
    hormone receptors and steroid-binding serum proteins
    by agar gel electrophoresis at low temperature. Hoppe
    Seyler's Z Physiol Chem 353: 1235.
Wittliff JL,Lewko WM, Park DC, Kute TE, Baker DT, Kane
    LN (1978). Steroid binding proteins of mammary tissues
    and their clinical significance in breast cancer. In:
    Mc Guire WL (ed): "Hormones, receptors and breast can
    cer. Progress in cancer research and therapy", vol 10,
    New York, Raven Press, p 325.

Hormones and Cancer, pages 109–117
© **1984 Alan R. Liss, Inc., 150 Fifth Avenue, New York, NY 10011**

PROLACTIN AND PROLACTIN BINDING SITES IN HUMAN BREAST
CANCER CELLS

Elisabetta Marchetti, Anna Paola Rimondi,
Patrizia Querzoli, Guidalberto Fabris, Italo Nenci

Istituto di Anatomia e Istologia Patologica
University of Ferrara, 44100 Ferrara, Italy

The well recognized prolactin dependence of some experimental mammary tumours has prompted for the investigation
of prolactin dependence also of human breast cancer, through
the demonstration of specific receptors (Nagasawa, 1979).
Immunocytochemical techniques have already been success-
fully exploited to trace steroid hormone receptors in target
tissues, thus contributing to the understanding of their mechanism of action (Nenci, 1981).
A study has been undertaken to trace prolactin binding
sites in breast cancer by immunocytochemical techniques, to
contribute to the understanding of the mechanism of action
of prolactin and of its role in tumour growth.

MATERIALS AND METHODS

Reagents

Lyophilized human Prolactin (hPrl) was diluted 5 x 10^{-10}
to 1 x 10^{-7}M in phosphate buffered saline pH 7.2, 0.1 M (PBS).
Rabbit anti hPrl immunoglobulins were diluted 1:100 to
1:800 in PBS. Human Prolactin and hPrl antibody were obtained from the National Institute of Arthritis, Metabolism and
Digestive Diseases, NIH, Bethesda).
Fluorescein-labelled goat anti rabbit Ig antiserum
(Behring) was used at 1:20 dilution in PBS. Sera for the
peroxidase-anti peroxidase technique (PAP) (Dako) were diluted in PBS.

Tissue sections

Breast cancer specimens were utilized soon after surgical removal. Whenever possible, specimens were cut in two fragments, which were respectively frozen or immersed in Bouin fixative. Cryostatic sections obtained from frozen fragments were air dried at 4°C for 1 h. Fixed specimens were processed according to standard procedures and paraffin embedded.

Tissue sections were also obtained from a human acidophilic pituitary adenoma clinically responsible for hyperprolactinemia.

Cell Suspensions

Cell suspensions were obtained from human breast cancer immediately after surgical removal by mincing tissue fragments in PBS, without any enzymatic treatment.

Labelling Procedure

Cryostatic tissue sections were rehydrated in PBS and incubated with hPrl for 1-3 hours at room temperature. After several washes in PBS, sections were reacted with rabbit anti hPrl antibodies for 1 h at room temperature. Lastly, an incubation was performed with fluorescein-conjugated goat anti rabbit Ig antiserum for 30' at room temperature. After the final washes, sections were mounted in glycerin-PBS (1:1).

Sections from the human pituitary adenoma were deparaffinized, rehydrated in PBS and processed with hPrl antibody by immunofluorescence and by PAP technique.

Sections from fixed and paraffin embedded blocks of human breast cancer were deparaffinized, rehydrated in PBS and incubated with hPrl at room temperature for 24 hours. After several washes in PBS, sections were reacted with hPrl antibodies for 24 hours at room temperature. Sections were then thoroughly washed in PBS and incubated with swine anti rabbit Ig antibodies for 30' at room temperature, washed, and covered with rabbit PAP for 30' at room temperature. After several washes in PBS sections were reacted for 4-5' with 3,3'-diaminobenzidine tetrahydrochloride in 0.05 M Tris-HCl buffer, pH 7.6, containing 0.03% H_2O_2. After a wash in tap water, sections were counterstained for 1' with Meyer Hematoxylin, dehydrated and mounted in Eukitt.

<u>Cell suspensions</u> from human breast cancer were collected in PBS, washed and resuspended in hPrl 5×10^{-10}, 5×10^{-9}, 5×10^{-8} in PBS containing $CaCl_2$ 10^{-2}M. The incubation was carried out at 4 and 25 °C for 15, 30, 60'. After a thorough wash, cells were resuspended in PBS, dropped on slides and allowed to dry at 4°C. After having being rehydrated in PBS cell preparations were incubated with hPrl antibodies for 30' at room temperature. Slides were then processed by immunofluorescence and by PAP (see above).

<u>The following control experiments</u> were performed on cell and tissue preparations:
- The incubation with hPrl was omitted;
- The exposure to hPrl antibody was left out;
- An incubation was performed with hPrl antibody 1:400 absorbed with hPrl 50 ug/ml;
- A rabbit immune serum was substituted for hPrl antibody.

RESULTS

Pituitary adenoma

Sections from the human pituitary adenoma treated with hPrl antibody displayed a cytoplasmic staining of most cells, when processed either by immunofluorescence or by PAP technique. Fluorescent labelling or specific peroxidase reaction were not observed in sections treated according to controls.

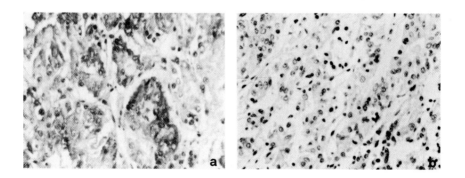

Fig 1. Human prolactinoma. hPrl antibody strongly decorates the cytoplasm of hPrl-containing cells (a). Lack of staining by hPrl antibody absorbed with hPrl (b).

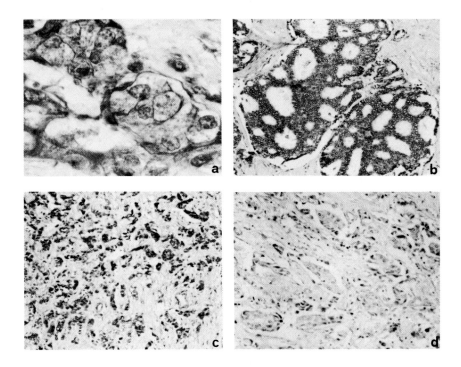

Fig 2. Breast cancer. Evident membrane binding of hPrl as
revealed by hPrl antibody in sections exposed to the hormone
in vitro prior to the PAP sequence (a). Endogenous hPrl is
detected by hPrl antibody in sections not pre-exposed to the
hormone (b, intraductal carcinoma; c, infiltrating ductal
carcinoma). The immunostaining is abolished when hPrl antibody has been absorbed with hPrl (d).

Breast cancer

In cryostatic sections incubated with hPrl and processed
with immunofluorescence, a cytoplasmic fluorescence was apparent in the majority of the cell population. Such a positivity, though of varying intensity in the different specimens and in cells of the same specimen, was usually quite
bright. Moreover, only seldom were negative cells evident. A
similar cytoplasmic fluorescence was also observed in sections

in which the incubation with hPrl had been omitted. On the o-
ther hand, a fluorescent staining was lacking in sections
treated according to the other controls.

In sections obtained from fixed and paraffin embedded
tissue specimens, incubated with hPrl and processed with the
PAP technique, a marked positivity was observed in a high proportion of neoplastic cells and, when present, also in normal,
non neoplastic tissue. The peroxidase reaction was diffusely
distributed on the cell cytoplasm with a granular pattern and
sometimes present on the plasma membrane, too.The plasma membrane was never decorated by hPrl antibody in tissue preparations not pre-exposed to hPrl. On the contrary, the diffuse cytoplasmic staining was appreciable also in sections not
exposed to hPrl prior to the PAP staining sequence. The immunostaining of all localizations was abolished in sections
processed according to the other control tests.

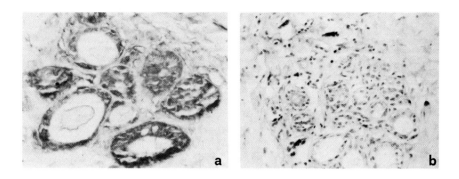

Fig 3. Normal mammary lobule. Endogenous hPrl is traced in
the cell cytoplasm by hPrl antibody (a). Lack of staining
with hPrl antibody absorbed with the hormone (b).

In cell preparations incubated with hPrl and processed by
immunofluorescence or by PAP technique, a diffuse membrane positivity could be appreciated. Immunostained cells were inter-
mixed with unstained cells and with cells displaying a cytoplasmic positivity only. The membrane positivity was evident
in cells incubated with hPrl 5×10^{-8}M at 25°C for 15, 30, 60';
however, a progressive increasing in staining intensity was
noted with longest incubation steps with hPrl. When higher
hPrl dilutions had been used or when the incubation with hPrl

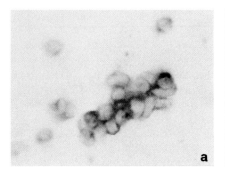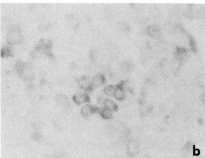

Fig 4. Breast cancer cell suspensions. Membrane binding of
hPrl as revealed by hPrl antibody in cells exposed in vitro
to the hormone (a). A faint cytoplasmic staining only is apparent in cells not pre-exposed to the hormone (b).

had been carried out at 4°C, the plasma membrane was no longer decorated by the antibody. Nevertheless, in these experimental conditions, a diffuse cytoplasmic positivity was apparent in the majority of the cells. It is worth noting that
also in cell preparations not pre-exposed to hPrl before the
immunostaining procedure, it was often possible to observe a
bright diffuse cytoplasmic staining, the plasma membrane ap-
pearing unstained. On the other hand, the immunostaining was
completely abolished by absorption of the anti hPrl antiserum
with hPrl, when incubation with hPrl antibody had been omitted, or when a rabbit immune serum had replaced the specific
hPrl antiserum.

DISCUSSION

In the present study the possibility has been tested of
localizing prolactin binding sites in human breast cancer.
For this purpose, breast cancer samples have been challenged
with prolactin in different experimental conditions; prolactin binding sites have then been traced by an immunocytochemical approach exploiting hPrl antibodies.
The cell surface positivity of cells exposed in vitro to
hPrl and reacted with specific antibodies shows that prolactin binding sites can be visualized by immunocytochemistry

on the plasma membrane of prolactin target cells. Present results are in accord with the mechanism of action of polypeptide hormones which, as a general rule, interact primarily
with the cell plasma membrane. Prolactin binding to the plasma membrane displays in the exploited vital cell system the
same characteristics as in cell-free membrane preparations
(Shiu, Friesen, 1974): it is time- and temperature-dependent
as it occurs at 25°C more than at 4°C and is enhanced by prolonged incubation steps. A high affinity binding of prolactin
to the plasma membrane can be inferred by the withstanding to
prolonged washing steps which are able to remove prolactin
from low affinity binding sites. Biochemical assay too exploits
extensive washing to distinguish high- from low-affinity binding sites (Frantz et al, 1974).

Prolactin binding sites on the plasma membrane appear
still available and reactive with the hormone in fixed and
paraffin embedded tissue sections. Actually, though not in
as many elements as in cell preparations, the cell membrane
was definitely stained by the antibody also in tissue sections, provided they had been exposed to prolactin before the
immunostaining reaction.

The hormone specificity can be held for certain by the
recognition of prolactin containing cells of the pituitary
adenoma by hPrl antibody and by the lack of staining of cell
and tissue preparations treated according to controls.

In contrast with the expected membrane binding and interestingly enough, an unexpected cytoplasmic positivity was
constantly present in both cell suspensions and tissue sections. This cytoplasmic staining was observed in cell and
tissue preparations also when incubation with prolactin had
been omitted and deserves some comments.

The possibility should be taken into account that the
cytoplasmic decoration by prolactin antibody is not dependent
on endogenous prolactin but on the presence of an antigenically related hormone, such as human placental lactogen,growth
hormone or chorionic gonadotropin. Though absorption tests
with these hormones have not been carried out in the present
study, recently reported immunocytochemical results (Purnell
et al, 1982) on breast tissue seem to rule out the dependence
of the positivity on the presence of these hormones.

The presence of endogenous prolactin in breast cancer
has been ascribed to ectopic synthesis of the hormone (Horne
et al, 1976); however, the cytoplasmic positivity observed
also in normal, not neoplastic lobules does not seem to sub-
stantiate this hypothesis.

The intracellular localization of prolactin could result

from a process of hormone internalization, as it occurs for other polypeptide hormones, through a receptor-mediated endocytosis followed by an intracellular delivery to subcellular constituents by receptosomes (Pastan, Willingham, 1981). The internalization of the hormone could thus subserve a modulation of cellular functions through the binding to intracellular receptor sites. In this respect, it is worthy reminding that prolactin has been identified in the Golgi and microsomal fractions of rat hepatocytes (Josefsberg et al, 1979). Moreover, prolactin and its own receptor have been traced in prolactin target tissues with an intracellular coincident pattern (Dunaif et al, 1982).

The observed cytoplasmic positivity could also be dependent on a lisosomal localization of prolactin; the described inactivation of the hormone following its internalization by breast cancer cell lines in culture (Shiu, 1979) lends support to this hypothesis.

In conclusion, the presence of endogenous prolactin does not interfere with the possibility of tracing membrane binding sites by immunocytochemical methods. Moreover, though at present only some hypothesis can be put forward to account for the meaning of the intracellular localization of prolactin, it seems worthy of further investigation. In particular, a longer follow up of the membrane binding in vital cell suspensions could contribute to the understanding of the relation, if any, between membrane binding and intracellular localization of the hormone. In this respect, the seemingly positive correlation appears quite interesting between membrane binding and cytoplasmic positivity in tissue sections and cell preparations exposed to prolactin.

ACKNOWLEDGEMENTS

The experimental work was supported in part by Grant n. 82.00301.96 from the Progetto Finalizzato CNR "Controllo della Crescita Neoplastica" and by Ministero della Pubblica Istruzione.

REFERENCES

Dunaif AE, Zimmerman EA, Friesen HG, Frantz AG(1982). Intracellular localization of prolactin receptor and prolactin in the rat ovary by immunocytochemistry. Endocrinology 110: 1465.

Frantz WL, MacIndoe JH, Turkington RW (1974). Prolactin receptors: characteristics of the particulate fraction binding
activity. J Endocr 60: 485.
Horne CHW, Reid IN, Milne GD (1976). Prognostic significance
of inappropriate production of pregnancy proteins by breast
cancers. Lancet ii: 279.
Josefsberg Z, Posner BI, Patel B, Bergeron JJM (1979). The
uptake of prolactin into female rat liver. Concentration
of intact hormone in the Golgi apparatus. J Biol Chem 254:
209.
Nagasawa H (1979). Prolactin and human breast cancer: a review. Europ J Cancer 15: 267.
Nenci I (1981). Estrogen receptor cytochemistry in human
breast cancer: status and prospects. Cancer 48: 2674.
Pastan IH, Willingham MC (1981). Receptor-mediated endocytosis of hormones in cultured cells. Ann Rev Physiol 43: 239.
Purnell DM, Hillman EA, Heatfield BM, Trump BF (1982). Immunoreactive prolactin in epithelial cells of normal and
cancerous breast and prostate detected by the unlabeled antibody peroxidase-antiperoxidase method. Cancer Res 42: 2317.
Shiu RPC (1979). Processing of prolactin by human breast cancer cells in long term tissue culture. J Biol Chem 255: 4278.
Shiu RPC, Friesen HG (1974). Properties of a prolactin receptor from the rabbit mammary gland. Biochem J 140: 301.

Hormones and Cancer, pages 119–132

ESTROGEN AND PROGESTERONE REGULATION OF PROLIFERATION AND
DIFFERENTIATION OF RABBIT UTERINE EPITHELIUM

L.E. Gerschenson, M.D., C.J. Conti, D.V.M.,Ph.D.,
J.R. Depaoli, Ph.D., R. Lieberman, B.S.,
M. Lynch, B.S., D. Orlicky, M.S. and
A. Rivas-Berrios, Ph.D.

Department of Pathology, School of Medicine
University of Colorado Health Sciences Center
Denver, Colorado   80262   USA

INTRODUCTION

Endometrial carcinoma is one of the few human neoplasms for which a clear association has been found
between hormones and cancer: a connection has been
described among the estrogen-secreting ovarian granulosa-
theca cell tumors or estrogen administration and endometrial hyperplasia and cancer (MacMahon 1974). Also, an
association between carcinoma of the endometrium and poly-
cystic ovaries or Stein-Leventhal syndrome has been reported (MacMahon 1974) and it is thought to be due to a
constant estrogenic stimulus without the progestogenic
counterpart. Progesterone administration has been found to
be helpful in treating patients suffering from endometrial
hyperplasia and carcinoma (Greenblatt, Gambrell, Stoddard
1982).

Experimental work has shown that the occurrence of
endometrial hyperplasia and carcinoma is unusually high in
rabbits (Greene 1959). This is attributed to continuous
estrogen stimulus in animals which are induced ovulators.
The administration of estrogens was found to increase the
incidence of endometrial carcinoma induced by chemical
carcinogens in ovariectomized rabbits (Baba, von Haam
1967), while progestin administration inhibited such an
effect (Baba, von Haam 1967).

As described above, the effects of estrogens and progestins on human or experimental endometrial cancer are clear: estrogens appear to promote that neoplasm, while progesterone can be used with partial success for its treatment. However, the mechanisms by which those steroid hormones regulate the development of endometrial carcinoma are not known, probably because the cellular and molecular bases for the hormonal regulation of endometrium are not yet known in full.

Our laboratory has been involved for several years in the development and analysis of experimental models using either the whole rabbit or primary cell cultures of rabbit endometrium for the study of estrogen and progesterone regulation of the proliferation and differentiation of that tissue. This was done with the expectation that a better understanding of the normal biology of the endometrium would result in better comprehension of the etiology and pathogenesis of endometrial hyperplasia and cancer.

In this article we describe briefly our research and discuss several hypotheses and theories which have emerged from our work.

Cell Culture Studies

We have described a simple technique to isolate rabbit endometrial cells and to culture them in chemically defined medium (Gerschenson, Berliner, Yang 1974). The culture is enriched for uterine epithelial cells (>98%) which attach and proliferate actively, while the fibroblastoid cells, presumably stromal cells, attach and grow poorly.

Electron microscopy studies (Berliner, Gerschenson 1976) confirmed the epithelial origin of most of the cells. Cells treated with estrogens had the appearance of rapidly dividing cultures, having large euchromatic nuclei and prominent nucleoli with a cytoplasm containing many free ribosomes. Progesterone appeared to convert the cells to a more secretory type with large amounts of rough endoplasmic reticulum and smaller nucleoli. Mitochondrial enlargement was induced by both sex hormones, but not by hydrocortisone.

Estrogens and progesterone induced a significant increase in the incorporation of labeled uridine and amino
acids into trichloroacetic acid precipitable material.
These hormonal effects were rapidly reversed upon removal
of the hormones from the culture medium and were also
inhibited by actinomycin D and cycloheximide. Neither
steroid hormone altered the specific activity of alkaline
phosphatase, acid phosphatase, lactic dehydrogenase, or
the uptake of 3-O-methyl-D-glucose and α-aminoisobutyric
acid (Gerschenson, Berliner 1976).

The addition of estrogens to cultured rabbit endometrial cells increased the number of DNA-replicating cells
while progesterone had an antagonistic effect (Gerschenson, Berliner 1976; Gerschenson, Conner, Murai 1977). The
cultures were found to be made up of dividing cells (20-
40%) and quiescent cells (60-80%). The addition of estrogens had the effect of recruiting cells from the quiescent
(G_0?) compartment into the cell cycle (Gerschenson,
Conner, Murai 1977).

Using techniques designed to select for either the
quiescent or dividing cells, it was also found that the
quiescent cell population is the only target for the
growth-promoting effect of estrogens. Epidermal growth
factor and prostaglandin F-2α stimulated the proliferation
of both quiescent and dividing cell populations. Progesterone was found not to antagonize the effect of estrogen
on the quiescent cells unless the hormone was incubated
previously with a mixed cell culture. This finding suggested the existence of an estrogen inhibitor factor,
which is progesterone-induced or -dependent, resulting
from the interaction of progesterone and dividing cells
(Tables I and II). Two other progestins, R-5020 and
20α-hydroxy-pregn-4-en-3-one were found not to have the
same effect as progesterone, showing its specificity
(Gerschenson et al., 1979).

The estrogen-dependent increase in cell proliferation
was found to be present only in low density cultures.
Moderate increases in cell density resulted in disappear-
ance of the estrogenic effect. Prostaglandin F2-α and
epidermal growth factor were effective proliferation
effectors in either low or high density cultures, hence
suggesting a specific inhibition of the estrogen effect
(Table III). Conditioned-medium experiments suggest the

TABLE I

Effect of Hormones on Different Cell Populations of
Cultured Endometrial Cells

	Original Mixed Cell Culture	Quiescent Cells	Cycling Cells
Co	31.8 ± 3.4	4.9 ± 0.8	23.3 ± 4.8
10^{-7} M DES	46.0 ± 1.0*	18.0 ± 0.4*	13.2 ± 4.6
10^{-7} M P	22.2 ± 5.5	3.5 ± 0.7	33.5 ± 4.2
10^{-7} M DES + 10^{-7} M P	30.0 ± 2.7	17.2 ± 0.8*	24.4 ± 0.2
10^{-9} M EGF	52.5 ± 4.8*	9.2 ± 1.2*	46.9 ± 3.0*
5×10^{-7} M PGF	40.5 ± 1.1*	8.6 ± 1.2**	38.4 ± 3.3***

Co = no additions, DES = diethylstilbestrol, P = progesterone, EGF =
epidermal growth factor, PGF = prostaglandin F-2α.

Values are means ± s.e.m. of percentage of labeled epithelial cells per
total number of epithelial cells. Mean = average of 5 dishes.

* = statistically significant when compared with control using the
t test.

Description of Experiment Described in Table I: Day 1, endometrial
cells were obtained from rabbits and plated in dishes for quiescent cell
selection. Day 2, a) the above cultures were divided into two sets, one
for studies on original mixed cell cultures, and in the other, high
specific activity ^{3}H-Tdr and cytosine arabinoside were added for
quiescent cell selection, b) another group of fresh cells was isolated
and plated for selection of dividing cells. Days 3 and 4, cells were
incubated as indicated for day 2. Day 5, medium with Colcemid was added
to the cells cultured in flasks, cells from approximately 10 flasks were
used to obtain enough dividing cells for one dish, and these cells were
then collected 6 hr later and plated in dishes. Day 6, the medium of
all the dishes was changed to medium with or without hormones and with
0.2 µCi/ml ^{3}H-Tdr (Sp. Act. 10 Ci/mM, New England nuclear). Day 7, the
cells were fixed and processed for autoradiography as described
previously. DES was dissolved in absolute ethanol and added to the
culture in 50 µl aliquots per 100 ml. Addition of similar amounts of
ethanol alone to cultures was found repeatedly to have no effect upon
the cells. (Taken from Gerschenson et al., 1979).

TABLE II

Effect of Conditioning Media on the Estrogenic Effect
on Quiescent Cells

	Medium Conditioned with Mixed Cell Cultures		Medium Conditioned with Quiescent Cells	
	With 10^{-7} M Progesterone	Without Progesterone	With 10^{-7} M Progesterone	Without Progesterone
Co	2.7 ± 0.4	2.7 ± 0.1	2.9 ± 0.3	3.2 ± 0.1
10^{-7} M DES	3.0 ± 0.5	$17.1 \pm 0.8*$	18.4 ± 1.1	$19.0 \pm 1.2*$
10^{-7} M P	4.0 ± 0.2	3.0 ± 0.2	3.4 ± 0.2	4.0 ± 0.3
10^{-7} M DES + 10^{-7} M P	2.6 ± 0.2	$16.0 \pm 0.1*$	$17.9 \pm 0.8*$	$18.1 \pm 0.9*$

Data is expressed as in the previous table. Co = control, DES =
diethylstilbestrol, P = progesterone. * = $P > 0.01$ when compared with
control using the t test.

Description of Experiment Described in Table II: Quiescent cells were
selected as explained above. Media with or without 10^{-7} M P was conditioned for 48 hr with either mixed cell or quiescent cell cultures.
Then the media was collected, pooled, centrifuged for 30 min at
10,000 rpm at 5°C and kept at 5°C for 48 hr before being assayed for
antagonism to the estrogen effect upon proliferation on another culture
of quiescent cells for 24 hr. (Taken from Gerschenson et al., 1979).

TABLE III

Cell Density Influence on 17β-Estradiol Effect on Proliferation and Floating Cells

	Number of cells attached per dish (x 10^3)	Labeling Index of attached cells	Number of floating cells per dish	Labeling Index of floating cells
Low density cultures				
No addition	123.0 ± 10.8	17.9 ± 1.3	11.6 ± 0.5	0
17β-estradiol	172.0 ± 9.8*	25.1 ± 1.7*	9.6 ± 1.5	0
Epidermal growth factor		27.5 ± 1.4*		
Prostaglandin F2α		27.3 ± 1.9*		
High density cultures				
No addition	1,125.0 ± 84.0	25.1 ± 5.1	110 ± 5.1	0.3 ± 0.2
17β-estradiol	1,074.0 ± 39.0	22.6 ± 1.7	94 ± 2.4	0.4 ± 0.2
Epidermal growth factor		37.6 ± 2.0*		
Prostaglandin F2α		39.0 ± 2.4*		

Data is expressed as mean ± s.e.m. Mean = average of 5 dishes.

* = statistically significant when compared with No Addition group using the t test.

Description of Experiment Described in Table IV: Cells were plated in plastic dishes (dia. = 6 cm) at a concentration of 7.2 10^5 cells per dish (low density) or 6 x 10^6 cells per dish (high density) on day 1, then hormones and [^{3}H]-Tdr (SA 20 Ci/mmol, New England Nuclear) at a final concentration of 2 μCi ml was added on day 3 and experiment terminated on day 4. Volume of medium per dish was 5 ml. The concentration of the hormones was as follows: 10^{-7} M 17β-estradiol, 10^{-9} M epidermal growth factor and 5 x 10^{-7} prostaglandin F2α. (Taken from Gerschenson et al., 1981).

production of a heat- and trypsin-sensitive factor which
is nondialyzable, precipitable at high concentrations of
ammonium sulphate, and has an approximate molecular weight
of 10-20K. A similar inhibitory activity was detected in
homogenates of high density cultured cells but not of low
density cultures. In the culture medium a low molecular
weight factor appears to be present which has an
amplifying effect on the estrogen-proliferative effect.
Preliminary evidence suggests that these factors appear
not to involve changes in the number of whole cell
estrogen receptors (Gerschenson, Depaoli, Murai 1981).
These specific hormone binders were measured using a
described whole-cell technique which showed that the
estrogen receptors appear to be composed of at least two
components: one has high affinity but low capacity, while
the other has low affinity but high capacity. It was also
found that either estrogen or progesterone addition
resulted in a decrease of the number of estrogen receptors
in the cultured cells (Table IV); however, each hormone
brought about this decrease with different kinetics (Murai
et al. 1979).

Uteroglobin (UG) is a secretory protein produced by
the rabbit uterine epithelium and its production is
increased during the process of cell differentiation
occurring during early pregnancy or pseudopregnancy.
Therefore, it is an interesting marker for progesterone's
mechanism of action and cell differentiation (Murai et
al. 1981).

We have determined that our primary cultures of
rabbit endometrium secrete UG in the culture medium (Table
V). Accumulation of UG was found to be linear for at
least a period of 24 hr and metabolic labeling studies
using [^{35}S]methionine showed its incorporation into UG
molecules. The cells were found not to catabolize
exogenously added radiolabeled UG. When pseudopregnancy
was induced by administration of human chorionic gonadotrophin (hCG) and cultures prepared at different times
after its administration, it was observed that the UG
production by the cultures was parallel to the level of UG
in the whole animals. Cycloheximide was found to inhibit
the synthesis of UG by the cultured cells. It was also
observed that cell density had an effect on the UG production, at higher densities an increased production of UG
per cell was detected (Rajkumar et al. 1983a).

TABLE IV

Effect of Hormones on Estradiol Receptor Levels

Hormone Treatment (10^{-7} M each)	^{3}H-Estradiol Bound (cpm/mgm protein x 10^{-3})
Control	5.24 ± 0.21
Estradiol-17β	3.01 ± 0.22*
Progesterone	2.43 ± 0.09*
Estradiol-17β + Progesterone	1.99 ± 0.21*

Values are means $\pm$ s.e.m. Mean = average of 5 dishes.

* = statistically significant when compared with control using the
  t test.

Description of Experiment Described in Table III: Cells were plated at
1.5×10^6 cells per 60 mm culture dish and washed twice with SA solution
one day later. Control medium or medium containing unlabeled hormones
were added and incubated for 24 hr. After the incubation period, cells
were washed 5 times with SA solution to remove the hormones and control
medium was added to the cells to allow the bound hormones to egress from
the cells. After a 4-hr egress period (with a change of medium at
2 hr), the cells were assayed for receptors as described above. The
concentration of ^{3}H-estradiol used in the binding assay was 1×10^{-9} M.
(Taken from Murai et al., 1979).

TABLE V

Production of UG in 24 hr by Cultured Cells Taken at Different
Times Post hCG

Time in Culture (days)	UG production (μg UG/mg DNA•24 hr)		
	Estrous cells	2 days post-hCG cells	4 days post-hCG cells
3	30.34 ± 2.34	371.13 ± 15.15*	1150.00 ± 94.55**

Values are the mean $\pm$ s.e.m. (n = 5 petri dishes).

 * = difference from control, P < 0.001.

** = difference from 2 days post hCG, P < 0.001.

(Taken from Rajkumar et al., 1983a).

Progesterone (10^{-8} M) addition "in vitro" resulted in increased production levels of UG in cultures derived from either estrous animals or animals 2 days after injection of hCG. That stimulatory effect was better observed in cultured cells obtained from 2-day post-hCG animals and when progesterone was present from the time of cell plating. The progesterone effect was dose dependent and biphasic; lower doses had an inhibitory effect. Estradiol (10^{-10} M) by itself had an inhibitory effect on UG production by cultured cells from 2-day post-hCG animals during the first day of culture. However, if the cultures were incubated with the same concentration of estradiol alone or together with progesterone, the stimulatory effect of progesterone on UG production on the second day of culture was enhanced significantly (Table VI). In conclusion, it appears that both ovarian hormones play a role in regulating UG production in cultures of endometrial cells and that their concentration and presence in the culture media at the time of plating is critical for the regulation of that secretory protein production (Rajkumar et al. 1983b).

Whole Animal Studies

Our laboratory developed a technique using "in-vitro" pulses with [^{3}H]thymidine to determine the effects of ovarian hormones administered to rabbits on the proliferation of endometrial epithelium. It was observed that estradiol-17β administration stimulates the proliferation of endometrial glandular cells in intact or ovariectomized rabbits. Progesterone induced an increase mostly in the proliferation of luminal epithelium of intact rabbits. Foci of cells with nuclei labeled with [^{3}H]thymidine showing active hyperplasia were observed in the luminal uterine epithelium of progesterone-treated rabbits which would seem to be related to the formation of glands characteristic of secretory endometrium. Simultaneous administration of both ovarian hormones produced a mutually antagonistic effect (Conti et al. 1981).

Other experiments carried out in our laboratory explored the possibility that estrogens and progesterone could have as their target different uterine cell populations. These cell populations may differ with respect to location as described above or in their cell cycle stage. Therefore, rabbits were injected with [^{3}H]thymidine for 3

TABLE VI

Effect of Progesterone and Estradiol on Uteroglobin Production

Group	Treatment schedule		Regression analysis		Increase at 24 hr (%)
	Day of plating (M)	24 hr after plating (M)	Coefficient of correlation	Slope ± SE (% increase/hr)	
1	Control	Control	0.9822	14.75 ± 0.60	291.15 ± 15.00
2	10^{-10} P	10^{-10} P	0.9895	15.31 ± 0.59	310.42 ± 14.33
3	10^{-10} P	10^{-8} P	0.9983	17.84 ± 0.88*	380.64 ± 22.83*
4	10^{-8} P	10^{-8} P	0.9953	17.85 ± 0.65*	372.03 ± 20.59*
5	Control	10^{-8} P	0.9966	16.69 ± 1.78	349.05 ± 66.39
6	10^{-10} E	10^{-1} E + 10^{-8} P	0.9932	27.31 ± 1.16*,†	570.13 ± 36.35*,†
7	10^{-10} E	10^{-8} P	0.9887	29.26 ± 1.48*,†	603.08 ± 21.14*,†
8	10^{-10} E + 10^{-8} P	10^{-8} P	0.9952	30.48 ± 1.80*,†	654.82 ± 59.09*,†
9	Control	Cycloheximide	0.6443	0.47 ± 0.27*	110.38 ± 9.14*
10	10^{-8} P	10^{-8} P + cycloheximide	0.7519	0.85 ± 0.28*	117.46 ± 6.85*

N = 10 petri dishes; E, estradiol; P, progesterone.

* = difference from group 1, $P < 0.05$.

† = difference from group 4, $P < 0.01$.

(Taken from Rajkumar et al., 1983b).

days to label nuclei of dividing cells, then either 17β-estradiol, progesterone or vehicle were administered. The estrogenic hormone was found to induce a decrease in the percentage of cells with labeled nuclei of either luminal or glandular epithelium. Since 17β-estradiol has been shown to have a significant growth effect on glands, the data suggest that its effect is exerted on unlabeled quiescent cells which are then recruited into the cell cycle. On the other hand, progesterone was found to induce a significant increase in the DNA synthesis of luminal epithelium. From this finding, it was concluded that dividing cells are a target for progesterone. Furthermore, analysis of the number of nuclear grains according to cell location in luminal vs. glandular epithelia and the effect of hormone administration confirmed that each ovarian hormone acts on different target cell populations (Conti et al. 1983).

Administration of estrogens for short- or long-term resulted in larger internal circumference of the uterus due to an increase in the number of luminal cells, while the number of glands and glandular cells per section did not appear to change. These findings, in combination with previous research, suggest that endometrial gland cells migrate towards the lumen and that estrogen administration decreases the rate of cell loss or death in the luminal epithelium. It is interesting to point out that the proliferative effect of estrogens on glandular cells appears to be desensitized by continuous administration of those hormones, while the effect on cell loss or death is not (Conti et al. 1983).

The concept of cell migration is supported by experiments in which a single administration of [^{3}H]thymidine for rabbits was followed by determination at different times of the geographical distribution of cells with labeled nuclei in longitudinal sections of glands. There was observed, as a function of time, a decrease in the number of labeled cells in the bottom of the glands with a concomitant increase in the same parameter in the upper part of the glands and luminal epithelia. The neck of the glands appear to function as a "decision zone" where the fate of the migrating cells is settled, they either are sloughed off or continue migrating towards the lumen. This decision is regulated by estrogens which favor cell migration vs. loss (Conti et al. 1983).

Using similar techniques as above, we determined the close relationship between progesterone-induced proliferation and differentiation in rabbit uterine epithelium, as measured by gland formation or arborization and uteroglobin secretion. Our results support the observation that it is nonproliferating, glandular epithelial cells that secrete uteroglobin (Murai et al. 1981).

CONCLUSIONS

It appears that in rabbit uterine epithelium, estrogen and progesterone act on different cell populations. Estrogens act on quiescent (G_0?, stem?) cells located in glands which function as a germinative source for dividing daughter cells that migrate towards the lumen where they become a target for progesterone. This latter hormone triggers further proliferation of these cells and forms new secretory glands which, when the cells become terminally differentiated, secrete uteroglobin.

Factors which appear to regulate (increase or decrease) the proliferative effect of estrogens appear to be made in culture and, at least in the case of the estrogen inhibitory activity, it is made by dividing cells under progesterone influence, but acts on quiescent cells.

We have described using cultured cells or whole animal models, the existence of intrinsic uterine epithelial growth mechanisms: cell proliferation–cell migration–cell loss (death and/or sloughing)–terminal differentiation. We have also shown how estrogens and progesterone modulate such phenomena and the possible involvement of cell-to-cell interaction through factors which regulate estrogen activity. It is thought that these findings could help to analyze further the postulate that derangement of the above described growth mechanisms or their hormonal regulation could result in endometrial hyperplasia or carcinoma (Gerschenson, Fennell 1982; Abell 1982).

FURTHER DIRECTIONS

Several important questions remain to be answered regarding the role of hormones in the biology and pathology of endometrium. 1) Characterization of the estrogen

regulating factors and their mechanism of action; 2) determination of the mechanism of action of the ovarian
hormones in modulating cell proliferation and differentiation; 3) study of the role of prostaglandins in the regulation of these phenomena; and 4) elucidation of the role
of different growth substrates on the ovarian hormone
effects.

ACKNOWLEDGEMENTS

This research has been supported by grants from the
NIH, ACS, and a departmental gift from R.J. Reynolds
Industries, Inc.

REFERENCES

Abell MR (1982). Adenocarcinoma (gland-cell carcinoma) in
  situ of endometrium. Pathol Res Pract 174:221.
Baba N, von Haam E (1967). Experimental carcinoma of the
  endometrium. Prog Exp Tumor Res 9:192.
Berliner JB, Gerschenson LE (1976). Sex steroid induced
  morphological changes in primary uterine cell culture.
  J Steroid Biochem 7:153.
Conti CJ, Gimenez-Conti IB, Conner EA, Lehman JM,
  Gerschenson LE (1983). Estrogen and progesterone
  regulation of proliferation, migration and loss in
  different target cells of rabbit uterine epithelium.
  Endocrinology. In press.
Conti CJ, Gimenez-Conti IB, Zerbe GO, Gerschenson LE
  (1981). Differential effects of estradiol-17β and
  progesterone on the proliferation of glandular and
  luminal cells of rabbit uterine epithelium. Biol Reprod
  24:643.
Gerschenson LE, Berliner JB (1976). Further studies on
  the regulation of cultured rabbit endometrial cells by
  diethylstilbestrol and progesterone. J Steroid Biochem
  7:159.
Gerschenson LE, Berliner JB, Yang J (1974). Diethylstilbestrol and progesterone regulation of cultured rabbit
  endometrial cell growth. Cancer Res 34:2873.
Gerschenson LE, Conner EA, Murai JT (1977). Regulation of
  the cell cycle by diethylstilbestrol and progesterone in
  cultured endometrial cells. Endocrinology 100:1468.

Gerschenson LE, Conner EA, Yang J, Andersson M (1979).
Hormonal regulation of proliferation in two cell popu-
lations of rabbit endometrial cells in culture. Life
Sci 24:1337.

Gerschenson LE, Depaoli JR, Murai JT (1981). Inhibition
of estrogen-induced proliferation of cultured rabbit
uterine epithelial cells by a cell density-dependent
factor produced by the same cells. J Steroid Biochem
14:959.

Gerschenson LE, Fennell RH Jr (1982). A developmental
view of endometrial hyperplasia and carcinoma based on
experimental research. Pathol Res Pract 174:285.

Greenblatt RB, Gambrell RD, Stoddard LD Jr (1982). The
protective role of progesterone in the prevention of
endometrial cancer. Pathol Res Pract 174:297.

Greene HSN (1959). Adenocarcinoma of the uterine fundus
in the rabbit. Ann NY Acad Sci 75:535.

MacMahon B (1974). Risk factors for endometrial cancer.
Gynecol Oncol 2:122.

Murai JT, Conti CJ, Gimenez-Conti I, Orlicky D,
Gerschenson LE (1981). Temporal relationship between
rabbit uterine epithelium proliferation and uteroglobin
production. Biol Reprod 24:649.

Murai JT, Lieberman RC, Yang J, Gerschenson LE (1979).
Decrease of estrogen receptors induced by 17β-estradiol
and progesterone in cultured rabbit endometrial cells.
Endocr Res Commun 6:235.

Rajkumar K, Bigsby R, Lieberman R, Gerschenson LE
(1983a). Uteroglobin production by cultured rabbit
uterine epithelial cells. Endocrinology 112:1490.

Rajkumar K, Bigsby R, Lieberman R, Gerschenson LE
(1983b). Effect of progesterone and 17β-estradiol on
the production of uteroglobin by cultured rabbit uterine
epithelial cells. Endocrinology 112:1499.

Hormones and Cancer, pages 133–144

ESTRADIOL, PROGESTERONE. AND TAMOXIFEN REGULATION OF ORNITHINE DECARBOXYLASE (ODC) IN RAT UTERUS AND CHICK OVIDUCTS.

Carlos Levy, Patricia Glikman, Irene Vegh, Jan Mester*, Etienne Baulieu* and Roberto Soto.

División Endocrinología. Hospital Ramos Mejía. Urquiza 609. (1221) Buenos Aires. Argentina. *U33 INSERM. Lab. Hormones. 94270 Bicetre. France.

Putrescine, spermidine and spermine are small aliphatic amines, fundamentally associated with growth and cell differentiation.

The increase in enzyme activities involved in the biosynthetic pathway of these polyamines, is a good marker for cell proliferation.

ODC, the enzyme which converts ornithine into putrescine , is the limiting step of polyamine synthesis.

The increase in polyamine concentration and thus, in ODC activity, has been demonstrated in embrionary tissues, in regenerating liver after partial hepatectomy, in tumoral growing tissues and in target organs after hormone administration (Janne et al, 1978; Tabor, Tabor, 1976).

Although the exact knowledge of the polyamine function in cell growth and differentiation is still to be elucidated, there is enough evidence to believe that these polycations are involved in DNA, RNA and protein synthesis regulation (Cohen, 1982; Russel et al, 1976).

Apart from using changes in polyamine concentrations to evaluate modifications in rapidly growing tissues, the fact that these organic cations increase dramatically in response to hormone stimulation on their target tissues, suggests that variations in polyamine level may be accepted as a useful model for the better understanding of the hormone and antihormone mechanism of action (Janne et al, 1981; Perin, Sessa,1978)

Moulton and Leonard (1969) have reported increase in spermidine concentration in ovariectomized rat uterus, 24 hours after intravenous estradiol injection.

A rapid increase in ODC activity has been found "in vivo" and "in vitro", in chick oviduct and in castrated or hypophysectomized rat uterus, after estradiol or DES administration (Cohen et al, 1970; Kaye et al, 1971).

Since progesterone inhibits estrogen-induced growth and differentiation on target tissues (Bo et al, 1971; Moulton, Leonard, 1969; Socher, O'Malley, 1973) and, furthermore, antiestrogens have been shown to modify ODC activity (Bulger, Kupfer, 1976; Bulger, Kupfer, 1977), our aim was to study ODC regulation by estradiol, progesterone and tamoxifen.

Chick oviducts were obtained from animals pre-treated with 10 i.m. injections of estradiol benzoate (1 mg/day), beginning at 8 days of age. Experimental treatment was started 4 to 8 weeks after this priming was withdrawn.

Twentyone to 25 days old Sprague-Dawley rats were used.

Techniques and experimental methods employed have previously been published (Levy et al, 1981; Pegg et al, 1970).

CHICK OVIDUCT

Figure 1a shows changes in ODC activity in the magnum portion of chick oviducts after i.m. injection of 1.5 mg/kg b.w. of estradiol benzoate. This stimulation was already significant after 2 hours, reaching its peak 6 hours following estradiol administration, and returning to base-line values after 24 hours.

Simultaneous progesterone administration (3 mg/kg b.w.) inhibited about 60 to 80% the maximal ODC estrogen-induced. Progesterone alone induced similar activity to that observed with estradiol plus progesterone.

Tamoxifen alone, in doses ranging between 0.1 to 10 mg/kg b.w., did not induce any ODC activity. Ten mg/kg b.w. dose produced complete inhibition of estrogen-induced ODC. As has been demostrated by Sutherland et al,(1977), in this experimental model tamoxifen behaves as a pure antiestrogen.

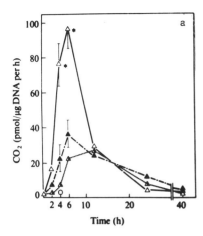 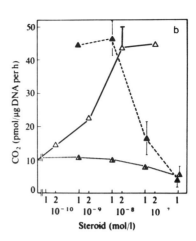

Fig.1- "In vivo" and "in vitro" studies in withdrawn
chick oviducts.

1a- "In vivo". ODC induced after administration of: 1.5
mg/kg b.w. estradiol benzoate in propylene glycol (△), 3 mg/
kg b.w. progesterone in sesame oil (▲), both hormones given
simultaneously (▲) or 10 mg/kg b.w. tamoxifen in 0.9% ClNa
plus estradiol (O). Points are the mean of at least two experiments. Vertical bars show SD of 4 experimental values.
(△) vs (▲) and (△) vs (O) *p<0.01 (Student's t-test)

1b- "In vitro". Dose related pattern of ODC induction.
Samples incubated with different concentrations of estradiol
(△), progesterone (▲) or with 20 nM estradiol plus increasing
concentrations of progesterone (▲). Values are means ± SD
of 4 to 6 experimental points.

ODC activity in the oviduct of inmature untreated chicken can be induced "in vitro" by estrogens, as has been shown
by Cohen et al (1970).

Figure 1b indicates that 20 nM estradiol concentration
produced a maximal response after 2 hours incubation in MEM
medium. The simultaneous progesterone addition, in increasing
concentrations, to the medium containing 20 nM of estradiol,
inhibited ODC induction in a dose related pattern, and an almost complete inhibition was achieved with 0.1 µM of proges-
terone·

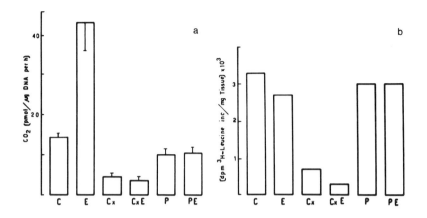

Fig.2- Withdrawn chick oviducts "in vitro".
ODC activity (2a) and ^{3}H-Leucine incorporation in acid precipitable fraction (2b) after 2 hours incubation with 20 nM estradiol (E), 25 µg/ml cycloheximide (Cx), cycloheximide plus
estradiol (CxE), 1 µM progesterone (P) or progesterone plus
estradiol (PE). Values are means ± SEM of 5 experimental
points (2a) or the mean of at least 2 experiments (2b)

Contrarily to what was observed "in vivo", progesterone
alone did not induce any ODC activity.

Estradiol had no detectable effect before the second
hour of incubation. At this time, it increased ODC activity
3 to 6 fold in comparison to chick oviducts incubated under
the same conditions but without estradiol (Figure 2a).

It should be pointed out that hormone free oviduct incubation, at 37°C for 2 hours, doubled ODC activity detected in
oviducts without incubation.

Cycloheximide (25 µg/ml) not only inhibited estradiol-
dependent ODC activity, but also the one induced by incubation in medium alone.

Figure 2b indicates that progesterone concentrations as
high as 1 uM had no toxic effect as regards leucine incorporation, rouling out non specific effect of progesterone. Cy-

cloheximide almost totally inhibited the aminoacid incorporation at the concentration employed.

Tamoxifen at concentrations between 20 nM to 20 µM did
not provoke any induction of ODC activity. At this highest
concentration it produced more than 50% inhibition of estradiol-induced enzyme activity (data not shown).

RAT UTERUS

Figure 3 shows ODC activity induced by estradiol administration (2.5 µg/rat) in rats previously treated with the
same dose 24 and 48 hours before. The maximal activity was
achieved 6 hours later, dropping to basal levels at 24 hours.

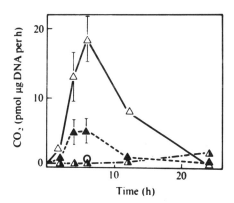

Fig.3- Time course of "in vivo" induction of ODC in rat
uterus.
Inmature rats were primed with 2 injections of estradiol
(2.5 µg/day) in NaCl:Ethanol (9:1), 48 and 24 hours before.
At time 0 they received 2.5 µg estradiol (△), 2.5 mg progesterone in sesame oil (▲) or both (▲), or 200 µg cyclohexi-
de in water plus estradiol (O) and were killed at different
times. Points are means of at least 2 experiments. Vertical
bars represent means $\pm$ SD of 4 experimental values. At 4 and
6 hours (△) vs (▲) $p < 0.05$ (Student's t-test).

Progesterone (2.5 mg/rat) significantly inhibited ODC

activity when injected simultaneously with estradiol. Progesterone alone did not increase enzymatic activity.

Cycloheximide (200 mg/rat) completely inhibited estradiol-induced ODC activity at 6 hours.

When rat uterus not previously treated with estradiol were used, progesterone did not significantly inhibit estradiol-induced ODC (Figure 4). This suggests that progesterone receptor or other estrogen-induced protein might be involved in the mechanism of progesterone inhibitory activity.

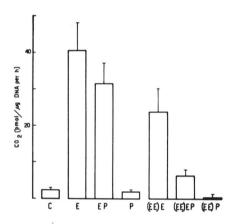

Fig.4- Inhibitory effect of progesterone on estradiol-induced ODC with or without estradiol priming.
ODC activity was measured 5 hours after estradiol, progesterone or both given simultaneously without or with (EE) estradiol pretreatment. Doses indicated in Fig. 3. Values are means $\pm$ SEM of 4 experimental points. (EE)E vs (EE)EP p<0.01 (Student's t-test)

Bulger and Kupfer (1976) reported maximal peak in ODC activity, in ovariectomized rat uterus, 6 hours after tamoxifen (1 mg/rat) injection. In unprimed inmature rats, we also found stimulation of ODC activity after tamoxifen (0.1 mg/rat). Figure 5 shows two peaks of ODC activity. The first one is seen at 6 hours, and the second one 24 hours after tamoxi-

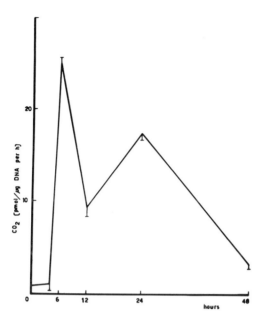

Fig.5- Time course of tamoxifen induced ODC in rat uterus.
Inmature rats without any previous treatment were injected
with a single dose of tamoxifen (0.1 mg/rat in 0.9% NaCl).
Vertical bars represent means ± SEM of 4 to 6 experimental
values.

fen administration, returning to base line values 48 hours
later. These peaks can not be interpreted as biological cir-
cadian rythms, since the same pattern was obtained when rats
were killed at the same time, but injected at different hours
of the day, or inversely.

Lavia et al(1981) also found two peaks in ODC activity
after estradiol injection in inmature rats. To explain this
effect, they consider that there is a possible correlation
between polyamine synthesis and mRNA association with poly-
ribosomes in uterus (Merryweather, Knowler, 1980).

When animals were treated with a daily tamoxifen injection for 3 days, no stimulation of ODC activity was observed

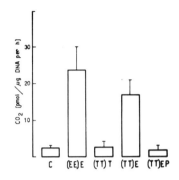

Fig.6- Effect of tamoxifen priming on ODC induction. Inmature rats pretreated 24 and 48 hours before with tamoxifen, were injected with estradiol (E), tamoxifen (T) or estradiol plus progesterone (EP), and were killed 5 hours after. Controls were injected with 0.9% NaCl. Values are means $\pm$ SEM of 4 to 10 experimental points.

5 hours after the last injection. On the contrary, if estradiol was administered after the rats were primed for two days with tamoxifen, ODC activity was induced. This activity was inhibited by the simultaneous administration of progesterone (Fig. 6). As previously reported, tamoxifen induces progesterone receptor (Jordan, Prestwich, 1978; Robel et al, 1978).

Estradiol can exchange with the receptor occupied by tamoxifen, either in the nucleus - where 24 hours after the injection, tamoxifen is found in its greatest proportion (Hsueh et al, 1976) - or in the cytoplasm. Furthermore, the functional integrity of this receptor seems to have been preserved.

Just as in the case of thymidine incorporation into DNA (Stormshak et al, 1976), ODC activity decreased significantly 5 hours after the third estradiol injection, in comparison with the activity 5 hours after the second administration (Fig. 7).

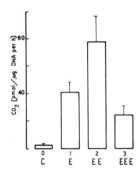

Fig.7- Effect of sequential injections of estradiol on ODC induction. Inmature rats were injected 1, 2 or 3 days with 2.5 µg/day estradiol. ODC activity was measured 5 hours after the last administration. Values are means $\pm$ SEM of at least 4 experimental points. EE vs E $p<0.05$; EE vs EEE $p<0.025$ (Student's t-test).

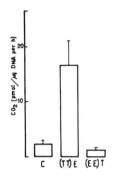

Fig.8- ODC activity in rat uterus after estradiol or tamoxifen priming.
Inmature rats pretreated 24 and 48 hours before with tamoxifen or estradiol, were injected with estradiol or tamoxifen. ODC activity was measured after 5 hours. Values are means $\pm$ SEM of at least 6 experimental points.

When tamoxifen was injected into rats previously treated with estradiol (48 and 24 hours before), the ODC activity found in the uterus after 5 hours, showed no significant difference with the controls (Fig. 8) whereas - as has been shown above - estradiol was able to induce enzyme activity in rats previously treated with two doses of tamoxifen.

It was impossible to induce ODC activity in rat uterus "in vitro" under the same incubation conditions used for chick oviducts, in accordance with Kaye et al (1971).

CONCLUSIONS

Progesterone has an early antiestrogenic effect on the estradiol-induced ODC. As has already been reported (Hsueh et al, 1976), progesterone administrated together with estradiol does not inhibit the translocation of the estradiol-receptor complex to the nucleus, neither the recycling and/or replenishment to the cytoplasm; later, progesterone inhibits the estradiol receptor neosynthesis. Hence progesterone inhibition of estradiol-induced ODC occurs before progesterone alters estradiol-receptor concentration.

Since progesterone inhibition is not observed in rats unless previously treated with estradiol, it would seem neccesary to reach threshold levels of progesterone receptor, or other estrogen induced protein, for this progesterone-inhibitory activity to occur.

Tamoxifen has an estrogen - antagonistic effect in chick oviduct (Sutherland et al, 1977). In rat uterus it behaves as agonist or antagonist with respect to ODC induction, as well as with other estradiol-induced functions, depending on the frequency of administration and previous treatment.

As in other experimental models, frequent or continuous administration of estradiol produces antiestrogenic effects, at least"in vivo" (Stormshak et al, 1976).

If the animals are previously treated with two doses of estradiol, a third injection induces activity - although this is lower than the one observed after two injections - whilst a third injection of tamoxifen does not.

Estradiol can induce ODC activity in animals previously treated with two injections of tamoxifen; on the contrary, tamoxifen does not. Estradiol can rescue the receptor ligated to tamoxifen in the nucleus or in the cytoplasm, and then induce ODC activity.

In rats previously treated with estradiol or tamoxifen, tamoxifen does not induce enzyme activity. On the other hand, it should be pointed out that a single dose of tamoxifen can induce ODC activity.

Finally, it could be postulated that the receptivity or refractoriness of an estrogen-sensitive cell, at least in the whole animal, does not depend on the alosteric or conformational changes of the hormone-receptor complex only, but that there might be regulatory changes of the acceptor activity at the genetic expression level.

ACKNOWLEDGEMENTS

We thank Dr. Paul Robel for his helpful discussion and Mrs. Elizabeth Silva Croome for her assistance in the translation of this manuscript.

REFERENCES

Bo WJ, Poteat WL, Krueger WA, Mc Allister F (1971). The effect of progesterone on estradiol-17β dipropionate induced wet weight, percent water and glycogen of the rat uterus. Steroid 18:389.

Bulger WH, Kupfer D (1976). Induction of uterine ornithine decarboxylase (ODC) by antiestrogens. Inhibition of estradiol-mediated induction of ODC: a possible mechanism of action of antiestrogens. Endocr Res Commun 3:209.

Bulger WH, Kupfer D (1977). Inhibition of the 1-(o-chlorophenyl)-1-(p-chlorophenyl)-2,2,2-trichloroethane(o,p'DDT)- and estradiol-mediated induction of rat uterine ornithine decarboxylase by prior treatment with o,p'DDT, estradiol and tamoxifen. Arch Biochem Biophys 182:138.

Cohen SS (1982). The polyamines as a growth industry. Fed Proc 41:3061.

Cohen S, O'Malley BW, Stastny M (1970). Estrogenic induction of ornithine decarboxylase in vivo and in vitro. Science 170:336.

Hsueh AJW, Peck Jr EJ, Clark JH (1976). Control of uterine estrogen receptor levels by progesterone. Endocrinology 98:438

Janne J, Alhonen-Hongisto L, Seppanen P, Siimes M (1981). Use of polyamines antimetabolites in experimental tumours and in human leukaemia. Med Biol 59:448.

Janne J, Poso H, Raina A (1978). Polyamines in rapid growth and cancer. Biochim Biophys Acta 473:241.

Jordan VC, Prestwich G (1978). Effect of non steroidal antiestrogens on the concentration of rat uterine progesterone receptors. J Endocr 76:363.

Kaye AM, Iceckson I, Lindner HR (1971). Stimulation by estrogens of ornithine and S-adenosylmethionine decarboxylases in the inmature rat uterus. Biochim Biophys Acta 252:150.

Lavia LA, Lemon HM, Stohs SJ (1981). Possible role of polyamines in controlling membrane binding or function of ribosomes during estrogen stimulation. Proc Endocr Soc p 158.

Levy C, Mester J, Baulieu EE (1981). Early inhibition by progesterone of estrogen-induced ornithine decarboxylase activity in the chick oviduct and rat uterus. J Endocr 90:1.

Merryweather MJ, Knowler JT (1980). The kinetics of the incorporation of newly synthesized ribonucleic acid and protein into the ribosomes of the uterus of the estrogen-stimulated inmature rat. Biochem J 186:405.

Moulton BC, Leonard SL (1969). Hormonal effects on spermidine levels in male and female reproductive organs of the rat. Endocrinology 84:1461.

Oka T, Schimke RT (1969). Interaction of estrogen and progesterone in chick oviduct development. I. Antagonistic effect of progesterone on estrogen-induced proliferation and differentiation of tubular gland cells. J Cell Biol 41:816.

Pegg AE, Lockwood DH, Williams-Ashman HG (1970). Concentration of putrescine and polyamines and their enzymic synthesis during androgen-induced prostatic growth. Biochem J 117:17.

Perin A, Sessa A (1978). Changes in polyamine levels and protein synthesis rate during rat liver carcinogenesis induced by 4-dimethylaminoazobenzene. Cancer Res 38:1.

Robel P, Levy C, Wolff JP, Nicolas JC, Baulieu EE (1978). Reponse a un anti-oestrogene comme critere d'hormono-sensibilité du cancer de l'endometre. C R Acad Sc Paris, t 287:1353.

Russel DH, Byus CV, Manen CA (1976). Proposed model of major sequential biochemical events of a trophic response. Life Sc 19:1297.

Socher SH, O'Malley BW (1973). Estrogen-mediated cell proliferation during chick oviduct development and its modulation by progesterone. Develop Biol 30:411.

Stormshak F, Leake R, Wertz N, Gorski J (1976). Stimulatory and inhibitory effects of estrogen on uterine DNA synthesis. Endocrinology 99:1501.

Sutherland R, Mester J, Baulieu EE (1977). Tamoxifen is a potent "pure" anti-oestrogen in chick oviduct. Nature 267:434.

Tabor CW, Tabor H (1976). 1,4-Diaminobutane (putrescine), spermidine and spermine. Ann Rev Biochem 45:285.

Hormones and Cancer, pages 145–165
© **1984 Alan R. Liss, Inc., 150 Fifth Avenue, New York, NY 10011**

REGULATION OF ESTROGEN RECEPTOR LEVELS IN ENDOMETRIAL CANCER
CELLS

Erlio Gurpide, Rosalyn Blumenthal, Honorée Fleming

Department of Obstetrics, Gynecology and
Reproductive Science, Mount Sinai School of
Medicine, New York, New York   10029

The mitogenic influence of estrogens on human
endometrial tissue has been evident from early observations
made throughout the menstrual cycle and under conditions of
pathologic or pharmacologic hyperestrogenism.   Other
studies correlating hormonal environment and endometrial
morphology, as well as clinical results of hormonal
treatment of dysfunctional uterine bleeding, have shown
that progesterone and synthetic progestins antagonize the
effects of estrogens on the endometrium.

Estrogen receptors mediate the effects of estradiol
and synthetic estrogens by binding these compounds tightly,
i.e. with association constants of about 10^{10} M^{-1}, and
forming complexes of enhanced affinity for acceptor sites
in nuclear chromatin. Although under physiologic
conditions the number of receptor binding sites exceeds the
available endogenous estradiol the law of mass action
indicates that the concentration of biologically active
receptor-estrogen complexes should depend on both receptor
and estrogen intracellular levels. When large doses of
estrogens are administered for therapeutic reasons, the
amount of available receptor can be expected to determine
the response.

It follows from these considerations that physiologic
or pharmacologic regulation of estrogen receptor levels is
a topic of great relevance to a discussion of the effects
of hormones on the proliferation or involution of estrogen
sensitive tumors.

Measurement of estrogen receptor levels

In spite of the feasibility of applying
radioimmunoassay techniques to the measurement of estrogen
receptors, these procedures are not yet in use due to the
unavailability of antibodies prepared by a few research
laboratories and under development by commercial firms.

Levels of estradiol receptor in endometrial tissue,
normal or cancerous, are currently evaluated by measuring
the binding of isotopically labeled estradiol (e.g. pmols
per unit weight of tissue, protein or DNA) to high
affinity, low capacity binders present in the samples.
Most commonly, receptor levels are measured in cytosol by
the dextran-coated charcoal (DCC) method, using unlabeled
competitors to reveal specific binding and Scatchard plots
to calculate concentrations and affinity constants of
binding sites (Clark,Peck, 1979). Receptor levels are also
measured in cytosol by sucrose or glycerol density gradient
analysis, a procedure that distinguishes 8-9S specific
binders (considered to represent the "true" receptors) from
4S binders (Daxenbichler et al, 1980).

Since estrogen receptors are also found in the nuclei
of endometrial tissue, both in bound and available forms
(Fleming, Gurpide, 1980), nuclear receptor levels are often
measured by similar procedures, either after extraction
with KCl solutions or after exchange with labeled estradiol
(Clark, Peck, 1979).

In early studies on estrogen receptor levels in
endometrium conducted in our laboratory, intact tissue was
incubated with excess $^3H-E_2$ to translocate
receptor–estrogen complex to the nucleus and specifically
bound $^3H-E_2$ was measured in the nuclear pellet (Tseng,
Gurpide, 1972; Gurpide et al, 1976). In more recent
experiments described in this Chapter, specific estrogen
binding was measured by incubation of either whole cells,
cell homogenates, cytoplasm or cytosol with 80 nM $^3H-E_2$ in
the presence or absence of 8 μM diethylstilbestrol (DES),
followed by DCC analysis or glycerol density gradient
analysis. The high concentration of ligand chosen for this
work ensured saturation of specific binding sites.
Occasionally, labeling was carried out both at 80 and 10 nM
concentrations of $^3H-E_2$.

Heterogeneity of estrogen receptors

A variety of specific estradiol binders have been described in animal uteri as well as in human endometrium. In addition to the classical forms of the estrogen receptor described in the pioneering reports of Jensen and Jacobson (1962) and Gorski et al (1968), which included a native unbound receptor with sedimentation constants of approximately 8S or 4S according to the experimental conditions, and a transformed or activated 5S receptor-estrogen complex capable of binding to chromatin, other types have been described. Cytosolic estrogen binders differing in their affinity to estradiol, and perhaps in their translocability to the nucleus, have been found in rat uterus (Eriksson et al, 1980), human endometrium (Smith et al, 1979), and in the human endometrial adenocarcinoma cell line HEC-1 (Fridman et al, 1982). Heterogeneity in cytosolic binders have also been revealed by differences in binding of estradiol and synthetic compounds such as DES or Tamoxifen (Fishman and Fishman, 1979; Sato et al, 1981; Taylor, Smith, 1982). Analysis of nuclear binders at various concentrations of labeled estradiol, distinguished sets of binders differing in their affinity towards the ligand (Eriksson et al, 1980). A nuclear binder in monkey endometrium was reported to bind estrone and not estradiol (Kreitmann-Gimbel et al, 1981). Heterogeneity of nuclear binding was also made evident by extracting nuclei with solutions of increasing concentrations of KCl and the physiologic significance of high and low affinity binders, salt extractable, salt insoluble and matrix bound nuclear estrogen receptors (13) is still a matter of investigation. A microsomal estrogen receptor of pig uteri was found to have physicochemical characteristic distinct from those of the corresponding cytosolic binder (Jungblut et al, 1979). Specific estradiol binding have also been found in the cell membrane (Pietro and Szego, 1979).

We have previously reported (Fleming et al, 1982; Fleming et al, 1983) that specific estrogen binders may be present in cytosol of human endometrium and endometrial cancer cells in an "inactive" or "masked" form unable to bind estradiol which can be rapidly converted to an estradiol binding form by cGMPvarious other endogenous compounds. Data demonstrating the existence of these forms of estrogen binders in specimens of endometrial cancer is reported in this Chapter.

No receptor forms with characteristics that could be used to distinguish normal from cancerous endometrial tissue have been reported.

Changes in endometrial receptor levels during the menstrual cycle

The total amount of estrogen receptor found in the nucleus after translocation of cytoplasmic receptors during incubations of endometrial specimens with excess estradiol at 37 C showed a marked decline in receptor levels during the luteal phase (Tseng, Gurpide, 1972; Gurpide et al, 1976). Average values were found to be about 3 pmol/mg DNA during the follicular phase and to decline to about 0.5 pmol/mg DNA in mid-secretory endometrium. Bayard et al (1978) reported that the decline in receptor levels following the development of the corpus luteum occurred in both the cytosol and nuclear fractions. Similar observations were made by Whitehead et al (1981) for nuclear and total estrogen receptor levels, and by Pollow et al (1980), Martin et al (1979) and others for cytosolic levels. These findings suggested that progesterone, the dominant ovarian hormone during the luteal phase, might be responsible for the fall in estrogen receptors in secretory endometrium.

Effects of progesterone and progestins on endometrial estrogen receptor levels

The effect of progestins on estrogen receptor levels was demonstrated under a variety of experimental conditions. In one type of studies, medroxyprogesterone acetate (MPA) was administered for a few days to patients in the proliferative phase of the cycle and estrogen receptors were measured in endometrial curettings obtained before any elevation of endogenous progesterone in plasma was detectable. Receptor levels were found to be lower than those measured in proliferative endometrium from untreated subjects (Tseng, Gurpide, 1975). A reduction in estrogen receptor levels was also observed when a progestin was given to postmenopausal women or postmenopausal patients treated with estrogens (Pollow et al, 1980; Whitehead et al, 1981). In some patients, samples of endometrial adenocarcinoma obtained before and after a short treatment with progestins also showed the depressing effect of these compounds on the concentrations of total and cytosolic estrogen binders (Gurpide et al, 1977; Martin et al, 1979; Pollow et al, 1980; Jänne et al, 1980).

Effects of estrogens on estrogen receptor levels

Suggestive but still inconclusive evidence indicates that estrogens may increase the levels of their own receptor. Pollow et al (1980) have reported a weak but positive correlation between plasma estradiol levels and estradiol receptor levels in endometrial cytosol. Estrogen intake has also been associated with higher levels of endometrial estrogen receptor levels (Tseng et al, 1977; Martin et al, 1979; Whitehead et al, 1981).

An effect of estrogens on estrogen binding levels could be the result of an estrogen-induced increase in intracellular concentrations of cGMP, reported to occur in rat uteri (Kuehl et al, 1974; Kuehl et al, 1975; Flandroy, Galand, 1982), followed by a cGMP-stimulated generation of estrogen binding sites, demonstrated in human endometrial cells (Fleming et al, 1982; Fleming et al, 1983).

Estrogen receptor levels in endometrial cancer

Levels of estrogen receptor as high as those of proliferative normal endometrium have been found in specimens of endometrial adenocarcinoma obtained from postmenopausal patients (Tseng et al, 1977) but the variance and range of the receptor values is much larger in cancer tissue than in normal endometrium (Pollow et al, 1980). A significant proportion of tumors show no detectable levels of cytosolic estrogen receptor (McCarty et al, 1979).

In contrast to the well documented decline in progesterone receptor levels with loss of differentiation in endometrial adenocarcinoma (Pollow et al, 1980), average levels of estrogen receptors in poorly differentiated adenocarcinomas are found by various authors either not to differ or to be much lower than those in well differentiated tumors (Martin et al, 1979; Pollow et al, 1980). Degree of histologic differentiation of the tumor is not a good indicator of estrogen receptor content and may not be adequate for the prediction of responsiveness to estrogen related therapy. Several authors have shown that the presence of progesterone receptors in the tumor correlates well with the presence of estrogen receptors (Pollow et al, 1980; Heuson, Leclercq, 1980), as could be expected from observations indicating that synthesis of the progesterone receptor is regulated by estrogens (Pollow et al, 1980).

Estrogen receptor levels in endometrial cell cultures

A surprising finding, first reported by Fleming et al (1980) and described in more detail in 1982 (Fleming, Gurpide, 1982), revealed that levels of specific estrogen binders in primary cultures of epithelial or stromal cells derived from proliferative or secretory endometria varied remarkably from day to day.

This phenomenon was further studied in cultures of HEC-1 cells, derived by Kuramoto from a specimen of moderately papillary adenocarcinoma of a postmenopausal patient (Kuramoto et al, 1972). The availability of large numbers of these cells allowed hourly as well as daily examination of receptor levels after plating. Highest estrogen binding levels were detected during the first day in culture (Fridman et al, 1982) and, during that day, marked increases and decreases were noted within a 2 h period (Fleming, Gurpide, 1982).

These rapid changes in estrogen binding capacity may reflect changes in intracellular cGMP, cAMP or cGMP/cAMP ratios, which are known to be related to the cell cycle in synchronized cell cultures (Rochette-Egly et al, 1972), since we have shown that cGMP increases and cAMP decreases estrogen receptor levels in endometrial cells (Fleming et al, 1982; Fleming et al, 1983).

Effects of purine nucleotides on estrogen receptor levels

The rapidity of the observed changes in the estradiol binding capacity of cell cultures suggested to us that metabolic factors might be responsible for modifications of the affinity of binders to estradiol. Precedents for such hypothesis could be found in reports by Munck et al and Pratt et al. These authors have shown energy-dependent activation and inactivation of glucocorticoid binding sites in cytosol of rat thymocytes and mouse L-cells (Munck et al, 1972; Nielson et al, 1977; Pratt, 1978). They suggested the possibility that phosphorylation/dephosphorylation of the glucocorticoid receptor might affect its binding ability. Furthermore, Sando et al (1979) noted that sodium molybdate prevented the loss of binding of glucocorticoids by L-cell cytosol during incubations at 37 C and suggested that this stabilizing effect might be due to the known phosphatase inhibitory actions of molybdate.

We tested the effect of adding $MoO_4^=$ to a suspension of HEC-1 cells during labeling with 80 nM ^3H-E_2 ± 8 µM DES for 1.5 h at 4 C or 37 C. At both temperatures, estradiol binding measured in cytoplasm was remarkably higher than the binding obtained in parallel control incubations carried out in the absence of $MoO_4^=$ or adding $MoO_4^=$ after labeling, but before homogenization (Fig. 1).

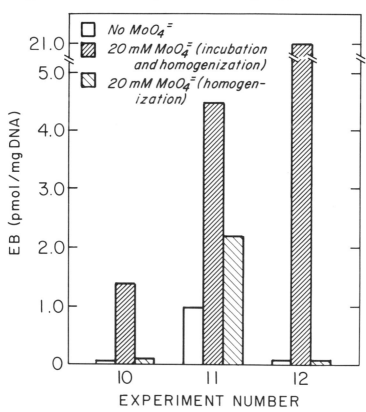

Fig. 1 Levels of specific E_2 binding to HEC-1 cells incubated for 1 h at 4 C with 80 nM ^3H-E_2 ± 8 µM DES in the

absence or presence of 20 mM Na_2MoO_4. Half of the cells incubated in the absence of $MoO_4^=$ were homogenized in medium containing 20 mM Na_2MoO_4.

Similar effects were obtained when $MoO_4^=$ was added to cell homogenates at the time of labeling with $^3H-E_2$. However, the effect was lost when cytoplasm (supernatant obtained after centrifugation of the homogenate at 500 x g pellet) or cytosol was used instead of whole homogenates. Addition of the 500 x g (nuclei + plasma membranes) to cytosol or cytoplasm restored the molybdate effect. Experiments carried out with nuclear plasma membranes separated by centrifugation in density gradients as described by Pietras and Szego (1979) showed that the particulate factors required to obtain the molybdate effect in cytosol resided in the plasma membrane fraction (Fleming et al, 1982).

The finding that cell membranes participate in the molybdate-induced generation of estrogen binding sites prompted us to test the effects of cAMP and cGMP, as well as those of ATP and GTP, on cell homogenates. As Fig. 2

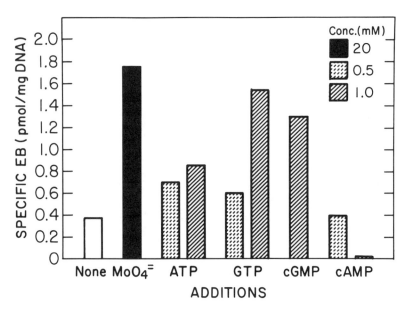

Fig. 2. Homogenates of HEC-1 cells were incubated with 80

nM ^{3}H-E$_2$ $\pm$ 8 uM DES for 2 h at 4 C in the presence of the compounds shown in the figure, at the indicated concentrations. Levels of specifically bound E$_2$ were measured in the 500 x g supernatant after dextran-coated charcoal treatment. (From Fleming et al, 1982, with permission).

shows, ATP, GTP and cGMP, at 1 mM levels, increased specific estradiol binding to about the same levels obtained with 20 mM Na$_2$MoO$_4$. Cyclic AMP, in contrast, reduced binding to almost undetectable levels.

As is the case with MoO$_4^=$, neither ATP nor GTP had an effect on estrogen binding in cytoplasm or cytosol, whereas cGMP maintained its full stimulatory activity in these fractions (Fig. 3). Cyclic AMP was also able to exert its inhibitory effect on estrogen binding when added to cytosol.

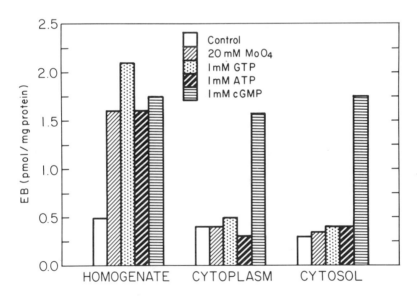

Fig. 3. Homogenates and cytoplasmic or cytosolic preparations from a specimen of secretory endometrium were labeled with 80 nM ^{3}H-E$_2$ $\pm$ 8 μM DES in the presence of the compounds shown in the figure, at the indicated concentrations. Levels of specific E$_2$ binding were measured as described in the Legend to Fig. 2. (From Fleming et al, 1983, with permission).

The effects of cGMP and cAMP on cytosolic estrogen binding were already noticeable at 10^{-9} M concentrations of the cyclic nucleotides and were maximal at 10^{-7} M in the presence of 0.01 M isobutylmethylxanthine (Fig. 4).

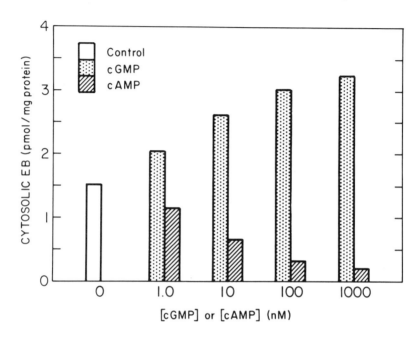

Fig. 4. Specific E_2 binding in HEC-1 cell cytosol in the presence of 0.1 mM isobutylmethylxanthine and cGMP or cAMP at the concentrations indicated in the figure. (From Fleming et al, 1983, with permission).

The importance of cyclic nucleotides as regulators of estrogen binding is made evident by the strong correlation observed to exist between cGMP/cAMP ratios and specific estrogen binding levels in cultures of HEC-1 cells at different times after plating (Fleming and Blumenthal, unpublished data). This correlation was maintained when cGMP/cAMP ratios were modified by addition of molybdate to HEC-1 cell homogenates.

Some characteristics of the processes of generation and inactivation of estrogen binding sites

Most of the observations described above can be interpreted by hypothesizing that MoO_4^-, ATP and GTP influence estrogen binding levels by increasing cGMP concentrations. Molybdate and ATP may exert their effect by increasing guanylate cyclase activity (Siegel et al, 1976) whereas GTP may serve as a precursor of cGMP (the non-hydrolyzable analog guanylylimidophosphate had no effect on estradiol binding).

Molybdate may also have a protective effect on estrogen binders and receptor estradiol complexes under destabilizing conditions, e.g. when cytosol is kept at 37 C for about 1 h (Nielsen et al, 1977) or at 4 C for several hours during sucrose or glycerol gradient analysis (Miller et al, 1981). However, most of the "stabilizing" effects of molybdate reported in the literature were observed under conditions in which the receptor-estrogen complexes are stable (short periods of time at 4 C during DCC analysis). In these cases, the higher values for estrogen receptors found when tissue was homogenized in the presence of molybdate or when molybdate was added to homogenates could have been due to generation of new sites rather than stabilization of existing binders.

Some experimental evidence indicates that both cGMP and cAMP influence estrogen binding by affecting processes involving phosphorylations. Thus, when ATP concentrations in HEC-1 cell homogenates were allowed to fall to undetectable levels by preincubation at 4 C for 3 h, the cyclic nucleotides had no effect on estrogen binding. Responsiveness was restored by addition of ATP to the depleted homogenate (Fleming et al, 1983). Furthermore, the influence of divalent cations (Mn^{++}, Mg^{++}, Ca^{++}) at varius concentrations on the magnitude of the effects of cyclic nucleotides on estrogen binding suggest that these effects are mediated by cGMP and cAMP-dependent kinases (Fleming et al, 1983). However, the evidence for phosphorylation as a mechanism of generation of new estrogen binding sites or inactivation of existing binders is still circumstantial. The possibility of allosteric interaction of cyclic nucleotides with actual or potential binders in the presence of ATP and divalent cations cannot be ruled out.

Recent interesting reports by Auricchio et al indicate that estrogen receptors isolated from calf uterus and inactivated by a nuclear phosphatase can be reactivated and radiolabeled during incubations with [$\int$-^{32}P] ATP and a Ca^{++} stimulated kinase, also isolated from calf uterus (Migliaccio et al, 1982). Similarities and differences between these observations on purified components of bovine uterus and those made in human endometrial cytosol remain to be established.

Low salt discontinuous glycerol density gradient analysis of specific estrogen binders in cytosol from HEC-1 cells incubated with 10 nM ^{3}H-E$_{2}$ $\pm$ 1 μM DES in the presence of 1 uM cGMP and 0.01 M isobutylmethylxanthine showed an enhancement of the number of both 8S and 4S binding sites (Fig. 5). Since 8S binders are usually considered to

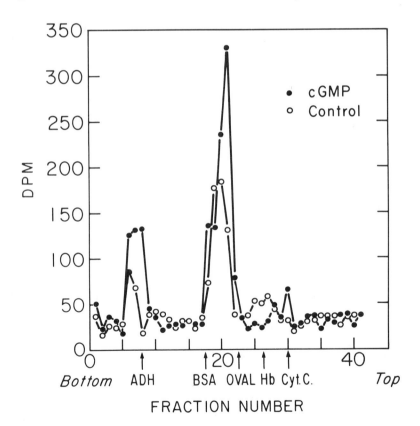

Fig. 5. Low-salt gradients of HEC-1 cell cytosol labeled with 10 nM ^{3}H-E$_2$ $\pm$ μM DES in the absence or presence of 1 uM cGMP and 0.1 mM isobutylmethylxanthine. (From Fleming et al, 1983, with permission).

represent "true" receptors (Daxenbichler et al, 1980) these finding points to the likelihood that at least some of the binders influenced by the cyclic nucleotides function as estrogen receptors.

Effects of purine nucleotides on estrogen binding by endometrial adenocarcinoma

All the effects of MoO$_4^=$, ATP, GTP, cGMP and cAMP described above have been documented in HEC-1 cells and in specimens of histologically normal endometrium. It remained to be shown that the same effects could be obtained on specimens of endometrial adenocarcinoma. Demonstration of these effects in cancerous tissue is of special interest since pharmacologic manipulation of estrogen receptor levels in tumors is a matter of considerable therapeutic relevance.

Figure 6 shows results obtained with a specimen of well differentiated endometrial adenocarcinoma taken from the uterus of a postmenopausal patient. As expected, Na$_2$MoO$_4$, ATP, GTP and cGMP increased specific estradiol binding when added at 1 mM concentrations to tissue homogenates and only cGMP was effective on cytosol. Cyclic AMP lowered estrogen binding to almost undectable levels when added to either homogenate or cytosol.

Figure 7 illustrates an interesting case in which the tumor showed nondetectable levels of estradiol binders (an ER$^-$ tumor) but became ER$^+$ when cGMP was added to the cytosol at the time of labeling, or when molybdate, ATP, GTP or cGMP was added to the homogenate together with the labeled ligand. These results indicate the potential of some tumors without detectable estrogen receptors to specifically bind estradiol under appropriate stimulation.

The Table presents data on effects of molybdate and nucleotides on various specimens of endometrial cancer tested. In average, levels of specific estrogen binders doubled when cGMP or other nucleotides were added to the

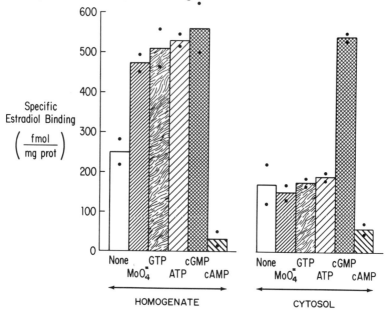

Fig. 6. Specific estrogen binding in homogenate or cytosol of a specimen or well differentiated endometrial adenocarcinoma (Exp. #267) in the absence or presence of Na_2MoO_4 (20 mM), GTP, ATP, cGMP or cAMP (1 mM), as described in the legend to Fig. 2.

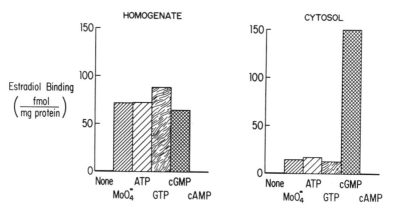

Fig. 7. Effects of Na_2MoO_4 (20 mM), ATP, GTP, cGMP or cAMP (1 mM) on the specific binding of E_2 in homogenate or cytosol of a specimen of endometrial adenocarcinoma with undetectable estrogen receptor levels under control conditions.

EFFECTS OF MOLYBDATE AND NUCLEOTIDES ON SPECIFIC ESTROGEN BINDING LEVELS

Exp. #	Histology	Cellular fraction	EB levels relative to controls				
			$MoO_4^=$ (1 mM)	ATP (1 mM)	GTP (1 mM)	cGMP (1 mM)	cAMP (1 mM)
[267]	Endo AC, grade I	Homogenate	1.9	2.1	2.0	2.2	0.2
		Cytosol	0.9	1.1	1.0	3.2	0.3
[295]	Adenosquamous carcinoma of the endometrium	Homogenate	1.3	1.6	1.3	1.3	0.5
		Cytosol	0.9	0.7	0.7	2.7	0.3
[262]	Endo AC, grade II (papillary features)	Homogenate	2.0	1.8	2.3	3.3	
[385]	Endo AC grade I	Homogenate	1.7	2.7	2.1	1.9	0.5
[379]	Endo AC grade III	Homogenate				1.9	0.1
[373]	Endo AC, well-differentiated omental metastasis	Homogenate				3.3	0
[386]	Endo AC, grade II	Homogenate				3.6	
		Cytosol				3.4	

homogenate and tripled when cGMP was added to cytosol during the binding assay. Cyclic AMP reduced estrogen binding levels to less than 1/3 of the control levels.

SUMMARY AND CONCLUSIONS

Recent experimental results from our laboratories revealed the following facts:

- Addition of GMP to homogenates or cytosol prepared from endometrial tissue or cultured endometrial adenocarcinoma cells during the assay for specific estrogen binders markedly increases specific binding levels. The effect is completed in about 15 min at 4 C (Fleming et al, 1983). Cyclic AMP has the opposite effect and in many cases lowers the number of binding sites to undectectable levels.

- ATP, a nucleotide that stimulates a particulate form of guanylate cyclase, Na_2MoO_4, a compound that can elevate cGMP levels (Fleming and Blumenthal, unpublished) and GTP, a metabolic precursor of cGMP, increase specific estradiol binding in the presence of plasma membranes and soluble factors.

- Cyclic AMP reduces the levels of estrogen binding when added to cell homogenates or to cytosol and counteracts the effects of cGMP, $MoO_4^=$, ATP and GTP.

- ATP is required for the expression of cGMP and cAMP effects on estradiol binding. It is therefore likely that phosphorylations are involved in the generation and inactivation of estrogen binding sites. Divalent cation requirements for these effects also suggest participation of protein kinases in these processes.

- The reported effects of nucleotides and molybdate have been observed in specimens of histologically normal endometrium, in specimens of endometrial carcinoma, in two endometrial adenocarcinoma cell lines, HEC-1 and HEC-50(Suzuki et al, 1980), and in two breast cancer cell lines, CG-5, a variant of MCF-7 obtained in Iacobelli's laboratory (Natoli et al, 1983), and in T47D) (Fleming et al, in press)

- Rapid changes in the levels of estrogen binding capacity observed in endometrial cells in culture can be associated with changes in cGMP/cAMP ratios shown, to vary during the cell cycle.

Although it has not yet been demonstrated that cGMP-induced increases in specific estrogen binding can enhance responses to available estrogens, such possibility is of potential importance. Reduction of estrogen receptor levels in patients with cancers of estrogen sensitive tissues may inhibit tumor growth promoted by endogenous estrogen. Cho-Chung et al have recently reported that cholera toxin causes a reduction in estrogen receptor levels and arrests hormone dependent growth of DMBA-induced mammary carcinoma in rats (Cho-Chung et al, 1983). They postulated that the effect of cholera toxin is mediated by a cAMP effect on the estrogen receptor, an hypothesis supported by the observation that only tumors containing receptor responded to treatment.

Conversely, cGMP-induced increases in specific estrogen binders may be useful in promoting a response of tumors to estrogen-related therapy, e.g. treatment with high doses of estrogens or with antiestrogens.

The heterogeneity of intracellular estradiol binders makes it difficult to evaluate which particular species are influenced by cGMP or cAMP. Although most of our studies were carried out at high concentration of ^{3}H-E$_2$ estradiol (80 nM) which can be expected to label both type I and II cytosolic binders (Fridman et al, 1982), clear elevations of 4S and 8S binders by cGMP have been detected by glycerol density gradient analysis after labeling with 10 nM ^{3}H-E$_2$.

Realization of the possibility of modulating estrogen receptor levels with drugs or hormones affecting cAMP and cGMP levels opens a promising new line of investigation. Much remains to be learned about the biochemical changes resulting in generation or inactivation of binders. Availability of the in vitro systems described here will facilitate these investigations.

REFERENCES

Barrack ER, Hawkins EF, Allen SL, Hicks LL, Coffey DS (1977). Concepts related to salt resistant estradiol receptors in rat uterine nuclei: nuclear matrix. Nuclear matrix. Biochem Biophys Res Commun 79:829.

Bayard F, Damilano S, Robel P, Baulieu EE (1978). Cytoplasmic and nuclear estradiol and progesterone receptor in human endometrium. J Clin Endocrinol Metab 46:635.

Cho-Chung Y, Clair T, Shepheard C, Berghoffer B (1983). Arrest of hormone-dependent mammary cancer growth in vivo and in vitro by cholera toxin. Cancer Res 43:1473.

Clark JH, Peck EJ, Jr (1979). Female Sex Steroids. Receptors and Function. In "Monographs on Endocrinology, Vol 14, Berlin-Heidelberg-New York, Springer-Verlag.

Daxenbichler G, Grill HJ, Geir W, Wittliff JL, Dapunt O (1980). Estrogen and progesterone receptors in normal and neoplastic uterine tissues. In Wittliff JL, Dapunt O (eds) "Steroid Receptors and Hormone-Dependent Neoplasia, New York, Masson Publishing USA, Inc, p 59.

Eriksson HA, Hardin JW, Markaverich B, Upchurch S, Clark JH (1980). Estrogen binding in the rat uterus: heterogeneity of sites and relation to uterotrophic response. J Steroid Biochem 12:121.

Fishman JH, Fishman J (1979). Differentiation of estradiol receptors in rat uterine cytosol by sensitivity to tamoxifen. Biochem Biophys Res Commun 87:550.

Flandroy L, Galand P (1982). Oestrogen-induced increase in uterine cGMP content in vitro: effects of inhibitors of protein and RNA synthesis. Mol Cell Endocrinol 25:49.

Fleming H, Namit C, Gurpide E (1980). Estrogen receptors in epithelial and stromal cells of human endometrium in culture. J Steroid Biochem 12:169.

Fleming H, Gurpide E (1980). Available estradiol receptors in nuclei from human endometrium. J Steroid Biochem 13:3.

Fleming H, Gurpide E (1981). Rapid fluctuations in the levels of specific binding sites in endometrial cells in culture. Endocrinology 108:1744.

Fleming H, Blumenthal R, Gurpide E (1982). Effects of cyclic nucleotides on estradiol binding in human endometrium. Endocrinology 111:1671.

Fleming H, Blumenthal R, Gurpide E (1983). Rapid changes in specific estrogen binding elicited by cGMP or cAMP in cytosol from human endometrial cells. Proc Natl Acad Sci USA 80.

Fridman O, Fleming H, Gurpide E (1982). Variability of levels of specific estrogen binding in a human endometrial adenocarcinoma cell line. J Steroid Biochem 16:607.

Gorski J, Toft D, Shymala G, Smith D, Notides A (1968). Hormone receptors: Studies on the interaction of estrogen with the uterus. Recent Progr Hormone Res 24:245.

Gurpide E, Gusberg SB, Tseng L (1976). Estradiol binding and metabolism in human endometrial hyperplasia and adenocarcinoma. J Steroid Biochem 7:891.

Gurpide E, Tseng L, Gusberg SB (1977). Estrogen metabolism in normal and neoplastic endometrium. Am J Obstet Gynecol 129:809.

Heuson JC, Leclercq G (1980). Quantitative aspects of estrogen receptors in the strategy of breast cancer treatment. In Wittliff JL, Dapunt O (eds): "Steroid Receptors and Hormone-Dependent Neoplasia", New York, Masson Publishing USA, Inc, p 239.

Jänne O, Kauppila A, Kontula K, Syrjälä P, Vierikko P, Vihko (1980). Female sex steroid receptors in human endometrial hyperplasia and carcinoma. In Wittliff JL, Dapunt (eds): "Steroid Receptors and Hormone-Dependent Neoplasia, New York, Masson Publishing USA, Inc, p 37.

Jensen EV, Jacobson HI (1962). Basic guides to the mechanism of estrogen action. Recent Progr. Hormone Res 18:387.

Jungblut PW, Hughes H, Gaues J, Kallweit E, Maschler I, Parl F, Sierralta E, Szendro PI, Wagner RK (1979). Mechanisms involved in the regulation of steroid receptor levels. J Steroid Biochem 11:273.

Kreitmann-Gimbal B, Bayard F, Hodges GD (1981). Changing ratios of nuclear estrone to estradiol binding in endometrium at implantation: regulation by chorionic gonadotropins and progesterone during rescue of the primate corpus luteum. J Clin Endocrinol Metab 52:133.

Kuehl FA, Ham EA, Zanetti ME, Sanford CH, Nicol SE, Goldberg ND (1974). Estrogen-related increases in uterine guanosine 3',5'-cyclic monophosphate levels. Proc Natl Acad Sci USA 71:1866.

Kuehl FA, Jr, Zanetti ME, Cirillo VJ, Ham EA (1975). Estrogen-induced alterations in cyclic nucleotide and prostaglandin levels in target tissue. J Steroid Biochem 6:1099.

Kuramoto H, Tamura S, Notake Y (1972). Establishment of a cell line of human endometrial adenocarcinoma in vitro. Am J Obstet Gynecol 114:1012

Martin PM, Rolland PH, Gammerre M, Serment H, Toga M (1979). Estradiol and progesterone receptors in normal and neoplastic endometrium: correlations between receptors, histopathological examinations and clinical responses under progestin therapy. Int J Cancer 23:321.

Migliaccio A, Lastoria S, Moncharmont B, Rontondi A, Auricchio F (1982). Phosphorylation of calf uterus 17 estradiol receptor by endogenous Ca^{2+}-stimulated kinase activating the hormone binding or the receptor. Biochem Biophys Res Commun 109:1002.

Miller LK, Tuazon FB, Niu EM, Sherman MR (1981). Human breast tumor estrogen receptor: effects of molybdate and electrophoretic analyses. Endocrinology 108:1369.

Munck A, Wira C, Young DA, Mosher KM, Hallahan C, Bell PA (1972). Glucocorticoid-receptor complexes and the earliest steps in the action of glucocorticoids on thymus cells. J Steroid Biochem 3:567.

McCarty KS, Jr, Barton TK, Fetler BF, Creasman WT, McCarthy KS, Sr (1979). Correlation of estrogen and progesterone receptors with histologic differentiation in endometrial adenocarcinoma. Am J Pathol 96:171.

Natoli C, Sica G, Natoli V, Serra A, Iacobelli S (1983). Two new estrogen-supersensitive variants of the MCF-7 human breast cancer cell line. Breast Cancer Res Treat 3:23.

Nielson CJ, Sando JJ, Vogel WM, Pratt WB (1977). Glucocorticoid receptor inactivaion under cell free conditions. J Biol Chem 252:7568.

Pietras RJ, Szego CM (1979). Estrogen receptors in uterine plasma membrane. J Steroid Biochem 11:1471.

Pollow K, Schmidt-Gollwitzer M, Pollow B (1980). Progesterone and estradiol binding proteins from normal human endometrium and endometrial carcinoma: a comparative study. In Wittliff JL, Dapunt O (eds): "Steroid Receptors and Hormone-Dependent Neoplasia, New York, Masson Publishing USA, Inc, p 69.

Pratt WB (1978). The mechanisms of glucocorticoid effects in fibroblasts. J Invest Dermatology 71:24.

Rochette-Egly C, Chouroulinkov I, Castagna M (1972). Cyclic nucleotide levels in rat embryo fibroblasts treated with tumor-promoting phorbol diester. J Cyclic Nucleotide Res 3:567.

Sando JJ, La Forest AC, Pratt WB (1979). ATP-dependent activation of L cell glucocorticoid receptors to the steroid binding form. J Biol Chem 254:4772.

Sato B, Maeda Y, Noma K, Matsumoto K, Yamamura Y (1981). Estrogen binding component of mouse Leydig cell tumor: an in vitro conversion from non-receptor to receptor-like molecule. Endocrinology 108:612.

Siegel MI, Puca GA, Cuatrecasas P (1976). Guanylate cyclase: existence of different forms and their regulation by nucleotides in calf uterus. Biochim Biophys Acta 438:310.

Smith RG, Clarke SG, Zalta E, Taylor RN (1979). Two estrogen receptors in reproductive tissue. J Steroid Biochem 10:31.

Suzuki M, Kuramoto H, Hamano M, Shirane H, Watanabe K (1980). Effects of oestradiol and progesterone on the alkaline phosphatase activity of a human endometrial cancer cell line. Acta Endocrinol (Kbn) 93:108.

Taylor RN, Smith RG (1982). Identification of a novel steroid binding protein. Proc Natl Acad Sci USA 79:1742.

Tseng L, Gurpide E (1972). Nuclear concentration of estradiol in superfused slices of human endometrium. Am J Obstet Gynecol 114:995.

Tseng L, Gurpide E (1975). Induction of human endometrial estradiol dehydrogenase by progestins. Endocrinology 97:825.

Tseng L, Gusberg SB, Gurpide E (1977). Estradiol receptor and 17β dehydrogenase in normal and abnormal human endometrium. Ann N Y Acad Sci 286:190.

Whitehead MI, Townsend PT, Pryse-Davies J, Ryder TA, King RJB (1981). Effects of estrogen and progestins on the biochemistry and morphology of the postmenopausal endometrium. New Engl J Med 305:1599.

This investigation was supported by grants CA-15648 from the National Cancer Institute and HD-07197 from the National Institutes of Health.

Hormones and Cancer, pages 167–179

FEMALE SEX STEROID RECEPTORS IN POST MENOPAUSAL ENDOMETRIAL
CARCINOMA. BIOCHEMICAL RESPONSES TO ANTIESTROGEN AND PROGESTIN

Paul Robel[1], Achille Gravanis[1], Lydie Roger-Jallais[2],
Maria-Grazia Catelli[1], Nadine Binart[1], Martine
George[3], Claude Laval[2] and Etienne-Emile Baulieu[1]

[1]CNRS ER 125 and INSERM U 33, Lab. Hormones, 94270
Bicêtre. [2]Centre René Huguenin, 92211 Saint Cloud.
[3]Institut Gustave Roussy, 94800 Villejuif, France.

Post-menopausal endometrial adenocarcinoma almost always contain estradiol receptor (ER) in varying, often large
amounts ; about two thirds of tumors also contain progestin
receptors (Mortel et al 1981). It is well accepted that pro-
gestational agents achieve objective remissions in only
about 30 to 35 % of patients with advanced or metastatic
endometrial cancer. Therefore it is unlikely that, based on
receptor assays, it will be possible to select those patients
likely to benefit from hormonal therapy.

Some attempts have been made to directly demonstrate
the effects of hormones on tumors, using incubations or
cultures of tumor explants in presence of steroid hormones
(Tseng et al 1977), or tumors grafted into nude mice (Satyaswaroop et al 1983). These approaches suffer from serious
limitations. We have tried to set up an in vivo biochemical
approach to relate receptor levels to hormone response in
endometrial cancers. The biochemical changes elicited in the
tumors might also be used to define the doses and combinations of hormones which produce optimal therapeutic responses.

Several compounds of the triphenylethylene series exhibit both estrogenic and antiestrogenic properties. This is
the case of tamoxifen (TAM), which, in the rodent uterus,
has been shown to increase progesterone receptor (PR) concentration, while it counteracts estrogen-induced uterine
growth (Jordan, Dix 1978). TAM behaves as a "pure antiestrogen" in the chick oviduct, as far as growth, ovalbumin
synthesis, or PR concentration are concerned (Sutherland et
al 1977). However, it was recently reported that combined

administration of TAM and progesterone to estrogen primed, withdrawns chicks, potentiates the effects of progesterone on egg white protein synthesis and produces estrogen-like growth-promoting properties (Binart et al 1982). Combination of an antiestrogen with steroid hormones may thus bring about novel and unpredictable types of responses. On theoretical grounds, we advocated the combination of antiestrogens and progestins for the treatment of endometrial (and breast) cancers (Robel et al 1983). This was based on the observation that PR in human endometrium seems to follow the same principles as in animal models (Milgrom et al 1973). It is induced by estrogens (Whitehead et al 1981), and it is decreased by progestins (Tseng, Gurpide 1975). We had shown that TAM given to post-menopausal women with endometrial carcinoma increased PR concentrations in the tumors, and may improve the responsiveness of the tumors to progestins (Mortel et al 1981). In the present work, three tumor samples could be obtained under acceptable ethical conditions, the first as a control, the second after administration of medroxyprogesterone acetate (MPA), and the third after administration of both MPA and TAM. Our purpose was to examine whether the antiestrogen could rescue the levels of progestin receptors. DNA polymerase α (DNA pol) activity was measured as a parameter related to the growth potential of the tumors. Plasminogen activator (PA) was also evaluated, because its activity was reported to be associated with steroid receptors (Thorsen 1982).

MATERIAL AND METHODS

Experimental Animals

    Newborn chicks were primed with estradiol benzoate and withdrawn for 4-6 weeks. After this period, they were reinjected in the upper leg muscle with the appropriate test compounds, as indicated in the Results section. Animals were killed 18 or 24 h after the last injection. The oviducts were removed, fragments of each oviduct magnum were pooled, and the relative rates of ovalbumin and conalbumin synthesis were measured as previously published (Binart et al 1982).

Patients

    We had previously reported ER and PR measurements in 43 cases of post menopausal endometrial cancer. Thirty five of these patients have been followed-up for 5 years or more, and we now discuss the relationship between receptor levels in the tumors and patient survival. Twelve more patients with histologically proven adenocarcinoma of the endometrium were seen in consultation and treated at the Centre René Huguenin, Saint-Cloud, France. They were treated with MPA alone, 100 mg daily per orally for 7 d, then with 100 mg of MPA and 40 mg of TAM daily for 7 d. Whenever possible, three partial uterine curettages were performed, before treatment, after MPA alone, and after combined MPA and TAM. Part of each biopsy specimen was processed for histology and the degree of tumor differentiation was recorded (data not shown). Receptor concentrations were determined in all biopsy samples and, in addition, the activities of DNA pol and PA were evaluated before and after hormone treatment.

Homogeneization

Tumor biopsy samples weighing 40 to 60 mg were kept in liquid nitrogen. They were homogenized in 20 vol of chilled TDS buffer [10 mM Tris-HCl pH 7.8, 1 mM dithioerythritol (DTE), 0.25 M sucrose]. Hundred μl of the homogenate were kept for the assay of DNA, two 50 μl samples were used for the assay of DNA pol and PA activities, and the remainder (∿ 650 μl) was used for the assay of ER and PR.

Receptor Measurements

The homogenate was diluted to a final concentration of 2 mg protein/ml, 20 mM molybdate, 0.5 mM PMSF, 20 % glycerol, pH 7.8. The technique utilized allowed measurements of total (filled and unfilled) ER and PR sites in the cytosol and nuclei as reported in detail by Bayard et al (1978). Total receptor concentrations were measured directly in the homogenates using hydroxylapatite (HAP) batch adsorption procedure to separate bound ligands (Erdos, Bessada 1979; Hechter et al 1983).

Aliquots of the homogenate were measured for protein using the technique of Bradford (1976) and for DNA using the technique of Burton (1968). All results were expressed in pmol of hormone binding sites per mg of DNA. Assay sensitivity was such that any value < 0.1 pmol of total receptors per mg of DNA was considered as not significantly different from zero.

DNA Polymerase α

The homogenate was diluted to 1.2 mg protein/ml, 20 mM Tris-HCl pH 7.6, 0.5 M KCl, 2 mM DTE, 0.5 % Triton X 100, sonicated, and kept at 0°C for 60 min. Thereafter, triplicate 20 µl samples were used for the assay of DNA pol activity according to Bertazzoni et al (1977). The results were expressed in pmol thymidine triphosphate incorporated per min per mg of protein.

Plasminogen Activator

The homogenate was diluted to 1.2 mg protein/ml, 10 mM Tris-HCl pH 7.6, 0.4 M KCl, 0.25 M sucrose, 0.1 % Triton X 100. Thereafter, 25, 50 and 75 µl samples were used for the assay of PA according to Searls (1980). This technique utilizes a chromogenic substrate, H-D-valyl-L-leucyl-L-lysine-p-nitroanilide-dihydrochloride, which in presence of plasminogen and activator liberates paranitroanilide. Results were expressed in terms of urokinase Units per hour per mg of protein.

RESULTS

Effects of Tamoxifen and Steroid Hormones on the Chick Oviduct

TAM alone has no effect on weight, DNA, or protein content of withdrawn chick oviduct. It does not induce ovalbumin synthesis and has minimal effects on the rate of conalbumin synthesis (Catelli et al 1980). It does not increase PR levels (Sutherland et al 1977). However, combined treatment with progesterone plus TAM increases conalbumin and ovalbumin synthesis more than progesterone alone and displays estrogen-like growth promoting properties (Binart et al 1982). Similar results have been obtained with the glucocorticosteroid dexamethasone (DEX). DEX alone has minimal effects on the weight, DNA and protein content of withdrawn chick oviduct. On the contrary, combined DEX + TAM increase the protein content of chick oviduct more than 7 fold, the weight and DNA content 2 to 3 fold after 4 d of treatment. The relative rates of ovalbumin and conalbumin synthesis are much larger after TAM + DEX than after DEX alone (Table I).

TREATMENT	OVALBUMIN	CONALBUMIN
Control	0.2	0.8
TAM	0.7	1.6
DEX	2.8	4.4
TAM + DEX	7.2	7.8

TABLE 1. Relative rates of ovalbumin and conalbumin synthesis. Withdrawn chicken received daily injections of TAM (10 mg) and DEX (2 mg) alone or combined for 4 d. Results are expressed in % of total protein synthesis.

DNA pol activity has also been measured in the chick oviduct 18, 24 and 96 h after treatment (Fig. 1). DNA pol activity was unchanged by progesterone and DEX treatment compared to controls, and tended to be decreased by TAM, whereas combined DEX and TAM markedly increased DNA pol activity to a level close to that produced by estradiol.

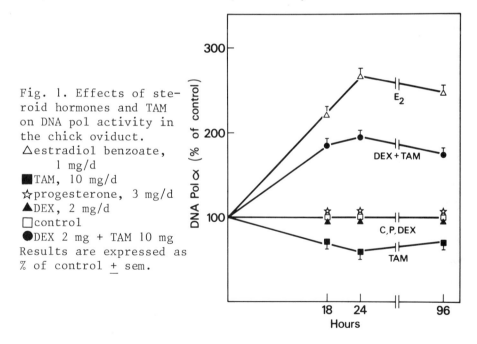

Fig. 1. Effects of steroid hormones and TAM on DNA pol activity in the chick oviduct.
△estradiol benzoate, 1 mg/d
■TAM, 10 mg/d
☆progesterone, 3 mg/d
▲DEX, 2 mg/d
☐control
●DEX 2 mg + TAM 10 mg
Results are expressed as % of control ± sem.

Effects of Medroxyprogesterone Acetate and Tamoxifen on Endometrial Cancer

Estradiol and progesterone receptors. Receptor amounts were undetectable or insignificant (< 0.3 pmol/mg DNA) in 1 tumor examined for estradiol and 6 tumors examined for progesterone. The mean values observed in this study confirmed our previous report and the findings of Tseng et al (1977) that, in postmenopausal endometrial carcinoma, the level of ER is similar to that in the endometrium of normal women in the proliferative phase of the cycle, whereas PR concentrations were generally low and similar to those observed in late secretory endometrium (Table 2).

	Control (n = 12)	MPA (n = 10)	MPA + TAM (n = 5)
ER[1]	$1.9 + 0.3$[2]	$0.7 + 0.2$[5]	$0.9 + 0.3$[5]
PR[1]	$0.5 + 0.1$	$0.4 + 0.1$[5]	$1.0 + 0.2$[6]
DNA pol[3]	$16.3 + 0.8$	$15.3 + 0.7$	$6.5 + 0.8$[6]
PA[4]	$1.3 + 0.1$	$0.8 + 0.1$[5]	$0.9 + 0.1$[5]

TABLE 2. Effects of MPA and of TAM on endometrial cancer. [1]pmol/mg DNA, [2]mean $+$ sem, [3]pmol thymidine triphosphate/min/mg protein, [4]urokinase units/h/mg protein, [5]$p < 0.05$ vs control, [6]$p < 0.05$ vs MPA.

Effects of medroxyprogesterone acetate. In the tumors of patients who had taken 100 mg of MPA daily for 7 d, there was a significant decrease of ER and of PA activity, whereas total PR was slightly decreased and DNA pol activity was unchanged.

Effects of tamoxifen. Forty mg of TAM were given together with MPA for 7 d. This combined regimen produced a significant increase of PR concentrations well above the control level, whereas ER values were only slightly increased above the low level reached under MPA. PA activity remained low. DNA pol activity was very markedly and significantly decreased to less than half the control and MPA induced levels.

Correlations between Receptors and Enzymes

A clearcut positive correlation was observed between ER concentrations and PA activity (Fig. 2).

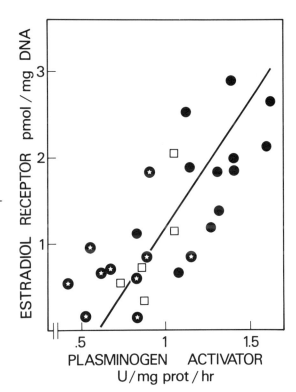

Fig. 2. ER and PA. PA activity was plotted vs ER concentrations in control (●), MPA (✪), and MPA + TAM (□) treated tumor samples.

Both parameters were correlated not only in control tumor samples, but also decreased coordinately after MPA treatment and tended to increase after MPA + TAM treatment. The coefficient of correlation between ER and PA was 0.71. Conversely a clearcut negative correlation occurred between PR concentrations and DNA pol activities (Fig. 3). This negative correlation was observed not only in control and MPA treated tumor samples, but also in tumor samples after combined MPA + TAM, in which PR concentrations and DNA pol activities were coordinately increased. The coefficient of correlation between PR and DNA pol was - 0.66.

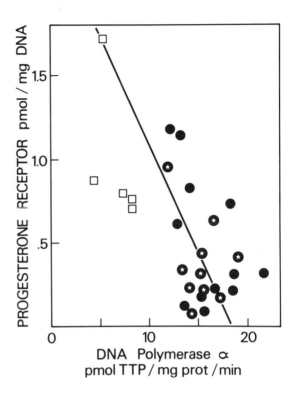

Fig. 3. PR and DNA
pol. DNA pol acti-
vity was plotted vs
PR concentrations
in control (●),
MPA (✪) and MPA +
TAM (□) treated
tumor samples.

Progesterone and Estradiol Receptors and Clinical Outcome

Thirty five patients have been followed up for 5 years
or more. The method of Kaplan was used to evaluate the relationship between patient survival and clinical or biological
criteria. The clinical criteria included the age and weight
of the patients, the grade and stage of the tumor ; the biological criteria included the concentrations of plasma estrone, estradiol and progesterone, and the concentrations of
PR and ER in control tumor biopsy samples. The only statistically significant correlate of patient survival was the
clinical stage of the tumor. Tumors with nuclear ER levels
> 0.4 pmol/mg DNA, or with total PR levels > 1 pmol/mg DNA
tended to have longer survival (Fig. 4).

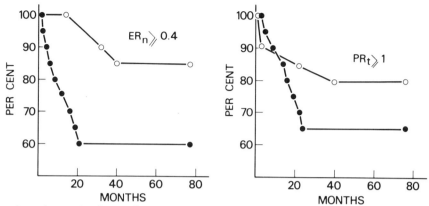

Fig. 4. Relationship between patient survival and receptor levels. Left panel : % patient survival is plotted vs nuclear estradiol receptor (ER_n). (◯), ER_n > 0.4 pmol/mg DNA ; (●), ER_n < 0.4 pmol/mg DNA. Right panel : % patient survival is plotted vs total progesterone receptor (PR_t) ; (◯), PR_t > 1 pmol/mg DNA ; (●), PR_t < 1 pmol/mg DNA.

DISCUSSION

When measurements are made on a small specimen of a malignant tumor, it is assumed that the results are representative of the whole tumor. It is quite likely that several samples of the same tumor may differ in terms of differentiation, cellularity, proportion of malignant cells, necrotic changes, and so forth. A critical point is the possibility that the biochemical responses to MPA and TAM might reflect the response of normal cells interspersed in the biopsy sample. However, careful histologic evaluation could be performed on most biopsies, and has shown with one exception that most if not all the cells were indeed malignant. It should also be recalled that sensitivity of endometrial cancer cells to hormones has been directly demonstrated in culture (Lippman et al, 1977), or in tumors grafted into nude mice (Satyaswaroop et al 1983).

In contrast to breast cancers, it is generally agreed that almost all endometrial cancers contain measurable and often relatively large concentrations of ER (Mortel et al 1981). PR on the contrary are practically undetectable

in about 30 % of cases, and are generally low, probably as
a consequence of the low plasma estradiol concentrations.
These observations underline the importance of a test chal-
lenging the hormonal responsiveness using a compound binding
to the ER, such as TAM. A several fold increase of PR had
been observed in about 60 % of cases, with poor correlation
with the level of ER in the control biopsy. Further investigations are needed to establish the predictive value of the
TAM challenge test for the selection of patients with endometrial carcinoma likely to respond to hormone therapy.

The measurement of ER and PR in endometrial cancer
tumors seems to provide reliable criteria for the prediction
of clinical outcome. Our own results confirm the conclusion
of Kauppila et al (1982) that the receptor-poor tumors tended to behave more aggressively than did receptor-rich malignancies in relation to patient survival. In our study, nuclear ER and total PR were most meaningful.

It is well established that progestagens are of definite
value in the treatment of patients with advanced or metastatic endometrial cancer (Kohorn 1976; Reifenstein 1974). However, one drawback of progesterone therapy is the decrease of
PR concentration (Billiet et al 1982; Jänne et al 1980). TAM
increases PR, even in face of continued progestagen treatment,
and therefore would be helpful in increasing the magnitude
and/or duration of response in patients with endometrial cancer.

The biological properties of antiestrogens can be profoundly altered by their association with some steroid hormones. This is exemplified by our experiments on the chick
oviduct, a species in which TAM has very little or no effect
on its own. However, when given together with progesterone and
DEX, TAM elicits growth and egg white protein responses similar to those produced by estrogens (Binart et al 1982). Therefore, the biological effectiveness of antiestrogen-progesta-
gen combinations on human tissues must be carefully evaluated before considering their use for the treatment of hormone dependent cancers. TAM and MPA have been simultaneously
added to the culture medium of CG 5 cells, a variant of the
MCF 7 cell line highly sensitive to estrogen (Iacobelli et
al 1983). The inhibition of cell proliferation was higher
than that obtained with MPA or TAM alone at the same dosage.
Our observations on the effects of TAM and MPA on endometrial
adenocarcinomas in vivo are in complete agreement with the

above observations : DNA pol activity was not changed by MPA alone, whereas it was markedly decreased when TAM was added. This effect may be related to the increase of PR induced by TAM, but may also be related to an effect proper of the drug combination.

Several clinical trials have suggested that TAM might potentiate the response of endometrial cancer to progestin therapy (Bonte 1983; Mortel et al 1981). Further investigations are needed to establish the therapeutic merits of combined progestagen-TAM therapy, which may more or less critically depend upon the respective doses of drugs and their continuous or sequential mode of delivery.

ACKNOWLEDGEMENTS

We thank Dr. Pejovic for statistical analysis, F. Boussac, J.C. Lambert and L. Outin for the preparation of manuscript. This work was supported in part by Inserm grant n° PRC 119027.

REFERENCES

Bayard F, Damilano S, Robel P, Baulieu EE (1978). Cytoplasmic and nuclear estradiol and progesterone receptors in human endometrium. J Clin Endocrinol Metab 46:635.
Bertazzoni U, Scovassi A, Brun G (1977). Chick embryo DNA-polymerase α. Eur J Biochem 81:237.
Billiet G, DeHertogh R, Bonte J, Ide P, Vlaemynck G (1982). Estrogen receptors in human uterine adenocarcinoma. Correlation with tissue differentiation, vaginal karyopycnotic index, and effect of progestogen or antiestrogen treatment. Gynecol Oncol 14:33.
Binart N, Mester J, Baulieu EE, Catelli MG (1982). Combined effects of progesterone and tamoxifen in the chick oviduct. Endocrinology 111:7.
Bonte J (1983). Hormone dependency and hormone responsiveness of endometrial carcinoma to estrogens progestogens, and antiestrogens. In Campio L, Robustelli Della Cuna G, Taylor RW (eds): "Role of Medroxyprogesterone in Endocrine Related Tumors", Vol II, New York: Raven Press, p 141.
Bradford M (1976). A rapid assay for proteins determination. Anal Biochem 72:248.
Burton K (1968). Determination of DNA concentrations with diphenylamine. In Grossman L, Moldave K (eds): "Methods of Enzymology", Vol XIIB, New York: Academic Press, p. 163.

Catelli MG, Binart N, Elkik F, Baulieu EE (1980). Effect of tamoxifen on oestradiol and progesterone-induced synthesis of ovalbumin and conalbumin in chick oviduct. Eur J Biochem 107:165.

Erdos T, Bessada R (1979). The hydroxylapatite-column assay of estrogen receptors : the routine analyses of many samples and the calculation of the equilibrium association constant. J Ster Biochem 10:267.

Hechter O, Mechaber D, Zwick A, Campfield LA, Eychenne B, Baulieu EE, Robel P (1983). Optimal radioligand exchange conditions for measurement of occupied androgen receptor sites in rat ventral prostate. Arch Biochem Biophys 224: in press.

Iacobelli S, Sica G, Natoli C, Gatti D (1983). Inhibitory effects of medroxyprogesterone acetate on the proliferation of human breast cancer cells. In Campio L, Robustelli della Cuna G, Taylor RW (eds): "Role of Medroxyprogesterone in Endocrine-Related Tumors", Vol II, New York: Raven Press, p 1.

Jänne O, Kauppila A, Kontula K, Syrjälä P, Vierikko P, Vihko R (1980). Female sex steroid receptors in human endometrial hyperplasia and carcinoma. In Wittliff JL, Dapunt I (eds): "Steroid Receptors and Hormone Dependent Neoplasia", New York: Masson Publishing, p 37.

Jordan VC, Dix CJ (1978). Effect of estradiol benzoate, tamoxifen and monohydroxytamoxifen on immature rat uterine progesterone receptor synthesis and endometrial cell division. J Ster Biochem 11:285.

Kauppila A, Kajansuu E, Vihko R (1982). Cytosol estrogen and progestin receptors in endometrial carcinoma of patients treated with surgery, radiotherapy, and progestin. Cancer 50:2157.

Kohorn EI (1976). Gestagens and endometrial carcinoma. Gynecol Oncol 4:398.

Levy C, Robel P, Gautray JP, deBrux J, Verma U, Descomps B, Baulieu EE (1980). Estradiol and progesterone receptors in human endometrium : normal and abnormal menstrual cycles and early pregnancy. Am J Obstet Gynecol 136:646.

Lippman M, Bolan G, Huff K (1976). The effects of estrogens and antiestrogens on hormone responsive human breast cancer in long term tissue culture. Cancer Res 35:4595.

Milgrom E, Thi L, Atger M, Baulieu EE (1973). Mechanisms regulating the concentration and the conformation of progesterone receptor(s). J Biol Chem 248:6366.

Mortel R, Levy C, Wolff JP, Nicolas JC, Robel P, Baulieu EE
(1981). Female sex steroid receptors in post menopausal
endometrial carcinoma and biochemical response to an antiestrogen. Cancer Res 41:1140.
Reifenstein EC (1974). The treatment of advanced endometrial
cancer. Gynecol Oncol 2:377.
Robel P, Mortel R, Namer M, Baulieu EE (1983). Progesterone
receptor as an indicator of the response of post-menopausal
endometrial carcinoma and metastatic breast cancer to an
antiestrogen. In Bardin CW, Milgrom E, Mauvais-Jarvis P
(eds): "Progesterone and Progestins", New York: Raven
Press, p 367.
Satyaswaroop PG, Zaino RJ, Mortel R (1983). Human endometrial adenocarcinoma transplanted into nude mice : growth
regulation by estradiol. Science 219:58.
Searls DB (1980). An improved colorimetric assay for plasminogen activator. Anal Biochem 107:64.
Sutherland RL, Mester J, Baulieu EE (1977). Tamoxifen is a
potent "pure" antiestrogen in chick oviduct. Nature 267:
434.
Thorsen T (1982). Association of plasminogen activator activity and steroid receptors in human breast cancer. Eur J
Cancer Clin Oncol 18:129.
Tseng L, Gurpide E (1975). Effects of progestins on estradiol receptor levels in human endometrium. J Clin Endocrinol Metab 41:402.
Tseng L, Gusberg S, Gurpide E (1977). Estradiol receptor and
17-beta-dehydrogenase in normal and abnormal human endometrium. Ann NY Acad Sci 286:190.
Whitehead MI, Townsend PT, Pryse-Davies J, Ryder TA, King
RJB (1981). Effects of estrogens and progestins on the
biochemistry and morphology of the post-menopausal endometrium. New Engl J Med 305:1599.

Hormones and Cancer, pages 181–194
© 1984 Alan R. Liss, Inc., 150 Fifth Avenue, New York, NY 10011

GLUCOCORTICOID ACTIONS ON LYMPHOID TISSUE AND THE IMMUNE
SYSTEM: PHYSIOLOGIC AND THERAPEUTIC IMPLICATIONS

Paul M. Guyre
Jack E. Bodwell
Allan Munck

Department of Physiology
Dartmouth Medical School
Hanover, New Hampshire 03756

The   therapeutic   value   of   glucocorticoids   as
immunosuppresive agents and in treatment of lymphocytic
leukemias and lymphomas is widely recognized, but the
mechanisms by which the hormones exert beneficial effects
are not understood. An action of glucocorticoids that has
often been considered to underlie their effects on both
normal and neoplastic lymphoid tissues is the direct
killing of lymphocytes, a phenomenon that has been studied
for decades and that can be reproduced with isolated cells
and cell lines. Cell killing probably plays an important
role in glucocorticoid therapy of some lymphoid
malignancies (Munck, Crabtree 1981). We believe, however,
that the effects on normal lymphoid tissues, and on the
immune system in general, are far more subtle and
multifaceted, and may have much in common with a variety
of physiological actions of glucocorticoids which seem to
be unrelated.

GLUCOCORTICOID PHYSIOLOGY, PHARMACOLOGY, AND THE IMMUNE
SYSTEM

According to the traditional view of glucocorticoid
physiology, schematized in Fig. 1, we can regard these
hormones as exercising a number of direct, primary effects
on peripheral target cells (cells characterized, among
other things, by having glucocorticoid receptors); in

addition, they regulate their own concentrations in blood through negative feedback control of the production of CRF and ACTH. This control can be overidden through the central nervous system by "stress" which, in myriad forms, causes elevation of blood levels of glucocorticoids. The elevated levels are thought in some way to protect against stress.

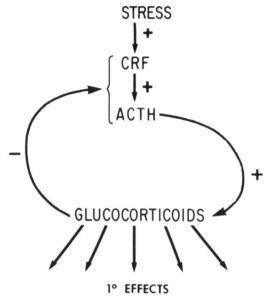

FIGURE 1. Traditional outline of glucocorticoid physiology

Prominent among peripheral effects are those on the immune system and the closely related antiinflammatory effects (Fahey et al. 1981). Perhaps because these effects are not evident under normal conditions, and because it is difficult to understand how they can protect against stress, endocrinologists have tended to relegate them to "pharmacological" status.

With regard to the immunosuppressive effects, what has become apparent during recent years is that many of them are indirect, and are due to inhibition by glucocorticoids of the production, and in some cases the actions, of a wide range of "lymphokines". These are substances - proteins or peptides in those cases where they have been characterized - that communicate between cells of the immune system, carrying messages that stimulate cells to proliferate, to differentiate, to manifest certain activities, etc. In many respects lymphokines resemble peptide hormones; as far as is known, for example, they act through high affinity receptors on the membranes of their target cells.

Glucocorticoids block the production of two important lymphokines, Interkeukin I and Interleukin II, also known respectively as lymphocyte activating factor (LAF) and T-cell growth factor (Gillis et al., 1979; Snyder, Unanue, 1982). These effects go a long way towards explaining why glucocorticoids are so effective in suppressing primary immune responses (Crabtree et al. 1980).

Another lymphokine of potentially great importance for glucocorticoid physiology and pharmacology is immune or gamma interferon, a product of antigenically stimulated T-cells. As we will show, one of the pleiotropic actions of immune interferon is to activate macrophages to express more receptors for IgG (Fc receptors). Glucocorticoids block the production but not the actions of immune interferon that we discuss here.

Functions of Macrophage Fc Receptors

Mononuclear phagocytes (monocytes and macrophages) have surface receptors which specifically bind the Fc portion of immunoglobulin G (IgG), and which are therefore called Fc receptors (FcR). (Unkeless et al. 1978). These receptors are important for recognition by the macrophage of particulate antigens which have been "antibody tagged" or opsonized. FcR are thus involved in the clearance by the reticuloendothelial system of immune complexes, bacterial pathogens, and, during the course of autoimmune disease, of antibody-tagged host cells (Fig. 2). FcR also appear to guide mononuclear phagocytes in the destruction of tumor cells (Shaw et al., 1978), in stimulation of immunoglobulin production (Morgan, Weigle 1981), and in the release of inflammatory mediators (Passwell et al. 1980). Griffin et al. (1975) have shown that, during phagocytosis, the macrophage membrane appears to "zipper" around the opsonized particle, guided by the binding of FcR to IgG (Fig. 3). It is reasonable, therefore, to suppose that the densities of both particle-bound IgG and of membrane FcR are important for this process.

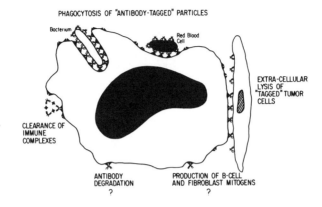

FIGURE 2. Fc receptor mediated functions on mononuclear phagocytes (Guyre, _et al_. 1982).

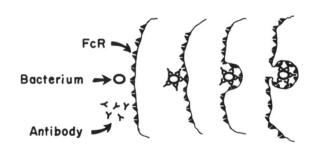

FIGURE 3. Interaction of IgG with Fc receptors during phagocytosis. (Griffin _et al_. 1975).

Augmentation of FcR By Immune Interferon

The FcR of human monocytes and of the human leukocyte cell lines HL-60 and U-937 have been widely studied (Crabtree, 1980; Anderson, Abraham 1980; Kurlander, Batker 1982; Fleit _et al_. 1982). In our own work we have measured FcR on these cells using binding of radiolabelled IgG, and more recently by flow cytometry using binding of fluorescein-labelled IgG.

Some years ago we found that a lymphokine activity produced by activated human lymphocytes causes a pronounced increase in the number of FcR on all three cell types mentioned (Guyre et al. 1981b). We referred to this lymphokine as FcR augmenting factor or FRAF. The increase in FcR induced by FRAF was maximal at about 48 h and was blocked by inhibitors of protein and RNA synthesis. Fig. 4 shows a Scatchard plot which demonstrates that the increased ^{125}I-IgG-binding was due to increased numbers of Fc receptors, and that the binding affinity remained about the same. Larrick et al. (1980) showed that similar lymphokine preparations increased FcR-dependent functions of the U-937 cell line.

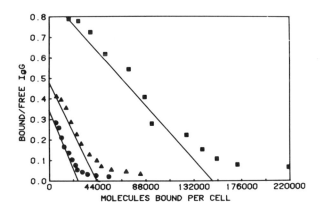

FIGURE 4. Scatchard analysis of ^{125}I-IgG binding to U-937 cells cultured for 40 h with 0% (●), 1% (▲) and 10% (■) FRAF. (Guyre, et al. 1981b).

Recently we have shown that immune interferon has the same effects as FRAF, and is probably the major active moiety which we detected in various crude lymphokine preparations. Fig. 5 shows the analysis by flow cytometry of human monocytes which were cultured for 40 h with and without 100 antiviral units per ml of immune interferon. The lymphocytes and monocytes were discriminated by correlated forward and right angle light scatter, and the fluorescence due to the binding of fluoresceinated IgG to monocytes only was measured. Fig 5B shows that immune interferon caused the number of FcR to increase 9-fold compared with controls (Fig. 5A), while the non-saturable binding was unaltered (Fig. 5 C,D).

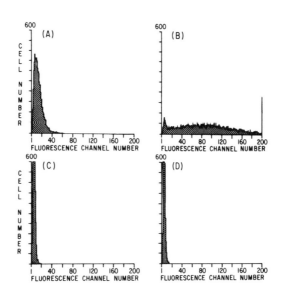

FIGURE 5. Immune-Interferon augmentation of human monocyte FcR. 1 x 10⁷ monocytes were cultured for 48 h in 120-ml teflon vessels (Scientific Specialties, Randallstown, MD) in 10 ml of RPMI 1640 plus 5 x 10⁻⁵ M 2-mercaptoethanol plus 10% autologous serum with (B and D) or without (A and C) 10 U/ml recombinant immune-interferon. FITC-IgG binding was assayed by flow cytometry as described. FcR increased from a mean of 18,000 sites/cell for control cultures (A) to 162,000 sites/cell following interferon treatment (B). Nonsaturable binding of the fluorescent IgG was identical for both treatments (C and D).

Fig. 6 shows the relationship between immune interferon concentration and FcR augmentation for U-937 cells. HL-60 and human monocytes gave identical responses. This figure also demonstrates the very low relative activities of alpha- and beta-interferons.

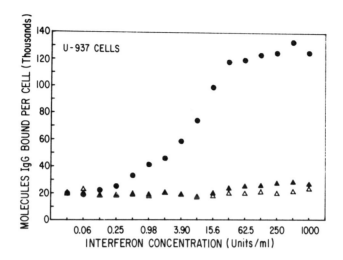

FIGURE 6. Concentration dependence of Fc receptor augmentation . 2.5 x 10⁵ U-937 cells/well were cultured for 16 h in 200 μl complete medium in 96-well microtiter trays (Costar, Data Packaging, Cambridge, MA). After incubation with interferons, cells were labeled with ^{125}I-IgG1 and the average number of IgG molecules bound per cell was determined. Figure 6 shows the response to α-(▲), β-(△), and γ-(●) interferon for U-937 cells.

Effects of Glucocorticoids on Immune Interferon and Fc Receptors

Atkinson and Frank (1974) were the first to suggest that the beneficial action of glucocorticoids in autoimmune hemolytic anemia involved a reduction of FcR-mediated clearance of the opsonized erythrocytes by the mononuclear phagocyte system. Crabtree et al. (1979) supported this hypothesis by showing that treatment of the HL-60 cell line with glucocorticoids in vitro resulted in a 30 - 50% reduction of plasma membrane FcR sites.

With normal human monocytes, however, while we have occasionally found a similar reduction of FcR following culture with glucocorticoids, we more commonly find no change. Kurlander (1981) has reported similar results. Direct effects of glucocorticoids on human monocyte Fc receptors may thus be either minor or non-existent.

Since immune interferon dramatically increases FcR sites, and is probably produced by T-lymphocytes during a normal immune response (Nathan et al. 1981), it is important to know whether glucocorticoids influence either its production or action. We have previously shown that glucocorticoids completely block the production of FRAF, which we now know to consist largely, if not entirely of immune interferon. Fig 7 shows the relationship between dexamethasone concentration and inhibition of FRAF production (Guyre et al 1981a). This effect is specific for glucocorticoids.

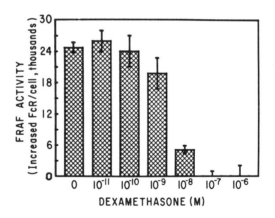

FIGURE 7. Effect of dexamethasone on FRAF production. Dexamethasone was added at the start of FRAF production to yield the final concentrations shown. FRAF supernatants (1% v/v) were tested in the FRAF assay. Results are the mean of triplicate FcR determinations per treatment, assayed as in Fig. 1.

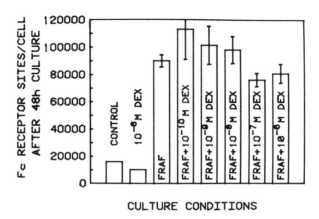

FIGURE 8. Glucocorticoid effect on FRAF action on HL-60 cells. Triplicate cultures of HL-60 cells containing 5% FRAF supernatant (v/v) and/or the indicated concentration of dexamethasone was incubated for 48 h. FcR sites/cell were determined as in Fig. 1, and are given as the mean ±SD.

Fig. 8 shows that in HL-60 cells glucocorticoids only slightly reduced the ability of FRAF to increase FcR. We have since shown that glucocorticoids similarly inhibit only slightly the augmentation of FcR and related functions induced by pure recombinant immune interferon.

Thus we conclude that as with TCGF, glucocorticoids inhibit the production, but not the action on FcR, of immune interferon. It should be noted the dose-response relations in Fig. 7 cover a range of dexamethasone concentrations that are equivalent to physiological concentrations of cortisol and corticosterone (under culture conditions the activities of dexamethasone and the natural glucocorticoids rarely differ by a factor of more than 10 or 20). Thus we can conclude that if these effects occur <u>in vivo</u> they do not require "pharmaco-logical" doses of glucocorticoids, but are likely to vary in intensity as glucocorticoid concentrations vary over their normal physiological range. In particular, the effects are likely to reach maximal levels (i.e. total suppression of lymphokine production) at concentrations of glucocorticoids achieved in stress, or under therapy.

GENERALIZED VIEW OF GLUCOCORTICOID PHYSIOLOGY: RELATION TO THERAPY AND STRESS

In addition to the examples given one could cite several other instances of inhibition (occasionally stimulation) of lymphokine production or action by glucocorticoids at physiological concentrations. We begin to perceive, therefore, a range of potential influences of the glucocorticoids that extends far beyond their primary target cells. These influences are carried by a secondary network of intercellular messengers exemplified by the lymphokines, but to which we can certainly add the prostaglandins and other hormone-like substances known to be under glucocorticoid control (c.f. Fahey et al. 1981). An outline of these ideas is shown in Figure 9, where lymphokines are symbolized by L_1, L_2 and prostaglandins and related compounds by PGs.

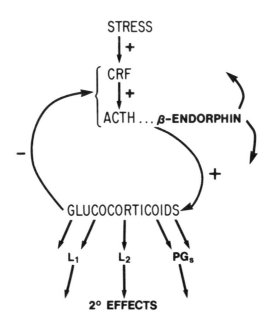

FIGURE 9. Proposed broader modern outline of glucocorticoid physiology.

Formally there is a similarity between the inhibitory influences exercised by the glucocorticoids peripherally over the lymphokines, and the classical inhibitory actions of glucocorticoids on CRF and ACTH. The latter "central" actions have been thought of until recently as exclusively part of the negative feed-back control system for glucocorticoids, quite separate from the peripheral actions. More and more, however, particularly after the discovery of the close link at the genomic level between ACTH and biologically active neuropeptides such as beta-endorphin (Nakanishi et al. 1979), the functions of these central and peripheral actions can be seen to overlap.

As we have discussed previously (Guyre et al. 1982), there are immediate therapeutic implications to the scheme in Figure 9. To the extent that some of the unwanted side-effects of glucocorticoid therapy - such as the increased susceptibility to infection - are due to inhibition of production of a particular lymphokine, it might be possible to selectively overcome that side-effect by administering the lymphokine along with the glucocorticoid. Now that pure lymphokines are being synthesized in large amounts through recombinant techniques, there may soon be opportunities to test such possibilities.

On a different plane, we have begun to consider what significance these widespread inhibitory effects of glucocorticoids on hormone-like intercellular messengers may have for the physiological functions of glucocorticoids in stress. Since the 1930's the accepted view has been that the function of stress-induced increases in glucocorticoid levels is to protect against stress. When, however, we look at lymphokines, prostaglandins, and many other substances, the production of which is inhibited by glucocorticoids, including ADH and even insulin, we discover that all these substances are components of basic physiological mechanisms designed to protect the organism against particular forms of stress - infection, tissue damage, hemorrhage, metabolic disturbances, pain, and so on. We are therefore faced with the paradox that rather than enhance normal defence mechanisms, glucocorticoids suppress them.

Our solution of this paradox is to suggest that, contrary to the traditional view, the real function of glucocorticoids in stress is to protect us not against stress itself, but against our normal reactions to stress, preventing those reactions from overshooting and causing damage. In relation to immunosuppressive and antiinflammatory effects the germ of such an idea is already to be found in the writings of Selye (1976), and more explicitely, in the work of Besedovsky and Sorkin (1977). What we propose is that this mechanism may explain a much wider spectrum of glucocorticoid actions involved in the response to stress.

ACKNOWLEDGEMENTS

The research of the authors has been supported by PHS Grant AM 03535, by PHS Grant CA17323 awarded by the National Cancer Institute, DHHS, by a grant from the Kroc Foundation and by the Core Grant CA23108 of the Norris Cotton Cancer Center.

REFERENCES

Anderson LL, Abraham GN (1980), Characterization of the Fc Receptor for IgG on a Human Macrophage Cell Line, U937. J Immunol 125:2735.

Atkinson JP, Frank MM (1974). Complement-Independent Clearance of IgG-Sensitized Erythrocytes: Inhibition by Cortisone. Blood 44:629

Besedovsky H, Sorkin E (1977) Network of immune-neuroendocrine interactions. Clin Exp Immunol 27:1

Crabtree GR (1980). Fc receptors of a human promyelocytic leukemic cell line: evidence for two types of receptors defined by binding of the staphylococcal protein A-IgG1 complex. J Immunol 125:448.

Crabtree GR, Gillis S, Smith KA, Munck A (1980). Mechanisms of glucocorticoid-induced immunosuppression: inhibitory effects on expression of Fc receptors and production of T-cell growth factor. J Steroid Biochem 12:445

Crabtree GR, Munck A, Smith KA (1979). Glucocorticoids inhibit expression of Fc receptors on the human granulocytic cell line HL-60. Nature 279:338

Fahey JF, Guyre PM, Munck A (1981). Mechanisms of anti-inflammatory actions of glucocorticoids. Adv. Inflammation Res 2:21.

Fleit HB, Wright SD, Unkeless JC (1982). Human neutrophil Fc receptor distribution and structure. Proc Natl Acad Sci USA 79:3275

Gillis S, Crabtree GR, Smith KA (1979). Glucocorticoid-induced inhibition of T-cell growth factor production – I. The effect on mitogen-induced lymphocyte proliferation. J Immunol 123:1624.

Griffin FJ, Griffin JA, Leider JE, Silverstein SC (1975). Studies on the mechanism of phagocytosis I. Requirements for circumferential attachement of particle-bound ligands to specific receptors on the macrophage plasma membrane. J Exp Med 142:1263.

Guyre PM, Bodwell J, Holbrook NJ, Jeffries M, Munck A (1982). Glucocorticoids and the immune system: activation of glucocorticoid-receptor complexes in thymus cells; modulation of Fc-receptors of phagocytic cells. In Lee HJ, Walker CA (eds): "Progress in Research and Clinical Applications of Corticosteroids, Philadelphia, Heyden and Sons, Inc., p. 14.

Guyre PM, Bodwell JE, Munck A (1981a). Glucocorticoid actions on the immune system: inhibition of production of an Fc-receptor augmenting factor. J Steroid Biochem 15:35.

Guyre PM, Crabtree GR, Bodwell JE, Munck A (1981b). MLC-conditioned media stimulate an increase in Fc receptors on human macrophages. J Immunol 126:666.

Guyre PM, Morganelli PM, Miller R (1983). Recombinant immune interferon increases immunoglobulin G Fc receptors on cultured human mononuclear phagocytes. J Clin Invest, in press.

Kurlander RJ (1981). The effects of corticosteroids on IgG Fc receptor and complement receptor-mediated interaction of monocytes with red cells. Clin Immunol Immunopathol 20:325.

Kurlander RJ, Batker J (1982). The binding of human immunoglobulin G1 monomer and small, covalently cross-linked polymers of immunoglobulin G1 to human peripheral blood monocytes and polymorphonuclear leukocytes. J Clin Invest 69:1.

Larrick JW, Fischer DG, Anderson SJ, Koren HS (1980). Characterization of a human macrophage-like cell line stimulated in vitro: a model of macrophage functions. J Immunol 125:6.

Morgan EL, Weigle WO (1981). Regulation of the immune response: III. The role of macrophages in the potentiation of the immune response by Fc fragments. J Immunol. 126:1302.

Munck A, Crabtree GR (1981). Glucocorticoid-induced lymphocyte death. In Bowen ID, Lockshin RA (eds): "Cell Death in Biology and Pathology", London: Chapman and Hall, p. 329.

Nakanishi S, Inoue A, Kita T, Nakamura M, Chang ACY, Cohen SN, Numa S (1979). Nucleotide Sequence of Cloned cDNA for Bovine Corticotropin-B-Lipotropin Precursor. Nature 278:423.

Nathan I, Groopman JE, Quan SG, Bersch N, Golde DW (1981). Immune interferon produced by a human T-lymphoblast cell line. Nature 292:842.

Passwell J, Rosen FS, Merler E (1980). The effect of Fc fragments of IgG on human mononuclear cell responses. Cell Immunol 52:395

Selye H (1976). "Stress in Health and Disease". London: Butterworth, p. 1119

Shaw GM, Levy PC, Lo Buglio AF (1978). Human monocyte cytotoxicity to tumor cells. I. Antibody-dependent cytotoxicity. J Immunol 121:573.

Snyder DS, Unanue ER (1982). Corticosteroids inhibit murine macrophage Ia expression and interleukin 1 production. J Immunol. 129:1803.

Unkeless JC, Fleit H, Mellman IS (1981). Structural aspects and heterogeneity of immunoglobulin Fc receptors. Adv Immunol 31:247.

Hormones and Cancer, pages 195–206

CHARACTERISTICS, STABILITY AND REGULATION OF GLUCOCORTICOID-RECEPTOR COMPLEXES IN NORMAL AND NEOPLASTIC CELLS AS STUDIED WITH A NEW MINI-COLUMN TECHNIQUE

Nikki J. Holbrook
Clara D.Bloomfield
Allan Munck

Department of Physiology (NJH and AM), Dartmouth Medical School, Hanover, NH 03755, and Section of Medical Oncology (CDB), Department of Medicine, University of Minnesota, Minneapolis, MN.

Most if not all physiologic and pharmacologic actions of the glucocorticoids are initiated through glucocorticoid receptors, protein molecules that the hormone encounters after traversing the cell membrane, and with which it initially forms complexes that are found in the cytosol after cell disruption. Whether these cytosolic complexes are in the cytoplasm or in the nucleus, or in both, has not been demonstrated unequivocally. Through a poorly understood process that we are currently studying in lymphoid cells, the cytosolic complexes become "activated", giving rise to complexes with affinity for DNA that are rapidly bound to the nucleus. Much indirect and some direct evidence indicates that the nuclear-bound complexes stimulate formation of mRNAs for particular effector proteins that are then responsible for the effects of the hormones in the cell.

As a prelude to more detailed studies of glucocorticoid-receptor complexes in normal and neoplastic tissues, we have characterized by standard physicochemical procedures the nonactivated and activated cytosolic complexes formed in rat thymus cells (Holbrook et al. 1983b). For this purpose we have made use of the remarkable stabilizing powers of molybdate (Nielsen et al. 1977, Sherman et al. 1982), which slows degradation and blocks activation of steroid hormone receptor complexes in cell-free systems.

Our principal conclusions from these studies are: (i) in cells at 37°C, the cytosolic complexes consist mainly of a nonactivated and an activated species, with perhaps traces of mero-receptor complex; (ii) in agreement with Sherman et al. (1982), the nonactivated complex has an apparent molecular weight of around 330,000; (iii) activation is accompanied by a reduction to about 100,000. This reduction in size may represent a dissociation of an oligomeric molecule - perhaps a tetramer - into monomers, as suggested recently by Raaka and Samuels (1983) and Vedeckis (1983).

By taking advantage of certain properties of the complexes found in cytosols, we have developed a mini-column method by which nonactivated, activated and mero-receptor complexes can be separated rapidly (Holbrook et al. 1983b). Three small columns in 1-ml plastic syringes are connected in series. The top one consists of DNA-cellulose, the next of DEAE-cellulose, and the bottom one of hydroxylapatite (HAP). When a cytosol is passed through the columns, activated complexes are retained with high efficiency by the DNA column, nonactivated complexes by the DEAE column, and mero-receptor and other complexes that do not bind to DNA or DEAE are retained on the HAP column. Each column bed is then assayed for radioactivity as a single sample.

The rapidity of the mini-column separation procedure (5-10 min, compared to hours by conventional methods) drastically diminishes the time during which degradation of complexes can take place. Furthermore, since the columns can be prepared and run simultaneously in large numbers, they afford the opportunity for experiments requiring analysis of many samples. Here we describe the results of a series of experiments designed to determine the stability of glucocorticoid-receptor complexes from various sources under several conditions. In addition, we illustrate the versatility of the technique by showing how a "reversed mini-column", with DEAE on top and DNA in the middle, can be used to separate complexes that bind to DNA but not to DEAE.

METHODS

The methods used throughout for preparing and incubating rat and chick thymus, chick bursa and human cells, and for mini-column analysis, are essentially those described in Holbrook et al. (1983a,b). Reversed mini-columns are prepared and used just as regular mini-columns, except that DEAE-cellulose is in the top syringe and DNA-cellulose in the middle syringe. Spleen cells were dispersed in the same way as thymus cells; the red blood cells in the preparation were lysed by incubation in 0.86% ammonium chloride at 0°C for 5 min., and then the remaining cells were washed and incubated in Krebs-Ringer bicarbonate buffer with 10mM glucose (KRBg). Cell lines were grown in RPMI 1640 with 10% fetal bovine serum. Before incubation with steroid they were washed with RPMI 1640 and left for 30 min at 37°C. All reagents were prepared fresh before each experiment, in Tris buffer at ten times the final concentrations used.

Glucocorticoid-receptor complexes were in all cases formed initially by incubating intact cells with approximately 30nM [^{3}H]triamcinolone acetonide ([^{3}H]TA) for about 2 h at 0°C, a procedure that yields mainly nonactivated complexes. Cells were lysed at 0°C in 1.5 mM $MgCl_2$ containing dextran-coated charcoal, and the broken-cell suspension was centrifuged to give the cytosols used for the experiments described. Cell-free activation was accomplished by warming cytosols to 25°C for 15 min.

RESULTS AND DISCUSSION

Stability of glucocorticoid-receptor complexes in cytosols from normal and neoplastic cells before and after cell-free activation.

TABLE 1. Stability of glucocorticoid-receptor complexes in cytosols of various normal and neoplastic cell types during and after cell-free activation. Numbers in parentheses indicate the number of samples tested. For other tissues, values are those of a representative experiment. PBL, peripheral blood leukocytes; PMN, polymorphonuclear cells; CLL, chronic lymphocytic leukemia; ANLL, acute non-lymphocytic leukemia.

| | PERCENT OF TOTAL COMPLEXES BOUND | | | | | | | | |
| Tissue | Before warming to 25°C | | | After warming to 25°C | | | After an additional 24h at 0°C | | |
	DNA	DEAE	HAP	DNA	DEAE	HAP	DNA	DEAE	HAP
Normal									
Rat thymus	1.7	94.8	4.2	70.8	14.5	14.7	5.8	12.0	82.0
Rat spleen	2.0	96.7	1.3	66.3	25.7	7.9	44.2	38.3	17.4
Chick thymus	4.2	93.9	1.9	56.0	25.0	18.9	4.3	20.1	75.8
Chick bursa	14.7	83.6	1.6	68.5	22.8	8.7	6.3	20.7	73.0
Human PBL(5)	4.2	90.6	5.1	55.0	29.5	15.4	–	–	–
Human PMN(3)	7.6	72.1	20.3	5.7	13.0	81.2	–	–	–
Leukemic Specimens									
Human CLL(9)	4.2	90.6	5.1	55.0	29.5	15.4	–	–	–
ANLL(15)	6.3	78.7	15.2	30.9	17.2	51.6	–	–	–
Cell Lines									
WEHI-7 mouse thymoma	9.7	87.2	3.0	63.0	30.9	5.3	61.1	33.1	5.8
K562 human erythro-leukemia	2.8	88.1	9.1	58.9	34.6	6.6	–	–	–
U937 human myelo-monocytic	5.5	79.1	15.4	58.5	28.5	13.0	–	–	–
HL60 human myelo-monocytic	7.6	79.1	12.8	65.4	23.7	10.9	–	–	–

In Table 1 we present results obtained with a variety of cell types. Complexes were formed by incubating the cells with [^{3}H]TA at 0°C for 2 h. The cells were then broken, and the resulting cytosols, which contained no molybdate, were immediately analyzed with mini-columns to give the results in the first three columns of numbers. DNA represents activated complexes, DEAE represents nonactivated complexes, and HAP represents mainly mero-receptor, along with other complexes that do not bind to DNA or DEAE. All these cytosols, as expected, contained predominately nonactivated complexes, which generally accounted for more than 80% of the total.

Aliquots of the same cytosols were warmed to 25°C for 15 min (cell-free activation), cooled, and analyzed again. This procedure causes negligible dissociation of [^{3}H]TA, so any changes observed can be ascribed to interconversion of complexes. The results are in the next three columns. All these cytosols had low levels of nonactivated complexes; most of them had over 50% activated complexes and less than 20% mero-receptor. The two clear exceptions were normal human PMNs and cells from ANLL patients. These cells, of similar lineage, apparently have high levels of enzymes that degrade receptors. Although the averages in Table 1 for preparations from ANLL cells suggest they are more stable than those from PMNs, the ANLL cytosols are highly variable from patient to patient; some are even more labile than those from PMNs and others are quite stable.

We should emphasize that none of our evidence, from these or other studies, suggests that the receptors from these two cell types have intrinsic defects that make them especially labile. In fact, as we show later, in certain circumstances the complexes formed by ANLL cells can be activated normally. It should also be noted that cytosols from the corresponding myelomonocytic cell lines, U937 and HL60, give normal activation, as do cytosols from cells of CLL patients.

In some cases, aliquots of the cytosols that had been warmed were left for an additional 24h at 0°C and analyzed again. These results are shown in the last three columns. The main points to note here are the lability of the preparations from all the normal cells tested except rat spleen cells, and the exceptional stability of the WEHI-7 preparation, which remained unchanged over the 24h.

Effects of various agents on stability of glucocorticoid-receptor complexes in rat thymus cytosols.

The experiments in Table 2 were performed in a similar way to those just described for Table 1, except that rat thymus cytosols were used throughout, and various reagents were added to the cytosols either before (Expts. 2,3,4) or after (Expt. 1) the 25°C activation step. The condition of the cytosols before warming can be assumed to be the same as for the rat thymus preparation in Table 1. The first set of results in Table 2 is from analyses performed immediately after warming, and the last three columns are from analyses after 8h at 0°C.

Experiment 1 illustrates how the well-known stabilizing influences of leupeptin and molybdate (Sherman et al. 1982) can be monitored with the mini-column procedure. The decrease in mero-receptor formation after 8h is particularly pronounced with leupeptin. Experiment 2 shows that the various protease inhibitors tested, here added before warming, do not block activation; we have also obtained this result with other inhibitors (Holbrook et al. 1983b). Furthermore, leupeptin and antipain can both be seen to prevent mero-receptor formation after 8h.

Experiment 3 shows that ATP, ADP and PPi apparently enhance activation, as measured simply by DNA binding. As will be seen later, PPi activates even without warming. These compounds have a remarkable ability to decrease mero-receptor formation. We return to these observations below. Finally, Experiment 4 shows that EDTA does not influence activation, but in these cytosols drastically reduces formation of mero-receptor.

Reversed mini-columns for detection of complexes that bind to DNA but not to DEAE.

From other experiments (Holbrook, Bodwell, Munck, unpublished) we have become aware that the enhanced DNA binding observed in Table 2 with ATP, ADP and PPi is not due to increased levels in the cytosols of the normal activated complex, which is characterized by a Stokes radius of 5-6 nm and binds to both DNA and DEAE (Holbrook et al. 1983b), but to the appearance of a complex with Stokes radius around 3 nm that binds to DNA but not to DEAE. We believe this complex is an intermediate in the

TABLE 2. Stability of rat thymus cytosolic glucocorticoid-receptor complexes in the presence of various reagents. Cytosols containing [³H]TA-receptor complexes were warmed to 25°C for 15 min either prior to (Exp. 1) or after (Exps. 2-4) treatment with the indicated reagents. Samples were then analyzed on the mini-columns immediately (Initial) and after an additional 8 h incubation at 0°C. PPi, sodium pyrophosphate.

Exp.	Cytosol treatment	Percent of total bound complexes					
		Initial			After 8 h at 0°C		
		DNA	DEAE	HAP	DNA	DEAE	HAP
1	none	66.6	18.6	14.8	34.5	11.6	53.9
	20 mM molybdate	76.9	14.1	9.0	42.7	21.9	35.4
	5 mM leupeptin	65.2	18.8	16.0	73.6	13.3	13.2
	20 mM molybdate + 5 mM leupeptin	75.4	14.6	10.2	79.8	10.8	9.4
2	none	66.6	24.9	8.5	30.0	24.0	45.9
	5 mM leupeptin	61.0	31.1	7.9	55.5	34.0	10.2
	2 mM antipain	68.3	26.4	5.3	61.2	29.3	9.6
	2 mM phosphoramidin	62.9	25.4	11.7	36.0	19.2	44.9
3	none	77.2	13.1	9.7	52.6	6.8	41.0
	10 mM ATP	90.6	4.7	4.7	90.5	5.4	4.1
	10 mM ADP	87.7	6.6	5.7	90.1	5.2	4.7
	10 mM AMP	80.5	11.6	7.8	62.8	6.5	30.7
	10 mM PPi	91.4	4.3	4.4	89.9	6.3	3.8
4	none	60.7	19.5	19.8	28.5	12.2	59.3
	4 mM EDTA	59.0	31.0	10.0	64.9	26.1	9.0

proteolytic conversion of the normal activated complex to
mero-receptor, and that the pyrophosphoryl compounds block
its further degradation.

To assay for this complex rapidly we have used
reversed mini-columns. When a cytosol is passed through
these columns the normal nonactivated and activated
complexes bind to the DEAE-cellulose, which is on top, and
only the 3 nm complex binds to the DNA cellulose. Thus, if
a cytosol is assayed by the standard and the reversed
mini-columns, in the standard mini-column DNA binding
measures the sum of normal activated and 3 nm complexes,
while DEAE binding measures only nonactivated complex;
whereas in the reversed mini-column DNA binding measures
only 3 nm complex, while DEAE binding measures the sum of
normal activated and nonactivated complexes.

TABLE 3. Generation and detection of non-DEAE binding,
DNA-binding glucocorticoid-receptor complexes in rat
thymus cytosols in the presence of 10 mM PPi. Cytosols
were treated with 10mM PPi and left at 0°C for the
indicated times before analysis on the mini-columns.
Numbers in parentheses indicate the percent of total
DNA-binding complexes (determined by the standard mini-
columns) which do not bind to DEAE (determined by the
reversed minicolumns)

| Hours treatment with PPi | Percent of total bound complexes | | | | | |
| | Standard mini-columns | | | Reversed mini-columns | | |
	DNA	DEAE	HAP	DEAE	DNA	HAP
0	3.1	88.5	8.4	98.0	0.7	1.3
2	63.3	27.9	8.8	62.5	29.3 (50)	8.2
6	80.1	10.2	9.0	39.6	47.1 (60)	13.3
24	76.5	6.1	18.0	32.6	50.6 (66)	16.8

Table 3 shows how treatment of a rat thymus cytosol
at 0°C with 10 mM PPi affects the distribution of these
complexes as a function of time up to 24h. Within 2h, 63%

of total complexes are in DNA-binding form, but half of these are 3 nm complexes. By 24h about 80% bind to DNA, and two thirds are in the 3 nm form. Even by 24h there is little formation of mero-receptor. Thus, by using both the standard and the reversed mini-columns we are able to gain insight into the mechanisms of these transformations.

A moral to be drawn from these results is that what binds to DNA (and presumably nuclei) is not just the normal activated complex. That is important to keep in mind, particularly when activation is studied under cell-free conditions.

Receptor-stabilizing factor in CLL cells.

The results in Table 1 showed that complexes in cytosols from cells of ANLL patients are degraded to mero-receptors much faster than those from CLL patients. The usual interpretation of this kind of result is that ANLL cells contain high levels of receptor-degrading enzymes, and CLL cells contain low levels. To test this interpretation we conducted the mixing experiments shown in Table 4. The two types of cells, one labelled with [^{3}H]TA, and the other treated with the same concentrations of TA to control for any possible hormone effects, were mixed and then broken to yield a mixed cytosol. The cytosol was analyzed with mini-columns before and after warming to 25°C. The first two mixtures in Table 4 are controls. They show that, as in Table 1, warming to 25°C causes much more mero-receptor formation with cytosols from ANLL cells than from CLL cells.

The third and fourth mixtures are designed to test the standard interpretation, according to which the presence of cytosol from ANLL cells in both these sytems should cause the [^{3}H]TA-labelled receptors to be degraded to mero-receptor. In neither case, however, does this happen; the preparations appear to be as stable as those from CLL cells.

Our conclusion from these results, supported by a number of other experiments, is that CLL cells contain a stablizing factor which can protect receptors in any cytosol to which it is added. The WEHI-7 cells, shown in Table 1 to give very stable preparations, also turn out to contain a stabilizing factor.

TABLE 4. Distribution of [^{3}H]TA-receptor complexes in cytosols from mixed ANLL and CLL cell preparations before (0°) and after (25°) cell-free activation. Cells from ANLL and CLL patients were incubated separately with approximately 30nM TA or [^{3}H]TA for 2h at 0°C. Equal volumes of the cell suspensions were mixed at 0°C and the cells lysed. The resulting cytosols were analyzed immediately and after activation by warming 15 min at 25°C.

Cell mixture	Treatment	Percent of total receptor-bound cpm retained on column		
		DNA	DEAE	HAP
[^{3}H]TA-ANLL + TA-ANLL	0°	4	77	19
	25°	15	10	75
[^{3}H]TA-CLL + TA-CLL	0°	4	85	11
	25°	54	26	20
[^{3}H]TA-CLL + TA-ANLL	0°	6	76	18
	25°	55	21	24
[^{3}H]TA-ANLL + TA-CLL	0°	3	82	15
	25°	59	18	23

An incidental but important observation from Table 4 is that whereas in the first mixture the ANLL control cytosol produced only slight amounts of activated complexes on warming (as was also the case in Table 1), in the fourth mixture, where the CLL stabilizing factor is present, [^{3}H]TA-labelled receptors from ANLL cells undergo normal activation, giving a distribution of complexes indistinguishable from that of cells with stable cytosols. That is one of the main reasons we think that, despite evidence to the contrary (McCaffrey et al., 1982), the receptors in ANLL cells are normal.

Kinetics of glucocorticoid-receptor complexes in rat thymus cells at 37°C.

By using mini-columns we have been able to refine our earlier studies on rapid kinetics of glucocorticoid-receptor complexes (Wira and Munck, 1974; Munck and Foley, 1980). The mini-columns have made it possible, for example, to do a full time-course of association of [³H]TA at 37°C in a single experiment, with sampling at intervals of seconds or minutes and analyses of nonactivated, activated and nuclear complexes for every time point.

We have also developed a simple mathematical model of receptor kinetics that is in remarkably good agreement with these and other experimental results. The model has its origins in the energy dependent cycle, involving possible phosphorylation-dephosphorylation reactions, that we postulated to account for the apparent dependence of receptor binding on ATP (Munck et al. 1972). It is also a cyclic model, and assumes activation to be irreversible.

The behaviour of each steroid in the model is determined by its dissociation rate constant. Although no steroid-specific control of activation is assumed, the model predicts the different steady-state ratios of activated to non-activated complexes that we have found experimentally with different steroids (Munck and Foley, 1980). In addition, the model implies that steroids with high dissociation rate constants will behave as glucocorticoid antagonists. This model, therefore, provides explanations for hitherto puzzling observations, as well as independent support for the validity of a cyclic model.

ACKNOWLEDGEMENTS

This work was supported in part by Public Health Service Grants CA17323, AM03535 and CA26273, by ACS Grant

CA-167 and by the Core Grant (CA23108) of the Norris Cotton Cancer Center. N.J.H. was a recipient of National Research Service Award CA09367 and currently holds a Fellowship Award from the Leukemia Society of America.

REFERENCES

Holbrook NJ, Bloomfield CD, Munck A (1983a). Analysis of activated and nonactivated cytoplasmic glucocorticoid-receptor complexes from human leukemia cells by rapid DNA-DEAE mini-column chromatography. Cancer Res in press.
Holbrook NJ, Bodwell JE, Jeffries M, Munck A (1983b). Characterization of nonactivated and activated gluco-corticoid-receptor complexes from intact rat thymus cells. J Biol Chem 258:6477.
McCaffrey R, Lillquist A, Bell R (1982). Abnormal glucocorticoid receptors in acute leukemia cells. Blood 59:393.
Munck A, Foley R (1980). Activated and non-activated glucocorticoid receptor complexes in rat thymus cells:kinetics of formation and relation to steroid structure. J Steroid Biochem 12:225.
Munck A, Wira C, Young DA, Mosher KM, Hallahan C, Bell PA (1972). Glucocorticoid-receptor complexes and the earliest steps in the action of glucocorticoids on thymus cells. J Steroid Biochem 3:567.
Nielsen CJ, Sando JJ, Vogel WM, Pratt WB (1977). Glucocorticoid receptor inactivation under cell-free conditions. J Biol Chem 252:7568.
Raaka BM, Samuels HH (1983). The glucocorticoid receptor in GH_1 cells. J Biol Chem 258:417.
Sherman MR, Moran MC, Neal RM, Niu E-M, Tuazon FB (1982). Characterization of molybdate-stabilized glucocorticoid receptors in healthy and malignant tissues. In Lee HJ, Fitzgerald TJ (eds): "Progress in Research and Clinical Applications of Corticosteroids", Philadelphia:Heyden, p. 45.
Vedeckis WV (1983). Subunit dissociation as a possible mechanism of glucocorticoid receptor activation. Biochem 22:1983.
Wira CR, Munck A (1974). Glucocorticoid-receptor complexes in rat thymus cells. "Cytoplasmic"-nuclear transformations. J Biol Chem 249:5328.

Hormones and Cancer, pages 207–222
© **1984 Alan R. Liss, Inc., 150 Fifth Avenue, New York, NY 10011**

ON THE USE OF ANTIBODIES IN STUDIES ON
GLUCOCORTICOID RECEPTOR STRUCTURE

Jan-Åke Gustafsson, Jan Carlstedt-Duke, Sam Okret and
Örjan Wrange

Department of Medical Nutrition, Karolinska Institute,
Huddinge University Hospital F69, S-141 86 Huddinge, Sweden

SUMMARY

   Limited proteolysis of the glucocorticoid receptor has
proven to be a valuable tool for a functional analysis of the
receptor protein. With the help of these analyses, it has
been possible to describe three functional domains of the
receptor protein. The native glucocorticoid-receptor complex
contains a steroid-binding domain (A), a DNA-binding domain
(B) and an immunoactive domain (C). This form of the glucocorticoid receptor has a Stokes radius of 6.1 nm and a molecular weight of 94 K when purified. Two steroid-binding proteolytic receptor fragments can be found. The larger one has
a Stokes radius of 3.3 - 3.6 nm and a molecular weight of
39 K and contains both the steroid- and DNA-binding sites
(A + B). The smaller steroid-binding receptor fragment, with
a Stokes radius of 1.9 nm and a molecular weight of 27 K,
contains only the steroid-binding domain (A). Analysis of the
proteolytic fragments of the glucocorticoid receptor using
the specific anti-receptor antibodies revealed the occurrence
of a fragment with Stokes radius 2.6 nm following limited
proteolysis of the receptor by α-chymotrypsin. This fragment
contains neither the steroid-binding nor the DNA-binding
domains but consists only of the immunoactive domain (C).
Further proteolysis of this fragment results in an even
smaller form with Stokes radius 1.4 nm.

   The apparent identity of the larger of the two proteolytic forms of the glucocorticoid receptor (the 3.3 - 3.6 nm
form) with the receptor isolated from certain corticosteroid-
resistant cells, together with the lack of the immunoreactive

domain in these cells appears to indicate an important function of this domain with regard to the biological activity of the receptor.

INTRODUCTION

A vast number of metabolic processes in almost all tissues are influenced by glucocorticoid hormones. These effects are thought to be mediated via the binding of the hormone to the receptor protein, activation, translocation of the hormone receptor complex to the cell nucleus and interaction of this complex with DNA (for review see 1). Although a considerable amount of data about the glucocorticoid receptor has been published a detailed understanding of the mechanism of action of glucocorticoid hormones is far from complete. Several research groups have raised antibodies against more or less pure preparations of several classes of steroid hormone receptors (Fox et al 1976, Greene et al 1977, Greene et al 1979, Greene et al 1980, Coffer and King 1981, Govindan and Sekeris 1978, Govindan 1979, Eisen 1980, Logeat et al 1981, Weigel et al 1981). Immunological techniques might provide new approaches concerning steroid hormone receptor structure and function. In this article we describe the use of poly-clonal antibodies in the elucidation of the structure of the glucocorticoid receptor.

Preparation of antibodies

The glucocorticoid receptor used for immunization was prepared from rat liver cytosol as we have previously described (Wrange et al 1979). Antibodies against the purified rat liver glucocorticoid receptor were raised in two rabbits (G4 and G5) by immunization of the rabbits with trichloroacetic acid-precipitated receptor eluted from the second DNA-cellulose column, average purity 50% (Okret et al 1981). Antibodies were also raised in five other rabbits (A3, A4, 93, 94 and 95) by immunization with glucocorticoid receptor further purified to apparent homogeneity by SDS-polyacrylamide gel electrophoresis (Wrange et al 1979). The receptor band was localized by the staining of parallel tracks and the corre-sponding bands from the unstained tracks were cut out and homogenized in 1 ml of Freund´s complete adjuvant. The rabbits (2-year-old male or female mixed breed) were injected sub-cutaneously at 10-15 sites with a total of 10 µg receptor in

Freund´s complete adjuvant. B. pertussis vaccine, 0.5 ml, was injected subcutaneously in the thigh. After 4 and 6 weeks, the rabbits were boostered with 10 μg receptor in Freund´s incomplete adjuvant. 10-14 days after the last boostering blood was collected from the ear marginal vein and, after purification (see below) the antisera were tested for antibodies against the glucocorticoid receptor.

Purification of antisera

Purification of the antisera was performed by affinity chromatography using Staphylococcus aureus protein A-linked Sepharose CL-4B as previously described (Okret et al 1981). The purified preparations (10 mg/ml) were stored in 20 mM sodium phosphate buffer pH 7.4, 0.02% (w/v) with respect to sodium azide, at -70°C. Preimmune or normal rabbit serum was purified in the same way. In all experiments protein A-Sepharose purified antisera were used at a protein concentration of 10 mg/ml unless otherwise stated.

Methods for studying antibody-receptor interaction

Antibody-receptor interaction was studied using the labelled hormone-receptor complexes. Preparation and labelling of cytosol was performed as previously described (Okret et al 1981). For all experiments EPG buffer (20 mM sodium phosphate buffer, pH 7.4, 1 mM disodium EDTA, 2 mM mercaptoethanol, 10% (w/v) glycerol) was used unless otherwise stated. All incubations were performed in the absence or presence of a 100-fold excess of unlabelled steroid in order to determine unspecific binding. After treatment of the cytosolic labelled receptors with dextran-coated charcoal the antigenic solution was incubated in parallel incubations with purified antisera from immunized or nonimmunized rabbits and, in most experiments, with a buffer control (sodium phosphate buffer, 20 mM, pH 7.4) without antibodies.

Protein A-Sepharose chromatography. After dextran coated charcoal treatment, aliquots of labelled cytosol were incubated with varying amounts of purified antisera (10 mg/ml) for 90 min at 4°C. The incubation mixtures were chromatographed on 1 ml protein A-Sepharose columns equilibrated in EPG buffer. After allowing the antibodies to bind to protein A for 10 min, the columns were washed with 3x1 ml EPG buffer including 0.15 M NaCl and eluted with 3x1 ml 0.1 M acetic acid. Aliquots (0.3 ml) were taken from the flow through and eluate pools and assayed for radioactivity.

Glycerol gradient centrifugation was performed as previously described (Okret et al 1981).

ELISA (enzyme-linked immunosorbent assay). Indirect competitive ELISA was performed as described (Okret et al 1981) with a few minor changes. Samples to be analyzed (0.2 ml) for glucocorticoid receptor were incubated at 4°C overnight with 0.05 ml purified antiserum diluted 1:40. After incubation, the amount of antibodies not bound to antigen in the test sample was measured on micro-ELISA plates coated with 20 ng purified glucocorticoid receptor (Wrange et al 1979) in each well. Thus, color development in the well was inversely proportional to the amount of glucocorticoid receptor in the test sample. The assay of glucocorticoid receptor using specific antibodies against the receptor by indirect competitive ELISA has proven to be a very useful and sensitive method for detection of the receptor (Okret et al 1981). The minimum detection level is about 0.2 μM of glucocorticoid receptor with a sample volume of 0.2 ml. The assay is specific for the glucocorticoid receptor.

In order to assay antibody titers, direct non-competitive ELISA was performed by incubating varying dilutions of the antisera directly with antigen coated micro-ELISA plates (see above) for 60 min at 37°C. Dilution of the antisera was performed in phosphate buffered saline supplemented with 0.05% (v/v) Tween 20 and 1% (w/v) bovine serum albumin. The amount of bound antibodies was measured by a second peroxidase conjugated swine anti-rabbit antibody. Thus, in contrast to the indirect competitive ELISA described above, color development in the well was proportional to the amount of specific anti-receptor antibodies in the antisera.

Determination of titers of anti-glucocorticoid receptor antisera

The titers of the antisera against the rat liver cytosolic glucocorticoid receptor were assayed by a direct ELISA method. Serial dilutions of unpurified antisera showed a titer of between 1:30–1:100, defined as the dilution giving

50% of maximum absorbance in the ELISA. Protein A-Sepharose purified antisera, at a concentration of 10 mg/ml, generally had higher titers, 1:100-1:320, compared to unpurified antisera. All anti-glucocorticoid receptor activity was found to be of immunoglobulin G class. No large differences between titers were observed for the antisera raised in the different rabbits.

Cross-reactivity of anti-glucocorticoid receptor antisera

Cross-reactivity of several anti-receptor antisera against the glucocorticoid receptor from various species was tested. All four of four antisera tested (G4, G5, A3 and A4) bound to the receptor from mouse liver cytosol or rabbit lung cytosol. However, only two of the four antisera tested (G4 and A3) cross-reacted with receptor from human lymphocyte cytosol. The same two antisera cross-reacted with chick embryo (day 16) liver glucocorticoid receptor. Unlike the rat and mouse liver receptor-antibody complexes, which precipitated to the bottom in glycerol density gradients in the presence of 0.15 M KCl, receptor-antibody complexes from chick embryo cytosol or human lymphocyte cytosol did not when the same amount of antibodies was used. A shift from 4 S to about 7-8 S and 12-13 S for the chick embryo receptor and the human lymphocyte receptor, respectively, was observed (Okret 1983).

None of the antisera tested cross-reacted with the following steroid hormone receptors: the estrogen or progestin receptor from rat uterus cytosol (G4, G5, A3, A4 tested), the androgen receptor from rat prostatic cytosol (G4 tested) or the mineralocorticoid receptor from rat kidney or hippocampus cytosol (G4 and A4 tested) (Wrange and Yu 1983). All these tests were performed by glycerol density gradient centrifugation and/or protein A-Sepharose chromatography. With five antisera tested (G4, G5, A3, A4 and 95) no significant difference in avidity to the activated glucocorticoid receptor (25°C, 30 min), when compared to the non-activated receptor from rat liver cytosol was observed, as judged by the amount of receptor retained on protein A-Sepharose columns in the presence of varying concentrations of antibodies.

Characterization of antibody binding site(s) on the glucocorticoid receptor

We have earlier described two proteolytic fragments
(domains) of the glucocorticoid receptor with a Stokes radius
of 6.1 nm, namely a 3.6 nm and a 1.9 nm receptor domain,
respectively (Wrange and Gustafsson 1978, Carlstedt-Duke et al
1977, Carlstedt-Duke et al 1979). The 3.6 nm receptor domain
retains the capacity to bind the steroid and to bind to DNA.
The 1.9 nm domain only binds the steroid, but has no capacity
to bind to DNA. The 6.1 nm glucocorticoid receptor and the
two receptor fragments (3.6 and 1.9 nm), which were obtained
by α-chymotrypsin and trypsin digestion of the 6.1 nm glucocorticoid receptor (Fig. 1, upper panel), respectively, were
incubated separately with anti-glucocorticoid receptor antiserum or preimmune serum. As seen from Fig. 1, lower panel,
only the 6.1 nm glucocorticoid receptor reacted with the
antiserum, while both the 3.6 and the 1.9 nm receptor fragments had lost their ability to interact with the antiserum.
This means that the antibody-binding part of the glucocorticoid receptor is split off during proteolytic digestion with
α-chymotrypsin or trypsin. Antibody-binding did not, as judged
from these results, occur near the steroid-binding site.

In another experiment, the 6.1 nm receptor and the 3.6
nm steroid- and DNA-binding receptor domain were incubated
separately with anti-glucocorticoid receptor antisera from
different rabbits and assayed by protein A-Sepharose chromatography (all seven antisera) or glycerol density gradient
centrifugation (A3, A4, G4, G5). Only the 6.1 nm glucocorticoid receptor was retained on the protein A-Sepharose column,
while no radioactivity was retained after α-chymotrypsin
digestion. All of the seven antisera tested behaved identi-
cally suggesting that the antibodies were directed against
the 6.1 nm receptor but not against the 3.6 nm steroid- and
DNA-binding proteolytic domain. These findings indicate that
the antibodies from all antisera recognize a certain domain
of the glucocorticoid receptor which is split off from the
steroid- and DNA-binding domain during proteolytic digestion
with α-chymotrypsin. However, the antigenic determinant(s)
of this domain is preserved after digestion with α-chymotrypsin
or trypsin, since immunoactivity was still detectable by an
indirect competitive ELISA using the anti-glucocorticoid
receptor antibodies. These results indicate that the steroid-
and DNA-binding sites are located in domains distinctly separated from the antibody binding sites on the receptor. This

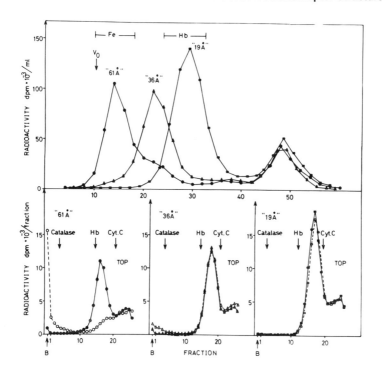

Fig. 1. Density gradient centrifugation and gel filtration chromatography of anti-glucocorticoid receptor-antiserum-treated native 6.1 nm glucocorticoid receptor and 3.6 nm and 1.9 nm fragments from rat liver cytosol. Rat liver cytosol was labelled with 100 nM [^{3}H]triamcinolone acetonide (spec. act. 45 Ci/mmol) for 1 h at 0°C and divided into three pools, two of which were treated so as to produce the proteolytic glucocorticoid receptor fragments (3.6 nm and 1.9 nm), respectively. After dextran-coated charcoal treatment, 3.5 ml of each pool was taken for analysis by Sephadex G-150 gel filtration (upper panel). 150 µl of each pool was incubated with 50 µl (5 mg/ml) antiserum (open symbols) or preimmune serum (filled symbols) for 2.6 h at 4°C in the presence of 0.15 M NaCl and analyzed with glycerol density gradient centrifugation (lower panel). The reference protein horse heart cytochrome c has a sedimentation coefficient of 1.7 S, hemoglobin 4.1 S and catalase 11.3 S. (o---o, ●——●) 6.1 nm; (△---△, ▲——▲) 3.6 nm; (□---□, ■——■) 1.9 nm.

is further supported by the finding that binding to DNA-
cellulose of the activated (25°C, 30 min) glucocorticoid
receptor was not influenced by prior formation of antibody-
receptor complex. Neither did preincubation with antibodies
reduce the amount of [^{3}H]-triamcinolone acetonide binding to
the receptor.

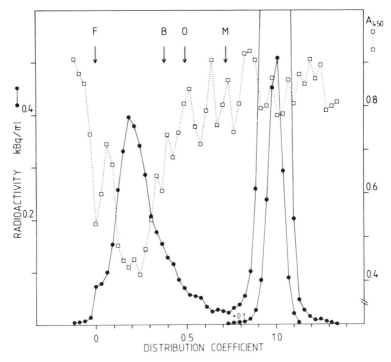

Fig. 2. Gel filtration of cytosol labelled with [^{3}H]-triam-
cinolone acetonide on Agarose A-0.5m. After incubation with
triamcinolone acetonide, the concentration of NaCl was ad-
justed to 0.15 M and the sample applied on the column which
was eluted with EPG buffer containing 0.15 M NaCl and 0.02%
NaN$_3$. After chromatography, the fractions were analysed for
radioactivity and for immunoactivity by ELISA (A$_{450}$). F =
ferritin; B = bovine serum albumin; O = ovalbumin; M = myo-
globin.

When labelled cytosol was analysed by gel filtration on
Agarose A-0.5m and the fractions were assayed for radioactivity
and immunoactivity using ELISA, both the radioactivity and immuno

activity were eluted together close after the void volume (Fig. 2). The elution volume corresponded to a Stokes radius of 5 - 6 nm.

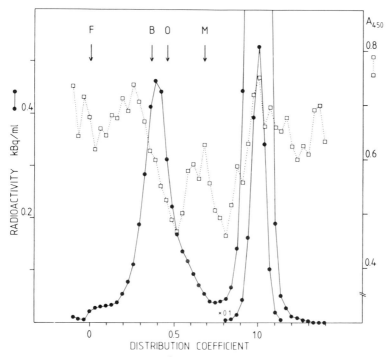

Fig. 3. Gel filtration of [³H]-triamcinolone acetonide-labelled cytosol treated with α-chymotrypsin. After incubation of the cytosol with triamcinolone acetonide, the labelled cytosol was incubated with α-chymotrypsin and the incubation was terminated by the addition of lima bean trypsin inhibitor. Chromatography on Agarose A-0.5m was performed as described in the legend to Fig. 2.

If the labelled cytosol was incubated with α-chymotrypsin prior to chromatography on Agarose A-0.5m, the immunoactivity eluted later than the radioactivity (Fig. 3). The radioactivity eluted at a volume corresponding to a Stokes radius of 3.3 nm whereas the immunoactive fragment eluted at a volume corresponding to a Stokes radius of 2.6 nm. Thus, treatment of the glucocorticoid receptor with α-chymotrypsin appeared to cleave the complex into two specific fragments. The larger, with a Stokes radius of 3.3 nm, contains the steroid- and DNA-binding sites (cf. above). The smaller, with a Stokes radius of 2.6 nm, contains the immunological determinant(s) (Carlstedt-Duke et al 1982). That the DNA-binding site was separated from the immunological determinant(s) can be seen in Fig. 4. When labelled cytosol was heat-activated and analysed by DNA-cellulose chromatography, the radioactivity was eluted simultaneously with the immunoactivity, at 0.17 M NaCl (Fig. 4). However, treatment of the labelled heat-activated cytosol with α-chymotrypsin resulted in the separation of the peak of immunoactivity, eluting at 0.06 M NaCl, from the peak of radioactivity, eluting at 0.25 M NaCl (Fig. 4).

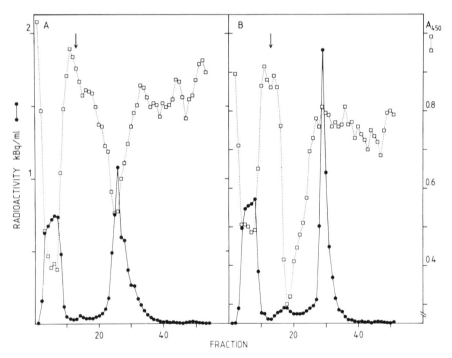

Fig. 4. DNA-cellulose chromatography of labelled cytosol treated (B) or not treated (A) with α-chymotrypsin. After application of the dextran-coated charcoal-treated samples, the columns were washed with EPG buffer and then eluted with a linear 0 - 0.5 M NaCl gradient. The arrow marks the start of the gradient. In A both the peaks of immunoactivity and of radioactivity were eluted at 0.17 M NaCl. In B the peak of immunoactivity was eluted at 0.06 M NaCl and the peak of radioactivity at 0.25 M NaCl.

Further proteolysis of the cytosol with α–chymotrypsin appeared to further reduce the immunoactive fragment to a smaller form with a Stokes radius 1.4 nm (Fig. 3). Prolonged proteolysis resulted in a reduction of the first of the immunoactive peaks on Agarose A-0.5m and an increase in the second immunoactive peak. Chromatography of the immunoactive peak eluted from DNA-cellulose at 0.06 M NaCl on Agarose A-0.5m resulted in a peak of immunoactivity eluting at a volume corresponding to a Stokes radius of 2.8 nm (Carlstedt-Duke et al 1982). The immunoactive peak eluting at 0.06 M NaCl on DNA-cellulose following α–chymotrypsin treatment of the cytosol was recovered irrespective of prior heat-treatment or not.

Absence of a glucocorticoid receptor domain responsible for biological effects in glucocorticoid-resistant mouse lymphoma P1798

Stevens et al (1979, 1978) have earlier described a mutant receptor-positive corticosteroid-resistant (CR) P1798 mouse lymphoma. Characterization of the glucocorticoid receptor from the P1798 lymphoma cells reveals in the corticosteroid-sensitive (CS) P1798 cells a glucocorticoid receptor with a Stokes radius of 6 nm and a calculated molecular weight of 90,000. However, the receptor from CR P1798 cells has a Stokes radius of 2.8 nm and a calculated molecular weight of 40,000. Furthermore, the receptor from CR P1798 cells has an increased affinity for DNA since higher ionic strength was needed for elution from DNA-cellulose when compared to the receptor from CS P1798 cells. A similar "resistant-like" form of glucocorticoid receptor could be obtained from CS P1798 cytosol by limited proteolysis with α–chymotrypsin (Stevens and Stevens 1981). This gave rise to a receptor fragment with Stokes radius of 2.8 nm and tighter DNA-binding, identical to the receptor from CR P1798 cells. No effect of α–chymotrypsin was seen on the receptor from CR cells.

The results of the limited proteolysis of the glucocorticoid receptor from CS P1798 cells might suggest that the receptor in CR cells may be synthesized as a larger precursor which then undergoes rapid intracellular processing (i.e. proteolysis) to the 3 nm form. This, however, is not very likely as experiments consisting of the mixing of CR and CS P1798 cytosol have shown no conversion of the 6 nm CS to a 3 nm form (Stevens and Stevens 1979, Stevens and Stevens 1981).

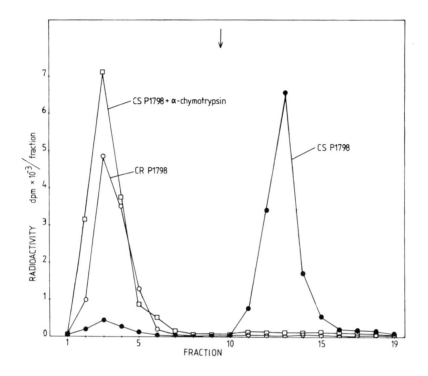

Fig. 5. Protein A-Sepharose chromatography of glucocorticoid receptor-antibody complexes from corticosteroid-sensitive (CS; ●), α-chymotrypsin-treated CS (□) and corticosteroid-resistant (CR; o) P1798 lymphoma cytosol. Preparation of cytosol, labelling with [^{3}H]-triamcinolone acetonide and treatment with α-chymotrypsin was performed as described by Stevens et al using EPG buffer. 100 µl of labelled cytosol was incubated with 50 µl purified antiserum for 1.5 h at 4°C. The incubation mixtures were then applied on two ml columns of Protein A-Sepharose and fractions of 0.5 ml were collected. The arrow indicates the start of elution with 0.1 M acetic acid. Incubation of CS cytosol with normal non-immunised rabbit serum gave no retention of radioactivity on the Protein A-Sepharose column.

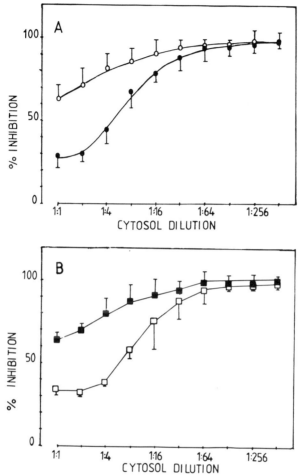

Fig. 6. ELISA of cytosol dilutions from corticosteroid-sensitive (CS; •) and corticosteroid-resistant (CR; o) P1798 cells (Fig. 6) and of α-chymotrypsin-treated CS (□) and CR (■) cytosol (Fig. 6). Cytosol preparation from P1798 tumours was performed in EPG buffer, pH 7.4 followed by centrifugation at 170,000 x g. Treatment with α-chymotrypsin was carried out as previously described. Cytosol (5 mg protein/ml) was diluted in EPG buffer and 200 μl aliquots of each dilution was incubated with 50 μl of purified antiserum solutions and assayed by indirect competitive ELISA. The bars represent 1 S.D.; CS (•) n = 3, CR (o) n = 5, α-chymotrypsin-treated CS (□) n = 2, and α-chymotrypsin-treated CR (■) n = 4.

Alternatively the CR P1798 receptor may be synthesized directly as a polypeptide corresponding to the 3 nm form because of a defect at the genome level permitting transcription of only a smaller receptor mRNA. A third alternative is that different domains of the glucocorticoid receptor are synthesized as separate polypeptides but fail to link up with each other.

Since our antibodies bind to a domain of the rat liver glucocorticoid receptor that is removed by limited proteolysis with α-chymotrypsin (see above) an immunocharacterisation of the receptor from CS and CR cells was deemed of great value. It has previously been reported that glucocorticoid receptor from CS P1798 cells interacts with specific antibodies against rat liver glucocorticoid receptor whereas the receptor from CR P1798 cells does not bind to these antibodies (Stevens et al 1981). The same is observed with our antibodies (Fig. 5).

In contrast to CS P1798 cytosol, both before and after limited proteolysis by α-chymotrypsin, no immunoactivity could be found in the cytosol from CR P1798 cells (Fig. 6). This was assayed by the indirect ELISA based on the specific anti-glucocorticoid receptor antibodies and purified glucocorticoid receptor as described above, both in whole cytosol and after gel filtration on Agarose A-0.5 m (Okret et al 1983). These results suggest that the domain normally removed by limited proteolysis by α-chymotrypsin appears to be missing in CR P1798 cells. It would seem, therefore, that this domain plays an important role in the mechanism of action of glucocorticoids. The evidence presented here for the apparent lack of the immunoactive domain in CR P1798 cells strongly suggests that this domain is completely missing in these cells and that a mutation has occurred affecting the genome resulting in a defect transcription of the receptor gene.

ACKNOWLEDGEMENTS

This work was supported by a grant from the Swedish Medical Research Council (No. 13X-2819).

REFERENCES

Baxter JD, Rousseau GG (1979) Glucocorticoid Hormone Action: An overview. In Baxter JD, Rousseau GG (eds): Glucocorticoid Hormone Action in Monographs on Endocrinology. Vol. 12. Springer-Verlag, Heidelberg, p. 1.

Carlstedt-Duke J, Gustafsson J-Å, Wrange Ö (1977). Formation and characteristics of dexamethasone-receptor complexes of different molecular weight. Biochim. Biophys. Acta 497: 507.

Carlstedt-Duke J, Wrange Ö, Dahlberg E, Gustafsson J-Å, Högberg B (1979). Transformation of the glucocorticoid receptor in rat liver cytosol by lysosomal enzymes. J. Biol. Chem. 254:1537.

Carlstedt-Duke J, Okret S, Wrange Ö, Gustafsson J-Å (1982). Immunochemical analysis of the glucocorticoid receptor: Identification of a third domain separate from the steroid-binding and DNA-binding domains. Proc. Natl. Acad. Sci. USA 79:4260.

Coffer AI, King RJB (1981). Antibodies to estradiol receptor from human myometrium. J. Steroid Biochem. 14:1229.

Eisen HJ (1980). An antiserum to rat liver glucocorticoid receptor. Proc. Natl. Acad. Sci. USA 77:3893.

Fox LL, Redeuilh G, Baskevitch P, Baulieu E-E, Richard-Foy H (1976). Production and detection of antibodies against the estrogen receptor from calf uterine cytosol. FEBS Lett. 63:71.

Govindan MV, Sekeris CE (1978). Purification of two dexamethasone-binding proteins from rat liver cytosol. Eur. J. Biochem. 89:95.

Govindan MV (1979). Purification of glucocorticoid receptors from rat liver cytosol. Preparation of antibodies against the major receptor proteins and application of immunological techniques to study activation and translocation. J. Steroid Biochem. 11:323.

Greene GL, Closs LE, Fleming H, DeSombre ER, Jensen EV (1977). Antibodies to estrogen receptor: Immunochemical similarity of estrophilin from various mammalian species. Proc. Natl. Acad. Sci. USA 74:3681.

Greene GL, Closs LE, DeSombre ER, Jensen EV (1979). Antibodies to estrophilin: Comparison between rabbit and goat antisera. J. Steroid Biochem. 11:333.

Greene GL, Closs LE, DeSombre ER, Jensen EV (1980). Estrophilin. Pro and anti. J. Steroid Biochem. 12:159.

Logeat F, Hai MTV, Milgrom E (1981). Antibodies to rabbit progesterone receptor: Cross-reactivity with human receptor. Proc. Natl. Acad. Sci. USA 78:1426.

Okret S, Carlstedt-Duke J, Wrange Ö, Carlström K, Gustafsson J-Å (1981). Characterization of an antiserum against the glucocorticoid receptor. Biochim. Biophys. Acta 677:205.

Okret S (1983). Comparison between different rabbit antisera against the glucocorticoid receptor. J. Steroid Biochem., in press.

Okret S, Stevens Y-W, Carlstedt-Duke J, Wrange Ö, Gustafsson J-Å, Stevens J (1983). Absence of a glucocorticoid receptor domain responsible for biological effects in glucocorticoid-resistant mouse lymphoma P1798. Cancer Res., in press.

Stevens J, Stevens Y-W, Rhodes J, Steiner G (1978). Differences in nuclear glucocorticoid binding between corticoid-sensitive and corticoid-resistant lymphocytes of mouse lymphoma P1798 and stabilization of nuclear hormone receptor complexes with carbobenzoxy-L-phenylalanine. J. Natl. Cancer Inst. 61:1477.

Stevens J, Stevens Y-W (1979). Physicochemical differences between glucocorticoid-binding components from the corticoid-sensitive and -resistant strains of mouse lymphoma P1798. Cancer Res. 39:4021.

Stevens J, Eisen HJ, Stevens Y-W, Haubenstock H, Rosenthal RL, Artishevsky A (1981). Immunochemical differences between glucocorticoid receptors from corticoid-sensitive and -resistant malignant lymphocytes. Cancer Res. 41:134.

Stevens J, Stevens Y-W (1981). Influence of limited proteolysis on the physicochemical and DNA-binding properties of glucocorticoid receptors from corticoid-sensitive and -resistant mouse lymphoma P1798. Cancer Res. 41:125.

Weigel NL, Pousette Å, Schrader WT, O'Malley BW (1981). Analysis of chicken progesterone receptor structure using a spontaneous sheep antibody. Biochemistry 20:6798.

Wrange Ö, Gustafsson J-Å (1978). Separation of the hormone and DNA-binding sites of the hepatic glucocorticoid receptor by means of proteolysis. J. Biol. Chem. 253:856.

Wrange Ö, Carlstedt-Duke J, Gustafsson J-Å (1979). Purification of the glucocorticoid receptor from rat liver cytosol. J. Biol. Chem. 254:9284.

Wrange Ö, Yu Z-Y (1983). Mineralocorticoid receptor in rat kidney and hippocampus. Characterization and quantitation by isoelectric focusing. Endocrinology, in press.

Hormones and Cancer, pages 223–233

GLUCOCORTICOID RECEPTOR LEVELS PREDICT RESPONSE TO TREATMENT IN HUMAN LYMPHOMA

Clara D. Bloomfield, M.D.*, Allan U. Munck, Ph.D. and Kendall A. Smith, M.D.

Section of Medical Oncology, Department of Medicine, University of Minnesota, Minneapolis, MN and the Immunology Program of the Norris Cotton Cancer Center and the Department of Physiology, Dartmouth Medical School, Hanover, NH

SUMMARY

Neoplastic tumor masses from 47 adults with B cell malignant lymphomas were examined for glucocorticoid receptors and in vitro sensitivity to glucocorticoids. The patients were then treated with dexamethasone as a single agent for 5-14 days. Forty-seven percent of patients achieved at least a partial remission; 40% had no significant tumor response. Lymphoma cells from patients who responded had significantly more glucocorticoid receptor sites per cell and greater in vitro sensitivity as measured by glucocorticoid inhibition of incorporation of thymidine than did tumor cells from non-responders. Using a receptor level of 3000 sites/cell, response could accurately be predicted in 82% of patients. Our data suggest that study of tumor glucocorticoid receptors and glucocorticoid sensitivity in vitro may allow selection of those patients with lymphoma who should receive glucocorticoids as part of combination chemotherapy.

INTRODUCTION

Glucocorticoids are part of most treatment programs used for adults with non-Hodgkin's malignant lymphoma

---

*To whom correspondence should be addressed at Box 277, University of Minnesota Hospitals, Minneapolis, MN 55455

(Peterson, Bloomfield 1982). However, a number of early reports suggested that many patients have lymphomas which are not sensitive to glucocorticoids (Ezdinli et al. 1969; Fortuny et al. 1972; Jones et al. 1972; Livingston, Carter 1970). Our own preliminary studies suggest that only about 50% of newly diagnosed patients will achieve a partial remission from a two week course of dexamethasone therapy (Bloomfield et al. 1980). Moreover, glucocorticoids have many side effects, particularly in an elderly group of patients such as those with lymphoma (McClean et al. 1983). In our experiments, for example, undesirable side effects were seen in 63 (92%) of 68 patients with lymphoma who received 5-14 days of dexamethasone at a dose of 16 mg per day. Consequently, in vitro tests that would rapidly identify before treatment those lymphoma patients likely to benefit from steroids would be of considerable use clinically.

Glucocorticoid-receptor complexes seem to be required for hormone action in all glucocorticoid-sensitive tissues (Munck, Leung 1977). In addition, in vitro studies have shown that incorporation of radiolabelled leucine, uridine and thymidine is inhibited by glucocorticoids in sensitive lymphocytes (Smith et al. 1977). Consequently, we have undertaken a series of studies which have as their major objective the determination of the utility of measuring in tumor cells of adults with lymphoma glucocorticoid receptor number and in vitro glucocorticoid sensitivity to identify pretreatment those patients likely to respond to glucocorticoids. The current results from these studies are summarized in this paper. Our findings suggest that tumor glucocorticoid receptor levels may allow us to select before treatment those patients with lymphoma who should receive glucocorticoids in their chemotherapy regimens.

PATIENTS AND METHODS

Patients

The patients studied were 47 adults with a diagnosis of B-cell malignant lymphoma. Thirty-nine patients were first studied at diagnosis and eight at relapse. Four had received prior glucocorticoid therapy; these patients had been off glucocorticoid therapy for a minimum of six weeks when in vitro studies were performed.

The study protocol (Bloomfield et al. 1980) consisted of first obtaining informed consent in writing from each patient. Then each patient underwent biopsy of an involved lymph node for pathologic examination and in vitro glucocorticoid studies. Following biopsy, each patient was treated with dexamethasone at a dose of 4 mg every six hours. Single agent glucocorticoid therapy was administered for a minimum of five days, since that is the duration of glucocorticoid treatment in most combination chemotherapy regimens for lymphoma. In 39 of the 47 patients glucocorticoid alone was continued for at least two weeks.

Antitumor response to dexamethasone was measured by a single investigator who had no knowledge of the results of the in vitro glucocorticoid studies. At the end of single-agent glucocorticoid therapy patients were classified as responders, mixed responders or nonresponders. They were scored as responders if they had a partial remission defined as at least a 50% reduction in all measurable tumor and had developed no new disease. In a few patients, all tumor masses decreased by at least 50%, but this was accompanied by an increase in the number of circulating lymphoma cells. These patients were classified as mixed responders. Patients who demonstrated less than a 50% decrease of all tumor masses or developed any new mass were classified as nonresponders.

Preparation and Handling of Tissues

Lymph nodes or other tumor masses were the source of tissue studied in all cases. Different portions of the same tissue were used to obtain sections for histologic diagnosis, cryostat sections for immunologic analysis and single cell suspensions. Part of the cell suspension was utilized for glucocorticoid studies and part for immunologic (lymphocyte surface marker) analysis. Lymph nodes were classified histologically according to the International Working Formulation for Clinical Usage (The Non-Hodgkin's Lymphoma Pathologic Classification Project 1982) and immunologically as B-lymphomas or T-lymphomas using previously defined criteria (Gajl-Peczalska et al.

1982). In brief, lymphomas were defined as B-cell by the presence of surface and/or cytoplasmic monotypic immunoglobulin. The biopsy specimens were classified histologically and immunologically without knowledge of the in vitro glucocorticoid data.

In single cell suspensions prepared from neoplastic lympho nodes the percent of malignant cells was first determined by immunologic analysis (Bloomfield et al. 1980). When the single cell suspension demonstrated at least 50% malignant cells, the tissue was studied for glucocorticoid receptors and in vitro sensitivity. The majority of specimens studied contained at least 70% malignant cells.

Glucocorticoid Receptors and In Vitro Glucocorticoid Sensitivity

The methods used for determining receptor sites per cell have been previously described in detail (Bloomfield et al. 1980; Crabtree et al. 1981). Briefly, the cells were incubated with a near saturating concentration (40 nM) of [^{3}H]dexamethasone (SA 35 Ci/mol, New England Nuclear, Boston, MA) with (B) and without (A) an excess of unlabelled dexamethasone (2 μM) for 30 minutes at 37°C. The cell suspension was then cooled to 3°C. Cytoplasmic receptors were determined by lysing the cells with a rapid dilution into hypotonic $MgCl_2$ (1.5 mM) containing dextran-coated charcoal to adsorb free glucocorticoid. After centrifugation an aliquot of the released cytosol was removed and counted by liquid scintillation. Nuclear receptor sites were determined similarly by lysing cells in hypotonic $MgCl_2$. The released nuclei were then pelleted, the cytosol removed, and the nuclear pellet counted.

For both nuclear and cytoplasmic binding, receptor binding in counts per minutes (CPM) was calculated by subtracting the bound cpm obtained from incubation (B) (which estimates nonsaturable binding) from the cpm obtained from incubation (A), corrected for differences in the radioactive-steroid concentrations in the two incubations. These cpm were converted to bound steroid molecules per cell. Receptor sites per cell were then calculated from these values by extrapolating to infinite steroid concentrations, assuming dexamethasone has a dissociation constant from gluccorticoid receptors of 10 nmol/l. Total receptor sites per cell (R_T) were calculated as the sum of the cytoplasmic and nuclear receptor sites per cell.

In vitro sensitivity to glucocorticoids was measured by studying the effects of dexamethasone on incorporation of radiolabelled leucine, uridine, and thymidine (Bloomfield et al. 1980). Cells (1×10^6/ml) were incubated in quadruplicate without and with 100 nmol/l dexamethasone for 20 hours at 37^0C. Radiolabelled leucine, uridine, and thymidine were then added and the incubation was continued for four hours. The cells were then harvested on glass-fiber filter-paper, and isotope incorporation was determined by liquid scintillation counting. Results for in vitro sensitivity studies have been expressed as percent change from the values obtained when cells were incubated without dexamethasone.

Statistical Methods

Differences between groups were evaluated for significance at the p=0.05 level or less. Differences in percentages for discrete variables were tested with the Pearson chi-square statistic correcting for continuity in 2 x 2 tables. Differences in continuous variables between groups were tested with the Mann-Whitney test.

RESULTS

Of the 47 patients treated with single-agent glucocorticoid therapy, 22 (47%) achieved a partial remission, 6 (13%) had a mixed response and 19 (40%) demonstrated no significant antitumor effect. Clinical and histological characteristics of these three patient groups are shown in Table 1. The only significant difference among groups was that the mixed responders more frequently had blood involvement at diagnosis. Nonresponders tended to more frequently be male and more often had diffuse lymphoma. Patients in all three response groups received single-agent glucocorticoid therapy for comparable periods of time (median 14 days).

Table 1. Clinical Characteristics of Lymphoma Patients
          According to Response to Glucocorticoid Therapy

	Response to Glucocorticoid Therapy		
	Remission	Mixed	None
Number of Patients	22	6	19
Sex (M:F)	12:10	4:2	16:3
Median Age (yrs)	63	48	61
Diagnosis (IWF)			
Small Lymph (A)	23%	0	42%
Fol. Sm. Cleaved (B)	55%	50%	37%
Other Follicular (C,D)	14%	33%	10%
Other Diffuse (F,G,H,J)	9%	17%	10%
Treatment Status at Study			
Newly Diagnosed	91%	83%	74%
Prior Glucocorticoid	0	1	3
Disease Extent at Study			
"Stage" I-IIIA	13%	0	26%
"Stage" IVA	55%	50%	47%
"Stage" IIIB-IVB	32%	50%	26%
Blood Involvement	9%	83%	26%

The results of the in vitro glucocorticoid studies for the three response groups are summarized in Table 2 and Figure 1. Median total glucocorticoid receptor sites per cell were 4031 for patients who achieved a partial remission, 4024 for patients who had a mixed response and 2049 for the nonresponders. Receptors were significantly higher in responders than nonresponders ($p<.001$). The median inhibition of thymidine incorporation was also significantly greater in responders than nonresponders (23% vs 9%, $p=.02$). Significant differences between responders and nonresponders were not seen in dexamethasone inhibition of radiolabelled leucine or uridine incorporation.

No pretreatment clinical characteristics could be used to predict those patients who would respond to glucocorticoid therapy. However, using total glucocorticoid receptor levels (R_T) we could accurately predict response in 37 (82%) of 45 patients. Among 30 patients with nodal tumor R_T of more than 3000 sites per

Table 2. Correlation of In Vitro Glucocorticoid Studies
with Response to Glucocorticoid Therapy in
B-Cell Lymphoma

	Response to Glucocorticoid Therapy			
	Remission	Mixed	None	P*
No. pts	22	6	19	

Glucocorticoid Receptors (sites/cell)

Cytoplasmic	937	999 (.01)**	549	.002
Nuclear	3067	2411 (.07)	1500	.002
Total	4031	4024 (.01)	2049	.0006

Glucocorticoid Inhibition of Isotope Incorporation (%)

Leucine	27	29	17	NS
Uridine	35	32	22	.06
Thymidine	23	28	9	.02

*P value for response groups: remission vs. none
**Mixed vs. none

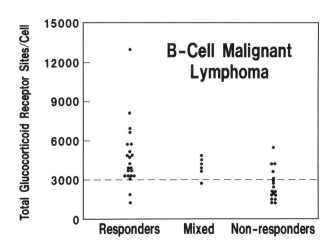

Figure 1. Glucocorticoid receptor levels according to
clinical response to dexamethasone therapy.

cell, 25 (83%) demonstrated more than a 50% decrease in nodal mass. Similarly among 15 patients with nodal tumor R_T of less than 3000, only 3 (20%) so responded.

DISCUSSION

Short courses of glucocorticoids (5-14 days) are included in almost all combination chemotherapy regimens used in treating malignant lymphoma. However, there are few data on either the antitumor effect or the toxicity of such glucocorticoid therapy. We have found that only about half of newly diagnosed adults with lymphoma will derive considerable antitumor benefit from such courses. However, almost all patients will experience toxic effects and in about 5-10% of patients these will be severe. Tests which would identify pretreatment those patients likely to respond to glucocorticoids would obviously be valuable.

Our findings suggest that measurement of tumor glucocorticoid receptor levels may enable us to select those patients who should receive glucocorticoid therapy. Lymphomas from patients who had at least a 50% reduction in measurable tumors after a short course of dexamethasone had significantly higher numbers of glucocorticoid receptors than tumors from patients with lesser responses. We could not identify any clinical or histologic characteristics that would allow us to predict which patients would respond to glucocorticoid therapy.

Our current results suggest that patients with more than 3000 total glucocorticoid receptor sites per lymphoma cell will demonstrate a significant antitumor response to glucocorticoid therapy. These results were achieved in patients with B-cell lymphomas who had primarily lymphocytic morphology. A different receptor level may discriminate between responders and non-responders in other types of lymphoma.

We know of no other studies correlating response of patients with lymphoma to glucocorticoid therapy with tumor glucocorticoid receptor levels. However, in acute lymphoblastic leukemia (ALL), we (Bloomfield et al. 1981b), Mastrangelo et al. (1980) and Ho et al. (1982) have found that glucocorticoid receptor level correlates with response to single-agent glucocorticoid therapy. Mastrangelo et al.

were able to predict response to a short course of steroid in 15 (79%) of 19 children with ALL. Eight of 12 patients with numbers of glucocorticoid receptors >4000 responded; 0 of 7 with glucocorticoid receptors <4000 responded. Our results in adult ALL are similar (Bloomfield et al. 1981b), as are more recent results of Ho et al. (1982). We have not found that tests of in vitro glucocorticoid sensitivity, such as inhibition of radiolabelled leucine, uridine or thymidine incorporation, improve our ability to predict response to glucocorticoid therapy over what we achieve with glucocorticoid receptors alone.

Our studies suggest that in patients with lymphomas, neoplastic cells found in marrow, blood and lymph nodes often have different numbers of receptors (Bloomfield et al. 1981a). Receptor levels in lymphoma cells from tumor masses (lymph nodes) allowed prediction of clinical response of tumor masses to glucocorticoid therapy in 82% of patients. Whether lymph node receptor levels will also accurately predict response of tumor in marrow and blood to glucocorticoid therapy is unknown. It may be that receptor levels in those tissues need also be determined to optimally predict the response of the patient in all sites.

Two additional practical implications of our studies deserve brief mention. First, if receptor levels are to be used to predict response to glucocorticoid therapy, they should not be measured until the patient has been off glucocorticoids for at least three weeks. We have demonstrated in both patients (Shipman et al. 1981) and normal volunteers (Shipman et al. 1983) that glucocorticoid administration rapidly results in a significant decline in receptor levels in lymphoid cells in most individuals. Receptor levels have required as long as 17 days to return to baseline. Second, our studies suggest that central reference laboratories for glucocorticoid receptor determinations are feasible. Our receptor determinations have all been done on specimens that have been shipped 1,300 miles in RPMI 1640 at ambient temperatures; the receptor assay was routinely performed 18 to 48 hours after tissue sampling. Our data clearly indicate that excellent prediction of response to glucocorticoid therapy can be achieved from receptor levels determined in this fashion.

To date we have correlated tumor receptor levels only with response to single agent glucocorticoid therapy.

Whether these results will be translatable to combination chemotherapy regimens which include glucocorticoid requires further study. If such is the case then determination of tumor glucocorticoid receptor level may become a necessary part of the evaluation of patients with lymphoma, just as estrogen receptor analyses are required in patients with breast cancer.

ACKNOWLEDGEMENTS

This research was supported in part by Public Health Service grants CA-26273 and CA-17323, American Cancer Society grant No. CH-167 and the Coleman Leukemia Research Fund.

REFERENCES

Bloomfield CD, Smith KA, Peterson BA, Hildebrandt L, Zaleskas J, Gajl-Peczalska KJ, Frizzera G, Munck A (1980). In vitro glucocorticoid studies for predicting response to glucocorticoid therapy in adults with malignant lymphoma. Lancet i:952.

Bloomfield CD, Smith KA, Peterson BA, Gajl-Peczalska KJ, Munck AU (1981a). In vitro glucocorticoid studies in human lymphoma: Clinical and biologic significance. J Steroid Biochem 15:275.

Bloomfield CD, Smith KA, Peterson BA, Munck A (1981b). Glucocorticoid receptors in adult acute lymphoblastic leukemia. Cancer Res 41:4857.

Crabtree GR, Smith KA, Munck A (1981). Glucocorticoid receptors. In Catovsky D (ed): "Methods in Hematology," Edinburgh, Churchill Livingstone, p. 252.

Ezdinli EZ, Stutzman L, Aungst CW, Firat D (1969). Corticosteroid therapy for lymphomas and chronic lymphocytic leukemia. Cancer 23:900.

Fortuny IE, Theologides A, Kennedy BJ (1972). Single, combined and sequential use of uracil mustard and prednisone in the treatment of lymphoreticular tumors. Minn Med 55:715.

Gajl-Peczalska KJ, Bloomfield CD, Frizzera G, Kersey JH, LeBien TW (1982). Diversity of phenotypes of non-Hodgkin's malignant lymphoma. In Vitetta E (ed): "B and T Cell Tumors," New York, Academic Press, p 63.

Ho AD, Hunstein W, Ganeshaguru K, Hoffbrand AV, Brandeis WE, Denk B (1982). Therapeutic and prognostic implications of glucocorticoid receptors and terminal deoxynucleotidyl transferase in acute leukemia. Leuk Res 6:1.

Jones SE, Rosenberg SA, Kaplan HS, Kadin ME, Dorfman RF (1972). Non-Hodgkin's lymphomas. II. Single agent chemotherapy. Cancer 30:31.

Livingston RB, Carter SK (1970). Prednisone and prednisolone. In "Single Agents in Cancer Chemotherapy," New York: IFI/Plenum, p. 337.

Mastrangelo R, Malandrino R, Riccardi R, Longo P, Ranelletti FO, Iacobelli S (1980). Clinical implications of glucocorticoid receptor studies in childhood acute lymphoblastic leukemia. Blood 56:1036.

McClean JW, Kiely-Grandbois K, Hurd DD, Peterson BA, Bloomfield CD (1983). Glucocorticoid toxicity in patients treated for non-Hodgkin's lymphoma. Proc Am Soc Clin Oncol 2:217.

Munck A, Leung K (1977). Glucocorticoid receptors and mechanisms of action. In Pasqualini JR (ed): "Receptors and Mechanism of Action of Steroid Hormones part II," New York: Marcel Dekker, p 311.

The Non-Hodgkin's Lymphoma Pathologic Classification Project (1982). National Cancer Institute sponsored study of classifications of non-Hodgkin's lymphoma-summary and description of a working formulation for clinical usage. Cancer 49:2112.

Peterson BA, Bloomfield CD (1982). Non-Hodgkin's malignant lymphomas. In Greenspan EM (ed): "Clinical Interpretation and Practice of Cancer Chemotherapy," New York: Raven Press, p 519.

Shipman GF, Bloomfield CD, Smith KA, Peterson BA, Munck A (1981). The effects of glucocorticoid therapy on glucocorticoid receptors in leukemia and lymphoma. Blood 58:1198.

Shipman G, Bloomfield CD, Gajl-Peczalska KJ, Munck A, Smith KA (1983). Glucocorticoids and lymphocytes. III. Effects of glucocorticoid administration on lymphocyte glucocorticoid receptors. Blood 61:1086.

Smith KA, Crabtree GR, Kennedy SJ, Munck AU (1977). Glucocorticoid receptors and glucocorticoid sensitivity of mitogen stimulated and unstimulated human lymphocytes. Nature 267:523.

Hormones and Cancer, pages 235–246
© 1984 Alan R. Liss, Inc., 150 Fifth Avenue, New York, NY 10011

GLUCOCORTICOID RECEPTORS AND STEROID SENSITIVITY OF HUMAN
ACUTE LYMPHOBLASTIC LEUKEMIA

Stefano Iacobelli, MD, Paolo Marchetti, MD, Giulio De Rossi°,
MD, Franco Mandelli°, MD.
        Catholic University S. Cuore,
        °State University
        Rome, Italy.

INTRODUCTION

Even though an association between hormones and cancer
was demonstrated nearly a hundred years ago when Beatson
obtained clinical remission of breast cancer patients following ovariectomy (Beatson 1896), only recently were the
scientific grounds of this discovery brought to light. It has
become increasingly clear that the mechanism by which steroid
hormones affect sensitive cells depends on the presence in
these cells of specific hormone binding proteins termed
receptors. In the case of hormone-dependent tumors, i.e. those
malignant diseases arising from hormone target cells, two
major applications related to hormone receptor physiology have
emerged: first, patients with receptor-positive tumors
frequently respond to therapeutic measures aimed at counter-
acting the effects of hormones on the tumor and second, the
presence of receptors is a biological-biochemical indicator
with prognostic significance. Hence, the measurement of
receptors may assist in selecting patients for therapy and
be used as a prognostic variable.

The application of knowledge of receptors to breast
cancer has in recent years been extended to those tumors
susceptible to aggression by chemical arms such as hormones.
These include endometrial and ovarian cancer and cancer of
the prostate (Iacobelli et al. 1980). To date little attention
has been focused on neoplasias arising in lymphoid cells,
primarily acute lymphoblastic leukemia. Although more than
90% remission is standard and expected, at least for childhood
leukemia, and as many as 50% of patients remain in complete

continuous remission for more than five years after diagnosis, some important problems in acute lymphoblastic leukemia are still to be solved. First, drug-induced deaths due to highly aggressive chemotherapy regimens, second resistance to therapy, third, early relapse and, finally, harmful side-effects of glucocorticoid treatment. Therefore, the aim of much hematological research is to identify new prognostic factors which would indicate a more suitable individualized treatment, thereby increasing therapeutic response and survival. The identification of patients with resistant disease, for example, will indicate the use of a more intensive therapy and reduce the toxic risks to patients who would sufficiently benefit from a less aggressive treatment.

The promising results obtained in breast cancer led some investigators to conduct analogous studies on glucocorticoid receptors in human leukemia. These studies were undertaken to demonstrate that the glucocorticoid-induced lysis of lymphoid cells is mediated by a specific receptor mechanism. In 1973 Lippman et al. first demonstrated that the leukemic lymphoblasts from twenty-two previously untreated acute lymphoblastic leukemia patients who were responsive to therapy retained high glucocorticoid levels, as did those from six other patients in relapse, whereas six patients who were resistant to the therapy showed low glucocorticoid levels Five years later the same group reported a positive correlation between the glucocorticoid concentrations in the cells of forty-five children with acute lymphoblastic leukemia and remission duration and survival rate (Lippman et al. 1978).

Here we summarize our studies on glucocorticoid receptors in acute lymphoblastic leukemia as related to sensitivity, therapy and prognosis.

Problems in Glucocorticoid Receptor Assay

Unlike in the solid tumor where it is only possible to measure receptor after homogenizing cells and extracting the receptor protein, in leukemic cells we can use either cytoplasmic assay (the same as for solid tumors) or whole-cell assay in which receptor measurement is on live cells. Whether it is preferable to measure receptor in cytoplasmic extracts or in intact cells is not simply a theoretical question related to the different geography in receptor evaluation – only in the cytoplasm or in the cytoplasm and nucleus – since the data reported in the literature (Table I) do demonstrate that the two assay methods are not interchangeable and give barely comparable results. Of course, these discrepancies in receptor values might have a profound influence on clinical studies aimed at correlating the receptor content of leukemic cells with in vivo sensitivity to drugs.

Table 1. Glucocorticoid receptors in human leukemias

Disease category	Whole-cell (sites/cell)	Cytosol (fmol/mg protein)
ALL	14,555+2,725 (8)	---
CLL	3,205+340 (4)	214+23 (27)
AML	6,375+845 (30)	347+121 (7)
CML (immature cells)	3,390+550 (17)	15+6 (14)
CML (mature cells)	3,110+755 (17)	2+1 (9)
ALL	17,106+13,737 (15)	5,434+6,817 (15)[a]
AML	14,954+10,083 (12)	6,536+6,822 (12)[a]
CLL	8,061+4,491 (14)	1,551+1,201 (12)[a]

Results are expressed as means + S.D. (no. of observations)
[a]Data are expressed as sites/cell
First series of data from Sloman, Bell 1980
Second series of data from Iacobelli et al. 1981

We therefore decided to effect a thorough comparison of glucocorticoid receptor measurement using both the cytoplasmic and the whole-cell assay. As shown in Fig.1, both assays detected saturable binding of ^{3}H-triamcinolone acetonide in various forms of leukemia including chronic lymphocytic, acute lymphoblastic and acute non-lymphocytic leukemia. From the analysis of 41 leukemic cell specimens it was found that the results of whole-cell assay, expressed as glucocorticoid receptor sites/cell, correlated well (p<0.01, Fig.1) with those of the cytoplasmic assay, calculated as fmoles/mg protein. However, for cells with low receptor content, i.e. those containing less than 10,000 sites/cell, the two assay procedures were more difficult to compare.

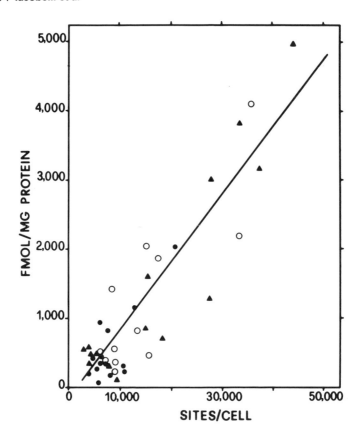

Fig. 1. Correlation between glucocorticoid receptor levels measured by whole-cell assay and cytosol assay in leukocytes from patients with chronic lymphocytic leukemia (●), acute lymphoblastic leukemia (▲) and acute non-lymphocytic leukemia (O). Methodological details are given in Iacobelli et al. 1981.

In agreement with previous reports (Galaini et al. 1973, Terenius et al. 1976), the cytoplasmic assay consistently underestimated the number of receptor sites with respect to the whole-cell assay, particularly in the case of lymphatic leukemia (Table II). Moreover, the extent of underestimation decreased for increasing levels of total cellular receptor (cf. chronic lymphocytic and acute non-lymphocytic leukemia (Table II).

Table II. Underestimation of glucocorticoid receptor content (cytosol assay versus whole-cell assay) in leukocytes from patients with various types of leukemia

	Sites/cell		
Leukemia type	Whole-cell	Cytosol	Underestimation (%)
CLL(14)[a]	8.061+4.491[b]	1.551+1.201	78.7+18.4[c]
ALL(15)	17.106+13.737	5.434+6.817	73.1+14.4[d]
ANLL(12)	14.954+10.083	6.536+6.822	57.8+22.3[e]

[a] Numbers in brackets, number of cases
[b] Mean + S.D.
[c,d,e] Mean difference (Student's t test): c versus e, p<0.05; d versus e, p<0.02; c versus d, not significant.

Among the causes which could account for a lower amount of receptor measured by cytoplasmic assay a major factor may be the release of factor(s) that partially inactivate the cytoplasmic receptor. In fact, previous data (Marchetti et al. 1981) have shown that the receptor binding capacity in cytoplasm from certain types of leukemia decreased rather rapidly, in less than 3h, suggesting that substances capable of inactivating the receptor molecule – probably enzymes – are active in these cells. Going by these and other similar observations (Crabtree et al.1978), our present opinion is that receptor assessments by cytoplasmic and whole-cell assays give non equivalent information and that one should not rely on one of these procedures alone, at least not until their precise clinical significance has been understood.

Glucocorticoid Receptor and Steroid Sensitivity of Human Leukemic Cells

It has long been known that glucocorticoids exert a widespread suppressive effect on lymphatic cells of many species. These effects, which in sensitive species result in cell lysis, form the basis for the use of glucocorticoids in the treatment of lymphoid cell neoplasias. As in other endocrine-related tumors, primarily breast cancer, it would

be undoubtedly of advantage to know in advance if a given
patient is sensitive to steroid therapy. In the case of
acute lymphoblastic leukemia, glucocorticoids have been a
valid therapeutic regimen for more than twenty years, first
alone and now in combination chemotherapy. Because of the
frequent and marked side-effects of glucocorticoid therapy,
along with the above-mentioned concept that clones of steroid
resistant cells may arise in some patients, various studies
have been devoted to relating glucocorticoid receptors to in
vitro steroid sensitivity (Crabtree et al. 1979, Ho et al.
1981, Kontula et al. 1980, Iacobelli et al. 1978, Homo et al.
1980). These studies have shown that the levels of glucocorticoid receptors were not correlated with any of the parameters of in vitro steroid sensitivity such as protein and DNA
synthesis or even cell lysis. On the other hand, at least
two groups - one working on acute lymphoblastic leukemia
(Mastrangelo et al. 1980) and the other on non-Hodgkin
lymphoma (Bloomfield et al. 1980) - established a positive
correlation between glucocorticoid receptors and short-term
response to glucocorticoids in vivo. Moreover, sequential
analysis of glucocorticoid receptors at diagnosis and at
relapse showed a decreased density of receptors after
treatment.

Glucocorticoid Receptors, Response to Polychemotherapy and
Prognosis

Although glucocorticoid receptors have now been
determined by several groups in approximately 250 patients
with acute lymphoblastic leukemia, attempts to correlate
the amount of receptors with response to polychemotherapy
and prognosis have been reported by only one group. As
mentioned above, using cytosol assay it was shown that the
lymphoblasts of twenty-two patients with previously untreated
acute lymphoblastic leukemia and those of six patients in
relapse but still responsive to treatment contained high
levels of glucocorticoid receptors while the cells of six
other patients no longer responding had barely detectable
receptor levels (Lippman et al.1973). Some years later the
same group (Lippman et al. 1978) reported that of forty-five
children with acute lymphoblastic leukemia those with
lymphoblasts containing more than 6,000 receptor sites/cell
had a longer remission duration and survival than those with
cells having less than 6,000 sites/cell. In 1978 we began a
prospective study on glucocorticoid receptors as indicators

of response to polychemotherapy and prognosis in acute
lymphoblastic leukemia. To date eighty-one patients with
previously untreated acute lymphoblastic leukemia have
entered the study. Seventy-one of these patients were found
to be evaluable. All patients received a four-drug combination
chemotherapy consisting of vincristine, methotrexate,
mercaptopurine and prednisone.

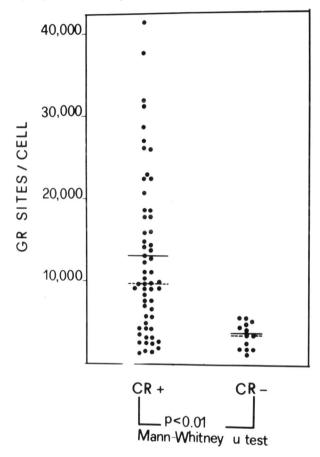

Fig. 2. Distribution of patients achieving (CR+) or not
(CR-) complete remission according to the number of
glucocorticoid receptors in lymphoblasts. Methodological
details are given in Iacobelli et al. 1981.

Of 71 patients treated, 58 achieved complete remission and 13 did not. Responders and non-responders to polychemotherapy did not differ significantly as regards sex, age, initial WBC, immunologic phenotype, presence of organomegalia, etc. As shown in Fig. 2, glucocorticoid receptors were significantly higher in patients achieving complete remission after induction polychemotherapy than in patients refractory to treatment ($p<0.01$). Moreover, patients with lymphoblasts containing more than 6,000 glucocorticoid receptor sites/cell, with only two exceptions, experienced complete remission (Table III). It is also evident that not all patients with lymphoblasts containing less than 6,000 sites/cell did not respond to therapy. The density of glucocorticoid receptor in leukemic cells appeared to be independent of the initial WBC, sex, age, Null, T or B phenotype and FAB classification.

Table III. Distribution of patients achieving or not complete remission (CR) as a function of the number of glucocorticoid receptors in lymphoblasts (less or more than 6,000 sites/cell)

GR (sites/cell)	CR+	CR−
<6,000	18	11
>6,000	40	2

Only newly diagnosed patients were included in the study

x^2 test, p<0.01

The relationship between remission duration and survival and glucocorticoid receptor content was also examined. These analyses were done in a highly homogeneous group of patients with null-cell leukemia (Fig.3). Although the actuarial curves did not reach a statistically significant difference in patients with lymphoblasts with more or less than 6,000 sites/cell, there was a clear trend towards a correlation between receptor density and remission duration in favour of patients with the higher receptor level ($p<0.06$).

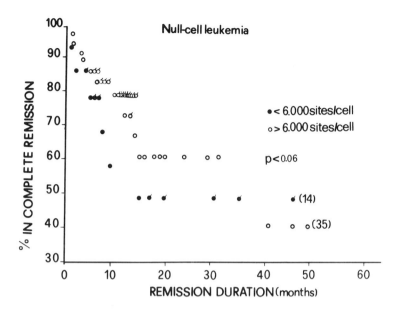

Fig. 3. Remission duration in patients with Null-cell
leukemia with respect to the number of glucocorticoid
receptors in lymphoblasts (less or more than 6,000 sites/
cell).

Finally, Fig. 4 shows that glucocorticoid receptor
measurement may provide valid information on patient survival.
Patients with lymphoblasts having more than 6,000 sites/cell
have a significantly longer survival than patients with
lymphoblasts containing less than 6,000 sites/cell (p<0.05).

Taken together these results support and extend
previous findings that glucocorticoid receptor measurement
in acute lymphoblastic leukemia may supply useful information
to distinguish those patients who are sensitive to
glucocorticoid therapy and those who respond to polychemotherapy. In addition they show that the presence of glucocorticoid receptor in leukemic cells is a biological-biochemical

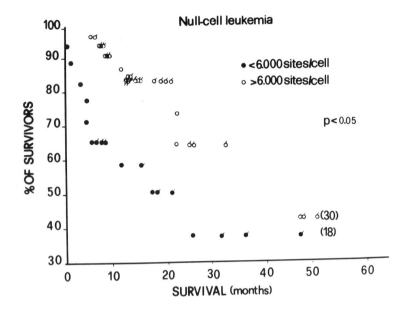

Fig. 4. Survival duration in patients with Null-cell leukemia with respect to the number of glucocorticoid receptors in lymphoblasts (less or more than 6,000 sites/ cell).

marker with prognostic significance. Further clinical trials on therapeutic procedures for acute lymphoblastic leukemia based on glucocorticoid receptor density in the cells are called for in order to establish whether or not glucocorticoids should be employed and a more or less aggressive form of treatment be adopted.

Beatson GT (1896). On the treatment of inoperable cases of carcinoma of the mamma: Suggestions for a new method of treatment, with illustrative cases. Lancet 2:104; 162.

Bloomfield CD, Smith KA, Peterson BA, Hildebrandt L, Zaleskas J, Gajl-Peczalska KJ, Frizzera G, Munck A (1980). In vitro glucocorticoid studies for predicting response to glucocorticoid therapy in adults with malignant lymphoma. Lancet 1:952.

Crabtree GR, Smith KA, Munck A (1978). Glucocorticoid
receptors and sensitivity of isolated human leukemia and
lymphoma cells. Cancer Res. 38:4268.

Crabtree GR, Smith KA, Munck A (1979). Glucocorticoid
receptors and in vitro sensitivity of cells from patients
with leukemia and lymphoma: a reassessment. In Bell PA,
Borthwick NM (eds.): "Glucocorticoid Action and Leukemias",
Seventh Tenovus Workshop, Alpha Omega Publishing Ltd,
Cardiff, p 191.

Galaini S, Minowada J, Silvernail P, Nussbaum A, Kaiser N,
Rosen F, Shimaoka K (1973). Specific glucocorticoid
binding in human hemopoietic cell lines and neoplastic
tissue. Cancer Res. 33:2653.

Ho AD, Hynstein W, Schmid W (1981). Glucocorticoid receptors
and sensitivity in leukemias. Blut 42:183.

Homo F, Duval D, Harousseau JL, Marie JP, Zittoun R (1980).
Heterogeneity of the in vitro responses to glucocorticoids
in acute leukemia. Cancer Res. 40:2601.

Iacobelli S, Ranelletti FO, Longo P, Riccardi R, Mastrangelo
R (1978). Discrepancies between in vivo and in vitro effects
of glucocorticoids in myelomonocytic leukemic cells.
Cancer Res. 38:4257.

Iacobelli S, King R.j.B., Lindner HR, Lippman ME (1980).
"Hormones and Cancer". New York: Raven Press.

Iacobelli S, Natoli V, Longo P, Ranelletti FO, De Rossi G,
Pasqualetti D, Mandelli F, Mastrangelo R (1981).
Glucocorticoid receptor determinations in leukemia patients
using cytosol and whole-cell assays. Cancer Res. 41:3979.

Kontula K, Andersson LC, Paavonen T, Myllyla G, Teerenhovi L,
Vuopio P (1980). Glucocorticoid receptors and glucocorticoid
sensitivity of human leukemic cells. Int. J. Cancer 26:177.

Lippman ME, Halterman R, Perry S, Leventhal B, Thompson E
(1973). Glucocorticoid binding proteins in human leukaemic
lymphoblasts. Natl. New Biol. 242:157.

Lippman ME, Yarbro GK, Leventhal BG (1978). Clinical
implications of glucocorticoid receptors in human leukemia.
Cancer Res. 38:4251.

Marchetti P, Natoli V, Ranelletti FO, Mandelli F, De Rossi
G, Iacobelli S (1981). Glucocorticoid receptor studies
in human leukemia. J. Steroid Biochem. 15:261.

Mastrangelo R, Malandrino R, Riccardi R, Longo P, Ranelletti
FO, Iacobelli S (1980). Clinical implications of
glucocorticoid receptor studies in childhood acute
lymphoblastic leukemia. Blood 56:1036.

Sloman PA, Bell PV (1980). L.J. de Asua, R. Levi-Montalcini,

R. Shields, S. Iacobelli (eds): "Control Mechanism in Animal cells", Raven Press, New York.

Terenius L, Simonsson B, Nilsson K (1976). Glucocorticoid receptors, DNA-synthesis, membrane antigens and their relation to disease activity in chronic lymphatic leukemia. J. Steroid Biochem. 7:905.

Hormones and Cancer, pages 247–259

ANDROGEN RECEPTOR ASSAY IN SMALL BIOPSIES OF HUMAN
PROSTATE. PRESERVATION OF NUCLEAR RECEPTOR FROM RAT
VENTRAL PROSTATE BY LYOPHILIZATION

Marie-Anne de Larminat[*], Carlos Scorticati[**],
Paul S. Rennie['] and Nicholas Bruchovsky['].
*Inst.Biol.y Med.Exp.,**Inst.Oncología Angel
Roffo,Buenos Aires, Argentina,'Cancer Control
Agency of B.C., Vancouver, Canada.

INTRODUCTION

Endocrine therapy is a valuable approach for the
treatment of prostatic carcinoma. In the advanced phases
of the disease, or when radical prostatectomy is not
advisable, orchidectomy, or administration of estrogen
and/or antiandrogens have proved to have a beneficial,
although temporary effect.

Since the probability of response to endocrine
therapy is relatively high amongst patients (60--80%),
(Bruchovsky, et al., 1980), a previous screening for
responsiveness through the detection of androgen receptor might not be essential. However, a negative receptor
test would direct the clinician to start without delay
another type of effective therapy, also avoiding side
effects and psychological impact caused by endrocrine
treatment. Furthermore, periodical tests in an initially responsive (receptor- +) subject will indicate when
the tumour becomes autonomous and thus the administration of hormones or antihormones ineffective.

It seems therefore important to determine androgen
receptor levels in the neoplastic prostate. However, in
this gland, where the available tissue is scarce, there
are several technical obstacles to overcome in order to
obtain a reliable receptor assay. The more serious
amongst these are: the lability of receptor protein, the
interference of both extracellular and intracellular
steroid-binding components (namely sex hormone binding
globulin and progesterone receptor), and the masking of
the sites by endogenous hormones.

Considering this, we have developed a technique which overcomes (or at least minimizes) the aforementio ned problems, and is suitable for the determination of androgen (and also estrogen or progesterone) receptors, in samples obtained from human prostates through needle biopsies, i.e., as small as 50 mg.

A stabilizing agent was included in the homogeniza tion buffer (Sirett and Grant, 1982) and endogenously bound hormone-receptor complexes were dissociated chemi cally prior to the assay, which consisted in the incuba tion of cytosols and nuclear extracts with ^{3}H - R-1881 plus an excess of triamcinolone acetonide.

The possibility of obtaining more stable forms of nuclear receptors was also investigated in another series of experiments. Extraction of purified nuclei from rat ventral prostate with the volatile buffer ammonium bicar bonate, followed by lyophilization, did not alter the characteristics of androgen receptor, and delayed consi derably its time-dependent inactivation.

EXPERIMENTAL PROCEDURES

A) Human Prostates

TISSUES: Samples were obtained from three different sources. From those patients affected with adenocarcino ma of the prostate, needle biopsies (50-100 mg) were ta ken at the time of histopathological examination,rinsed with homogenization buffer, transported on ice to the laboratory and stored within one hour at -70ºC. Hyperplastic tissue was obtained at the time of open surgery and treated similarly. Normal tissue was taken from two patients with cancer of the bladder and from a case of surgery after a severe accident. The average age was 70 for carcinoma (Ca), 67 for benign hyperplasia (BPH) and 44 for normal prostate (N). Processing of sam ples were performed between 1 and 4 weeks after obten tion. Only those patients lacking previous hormone the- rapy were selected.

HOMOGENIZATION PROCEDURES

All procedures were carried out at 0-4ºC. After thawing, prostate specimens were rinsed,blotted, weighed and finely minced with scissors. Homogenization was performed with a Polytron (3x10'' strokes at speed 5) in about 20 vol. of a Buffer made of 50 mM Tris pH 7.4 containing 0.25 M Sucrose, 1.5 mM EDTA, 10mM Na_2Mo O_4, 10% Glycerol (v/v) and 0.05% NaN_3. After filtering through nylon mesh, the homogenate was centrifuged at 800xg for 20 min. yielding a nuclear pellet and a supernatant. The latter was centrifuged at 105,000xg for one hour to obtain the cytosol, while the first pellet was re-suspended with homogenization buffer and recentrifuged at 800xg to yield a pellet of washed nuclei.

PRE-TREATMENT OF CYTOSOLS

In order to displace endogenously bound hormone from receptor sites prior to the assay, samples were treated with the mercurial reagent Mersalyl (Sigma Chemical Co. Missouri) (Coty, 1980; Traish, et al., 1981, De Larminat,et al., 1983).
After measuring cytosol volumes, aliquots were saved for protein determination, and fractions were added with Mersalyl (10mM solution, dissolved in .6M NaCl) to a final concentration of 0.1 mM of the reagent. Reaction was allowed to proceed over ice for exactly 30 min.,and was then stopped through the addition of an excess (25mM final conc.) sulfhydryl-reducing compound 2-Mercaptoethanol or DTT . This leads to inactivation of the mercurial and regeneration of the receptor,which is now depleted from its steroid ligand and can be incubated with the radioactive tracer.

INCUBATION WITH ^{3}H R_{1881}

200 ul cytosol aliquots were incubated with 10 nM ^{3}H-R_{1881} (New England Nuclear) in the presence of a 500 fold excess Triamcinolone Acetonide (to eliminate the interference of progesterone receptors present in human prostate); duplicate samples were also added with 500x Cyproterone Acetate, in order to evaluate non-specific binding. Incubation was carried out at 4ºC for 16 h. Bound ^{3}H-R_{1881} was separated from free ligand through Dextran Coated Charcoal absorption method (Tezón, et al. 1982). To each 200 ul sample, one volume charcoal-dextran 1%:.5% in homogenization buffer was added, at 4ºC. After incubation for 10 min. T-70 with vortexing every 2 min., tubes were centrifuged at 1000xg for 10 min. 150 ul aliquots were taken by duplicate and counted in Omnifluor (4g/liter) Toluene-Triton X-114 (7:3 v/v)

solution. Results were calculated as fmoles bound/mg pro
tein and pmoles/g tissue.

ASSAY OF RECEPTOR IN NUCLEAR FRACTIONS

Washed nuclei were added with 500 ul of a hypotonic buf
fer 2 (1mM Tris pH 8,0.1mM CaCl$_2$, 1mM DTT, 20 mM NaCl,
1.5 mM EDTA). After incubating for 30 min. over ice,the
suspension was sonicated (3x5'', setting 40), then added
with 500 ul Extraction Buffer (20 mM Tris, pH 7.4, 1.2M
NaCl, 10 mM MgCl$_2$, 1.5 mM EDTA, 1mM DTT) and sonicated
again. After 30 min. over ice, the samples were centrifuged at 12,000 g for 30 min. Supernatant was decanted
and used for receptor binding assay.
The conditions for the incubation were the same as for
the cytosol samples, except that the radioactive ligand
was 20 nM ^{3}H-R$_{1881}$. When pre-treatment of nuclear
extracts was performed, the time of incubation was only
15 min. and both hypotonic and extraction buffers did
not contain any sulfhydryl reducing compound (DTT).
After 20 h. incubation, samples were analyzed through
5 ml G-25 Sephadex columns (Pharmacia Chem., Upsala,
Sweden), equilibrated with 0.6M NaCl extraction buffer.
Bound radioactivity was recovered in the void volume and
counted as stated before. Results were expressed as
fmoles/mg protein in the nuclear extract and as pmoles/
g tissue. Total receptor content of a sample was the sum
of cytosol and nuclear specific binding, expressed as
pmoles/g tissue.

B) Rat Ventral Prostate

OBTENTION OF NUCLEAR EXTRACTS

The experimental procedure has been described in detail
by de Larminat et al, 1981.
Briefly, nuclei from rat ventral prostate were purified
through a discontinuous sucrose gradient, then sonicated
in a hypotonic medium, and digested partially with micro
coccal nuclease. Extraction of the particulate fraction
was performed sequentially with volatile 0.6 M and 1.2M
NH$_4$HCO$_3$ buffer, containing also 5 mM MgCl$_2$, 1.5 mM EDTA,
and 1 mM mercaptoethanol. Salt extracted samples were
then lyophilized and the resultant powdery residue containing androgen nuclear receptor was stored at -80ºC.

RECONSTITUTION OF THE LYOPHILIZED EXTRACTS AND ASSAY OF

NUCLEAR RECEPTOR

Lyophilized extracts from rat prostate nuclei were dis
solved in a small volume (0.2-1.2 ml) of extraction
buffer. The sample was then equilibrated for 30 min.
before being processed further.
To measure receptor, the reconstituted samples were
incubated with 20 nM ^{3}H-R1881 for 16-20 h at 4°C. After
incubation, the samples were analyzed by gel-exclusion
chromatography in a G-25 - G-100 Sephadex dual column
system, equilibrated with extraction buffer; 0.5 ml
fractions were collected automatically and counted.
Duplicate samples containing a 1000 fold excess non radioactive steroid were analyzed in parallel with the
above. The amount of non specific binding was calculated
as the difference between the total and non-specific
binding in the receptor containing fractions (17-33).
In these conditions, non-specific binding was found to
be minimal.

RESULTS AND DISCUSSION

A) Effect of mersalyl on the recovery of cytosol and
   salt extracted androgen receptor from human prostate.

The properties of the organomercurial compound mersalyl
had been previously described by Coty (1980) and Traish
et al 1981.
Sulfhydryl groups present in steroid receptor molecules,
which are apparently essential for the integrity of the
binding site (Jensen et al., 1967; Rice et al., 1982;
Coty 1980), react reversibly with mersalyl displacing
at the same time any pre-existing steroid ligand.
Through the addition of an excess sulfhydryl reducing
compounds, the mercurial can then be inactivated and the
SH groups of the receptor regenerated, allowing formation of new hormone-receptor complexes.
It seemed therefore of interest to try mersalyl as a dis
sociating agent, in order to unmask endogenously bound
sites of receptor that might cause underestimation of
the detectable levels in human prostate.

The effect of pretreatment of cytosol and nuclear extract
with 0.1 mM mersalyl for 30 min. and 15 min. respective
ly before the exchange assay is shown in TABLE 1.

Table 1 . EFFECT OF MERSALYL ON THE DETECTION OF ANDRO-
GEN RECEPTOR SITES

FRACTION	% of control[*] $\pm$ SE	(N)	Statistical analysis
CYTOSOL	202 $\pm$ 18	(7)	p< 0.005
NUCLEAR EXTRACT	33 $\pm$ 13	(5)	p< 0.005

*Data are expressed as percentage of receptor (pmoles/
g of tissue) found in controls from each subcellular
fraction.
Controls: Samples not treated with mersalyl prior to
the binding assay.

The recovery of measurable sites was greatly enhanced
in cytosol fractions (102% increase); it was therefore
decided to incubate all these fractions with mersalyl
prior to the receptor binding assay. It is worth noting
that the positive effect of this treatment was detected
even when the incubation with ^{3}H-R1881 was made in the
presence of both the inactivated mercurial and the free
endogenous hormone.
In the case of salt-extracted receptor, the chemical dis
sociation of hormone receptor complexes with mersalyl
lead to a different result, i.e., to a significant reduc
tion in the detectable binding sites. For that reason,
this step was omitted in further experiments. It might
be noted, however, that the specimens analyzed had been
stored for about three weeks at -70ºC before being processed. It is a known fact that the nuclear form of
androgen receptor obtained through salt extraction is
labile, especially after storage of tissue in the frozen
state, and that sodium molybdate lacks any stabilizing
effect on this form (de Larminat et al., 1981; Sirett and
Grant, 1982) contrary to what has been widely observed
with respect to cytosol receptor Therefore increased
instability of nuclear receptor might affect the revesi
bility of the reaction with mersalyl and explain the
lower recovery of the sites found in that case.
Moreover, when nuclear receptor from a fresh tissue sample was analyzed, the adverse effect of pre-incubation

with mersalyl disappeared, although no significant impro
vement in the recovery of binding sites could be detected in the experimental conditions used here.

B) Applicability of the technique to the determination
of androgen receptor in Normal, Hyperplastic and Ade-
no-Carcinomatous Prostate.

Using the experimental conditions described before, including a pre-incubation of cytosols with mersalyl, we
have determined total androgen receptor levels in small
prostatic biopsies from three different groups of patients.
Data from Normal, Hyperplastic and Carcinomatous tissues
are presented in TABLE 2.

Table 2. TOTAL ANDROGEN RECEPTOR LEVELS IN BIOPSIES FROM
HUMAN PROSTATE

Sample	Receptor levels (pmoles/g of tissue $\pm$ SE)	N
NORMAL	7.38 ± 1.47	3
HYPERPLASIA	2.03 ± 0.55 *	6
CARCINOMA	3.42 ± 0.80 *	15

*$p < 0.025$ with respect to NORMAL

Both hyperplasia and carcinoma values are significantly
lower than normal, although no statistical difference
was found between carcinoma and hyperplasia. The values,
when expressed in fmoles/mg protein ranged between 35-
250 for the cytosols, and between 200-600 for the nuclear
extracts.

The receptor found in the salt extracted fractions
amounted to about 30-50% of the total binding sites,but
had a tendency to decrease when tissue specimens had
been stored for long times (10% after 2 months storage).
In that respect, no differences were found in cytosol

receptors.

We can conclude from these studies that the method is
suitable for determining androgen receptors in prostatic needle biopsies; it is sensitive enough as for detecting differences between various pathologies.
However, it must be stressed that for screening purposes,
a careful histological analysis has been recommended
when using this type of biopsies, since cell heterogeneity in the specimens (for example stromal or hyperplas
tic components adjacent to neoplastic tissue) may cause
artifactic results concerning the potential of response
of the carcinoma to endocrine therapy.

C) Concentration and preservation or nuclear androgen
   receptor by lyophylisation.

Since the biological action of steroid hormones is
known to take place through the interaction of hormone-
receptor complexes with the chromatin, detection of
these entities within the nuclear compartment is of
great physiological importance.
Unfortunately, an important loss of nuclear binding sites occur during the storage of frozen tissue (from both
rat and human samples), rendering their detection somewhat unreliable.
Awaiting for widespread availability of the newly developed immunocytochemical techniques based on the use of
monoclonal antibodies to receptors we have explored the
possibilities of obtaining more stable forms of nuclear
androgen receptor through lyophilisation of salt extracts.
Although the experiments described here were performed
with rat prostate nuclei, it is hoped they may also be
applied to human samples.

C.1 - Extraction of nuclear androgen receptor with 0.6M-
      1.2 M ammonium bicarbonate

Extraction of purified nuclei from rat ventral prostate
was performed with ammonium bicarbonate buffer, which
can then be volatilized through freeze-drying. The reco
very of nuclear androgen receptor after extraction with
NH_4HCO_3 was compared with that of samples extracted with
the usual 0.6 M NaCl buffer.
No differences were found in the specific binding, as
it is shown in TABLE 3. Moreover, the use of 0.6 M NH_4

HCO₃ as equilibrating buffer in the Sephadex columns
did not alter the recovery or the elution profile of the
bound fraction (FIGURE 1 A).

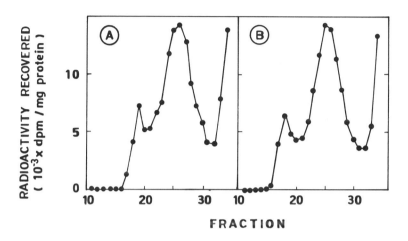

FIGURE 1. Lyophilization of androgen nuclear receptor.

Data were taken from Reference 3, with permission.

C.2 - Effect of Lyophilization

After reconstitution of a lyophilized extract with 0.6M
NH₄HCO₃ buffer and its incubation with 20 nM ³H-R1881
for 16-20 hours at 4ºC, the specific binding was analyz
ed by gel exclusion chromatography. The resulting profi
le is shown in FIGURE 1 B.
Since there is no change in the amount of radioactivity
associated with the void volume peaks (fractions 15-20),
lyophilization does not increase the tendency for agre-
ggation of nuclear androgen receptors.
The stability of the individual peaks of binding activi
ty described in Figure 1 was examined in the following
experiment: After a first lyophilization, a nuclear ex-

Table 3 - EXTRACTION OF NUCLEAR ANDROGEN RECEPTOR WITH
0.6-1.2M NH_4HCO_3

Extraction buffer	Chromatography buffer	No.Exp.	Recovery of Receptor dpm / mg protein
Tes-NaCl	Tes-NaCl	8	112,000 $\pm$ 18,300
NH_4HCO_3	Tes-NaCl	8	111,000 $\pm$ 19,700
NH_4HCO_3	NH_4HCO_3	15	110,000 $\pm$ 6,600

Data were taken from Reference 3 with permission.

tract was reconstituted with ammonium bicarbonate buffer
incubated with ^{3}H-R$_{1881}$, and chromatographed 20h later.

Fig. 2

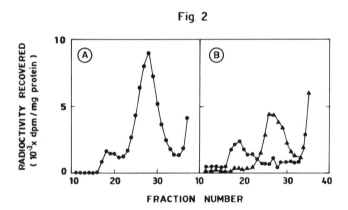

FIGURE II. Stability of Nuclear Androgen Receptor Peaks
after Lyophilization.

The profile of radioactivity is shown in FIGURE II A.
Excluded fractions (17-21) and receptor containing frac
tions (22-33) were pooled and subjected separately to a
second cycle of lyophilization and gel exclusion chroma

tography. The profiles are shown in FIGURE II 8, and
indicate that the identity of each peak is maintained.
The apparent decrease in the recovery of bound fraction
following the second lyophilization is probably due to
a partial dissociation of the steroid-receptor complex
during the procedures.

C.3 - Storage of Lyophilized Extracts

It was important to determine in what extent the time of
storage (at -80ºC) would affect the integrity of the re
ceptor once nuclear extracts had been lyophilized.
FIGURE III shows the recovery of lyophilized nuclear
androgen receptor after different periods of time, rang
ing from 12 hours to 105 days.

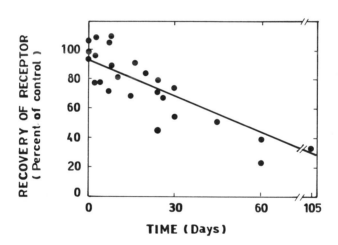

FIGURE III. Effect of time of storage on the recovery
            of androgen receptor.

During the initial 2-3 days, no loss of binding activity
is observed.
Thereafter, a gradual loss of binding takes place, and
was estimated through linear regression analysis (r=0.82)

in 6% per week.

On the other hand, it was observed that the addition of
MgCl$_2$ (5-10mM) and sulfhydryl reducing agents (10mM mer
captoethanol), had a beneficial effect upon recovery of
binding activity, while ammonium molybdate lacked any
effect.

It could be concluded from these experiments that lyophilization of nuclear extracts from rat ventral prosta
te, when obtained using NH$_4$HCO$_3$ buffer, preserves the
binding activity of androgen receptor, and its gross
molecular characteristics. The method appears therefore
suitable for the concentration and storage of nuclear
form of androgen receptor, for either analytical or puri
fication purposes.

REFERENCES

Bruchovsky N, Callaway T, Lieskovsky G, Rennie PS (1980)
    Markers of androgen action in human prostate:Potential
    use in the clinical assessment of prostatic carcinoma.
    In JL Wittliff and O Dapunt (eds): "Steroid Receptors
    and Hormone-Dependent Neoplasia", New York; Masson Pu
    blishing USA Inc p 121.
Coty WA (1980). Reversible dissociation of steroid hor-
    mone-receptor complexes by mercurial reagents. J biol
    Chem 255(1): 8035.
De Larminat MA, Bruchovsky N, Rennie PS (1981). Concen-
    tration and preservation of nuclear androgen receptor
    by lyophilization. J Steroid Biochem 16: 811.
De Larminat MA, Bruchovsky N, Rennie PS Sing Ping Lee,
    Tertzakian G (1983). Synthesis and evaluation of immo
    bilized androgens for affinity chromatography in the
    purification of nuclear androgen receptor.(Submitted).
Jensen EV, Hurst DJ, De Sombre ER, Jungblut PW (1967).
    Sulfhydryl groups and estradiol receptor interaction.
    Science 158: 385.
Rice RG, Madray S, Rocchio R, Vaughn CB (1982). The
    effect of dithiothreitol on the estrogen receptor.
    Anticancer Res 2: 141.
Sirett DAN, Grant JK (1982). Effect of sodium molybdate
    on the interaction of androgens and progestins with
    binding proteins in human hyperplastic prostatic
    tissue. J Endocrinol 92: 95.
Tezón JT, Vazquez MH, Blaquier JA (1982). Androgen-con

trolled subcellular distribution of its receptor in the rat epididymis: 5α -dihydrotestosterone-induced translocation is blocked by antiandrogens. Endocrinology 111: 2039.

Traish AM, Muller RE, Wotiz HH (1981). A new procedure for the quantitation of nuclear and cytoplasmic andro gen receptors. J biol Chem 256 (23): 12028.

Hormones and Cancer, pages 261–290

STUDIES ON STEROID RECEPTORS IN HUMAN AND RABBIT SKELETAL
MUSCLE - CLUES TO THE UNDERSTANDING OF THE MECHANISM OF
ACTION OF ANABOLIC STEROIDS

Jan-Åke Gustafsson[1], Tönu Saartok[1,2], Erik Dahlberg[1],
Marek Snochowski[1,3], Tom Häggmark[2] and Ejnar Eriksson[2]

[1]Department of Medical Nutrition, Karolinska Institute,
Huddinge University Hospital F69, S-141 86 Huddinge,
[2]Department of Surgery, Section of Trauma, Karolinska
Hospital, Box 60500, S-104 01 Stockholm, Sweden and
[3]Institute of Animal Physiology and Nutrition, Polish
Academy of Sciences, 05-110 Jablonna-near-Warsaw, Poland

SUMMARY

The mechanism of action of steroid hormones in target
tissues include the binding of the steroid molecule to
specific receptors in the cytoplasm. Steroid receptors may
therefore be regarded as mediators of hormone action. The
presence of such receptors in tissues reflects their hormone-
sensitivity and the receptor levels are indicative of the
relative potential for a direct hormonal action on the
tissue in question.

Using ^{3}H-labeled synthetic ligands and a charcoal
adsorption assay, the presence of specific androgen, glucocorticoid and estrogen (in rabbits only) receptors was
demonstrated in human and rabbit skeletal muscle cytosol.
These tissues can therefore be regarded as targets for these
steroids. Scatchard analysis was then used to quantitate the
receptors in muscle in different conditions.

In back muscle of scoliotic patients, the concentrations of androgen and glucocorticoid receptors were
similar on the convex and concave sides, except the concentration of glucocorticoid receptors (per g of wet weight),
which was higher on the convex side.

The tissue concentration (per g of wet weight) of glucocorticoid and estrogen receptors (but not of androgen receptor) was higher in rabbit soleus (slow-twitch) muscle than in the gastrocnemius/plantaris (fast-twitch) muscle complex. When the concentrations were related to the number of nuclei (i.e. expressed per mg of DNA), however, only the estrogen receptor concentration differed between the muscles (higher in soleus).

Muscle atrophy in rabbit gastrocnemius muscle was induced by tenotomy or denervation and led to similar changes with an increase with time in androgen and gluco-corticoid receptor levels (expressed per g of wet weight or per mg of protein) and a concomitant loss of muscle weight and protein. The total muscle content of receptors or the receptor concentration expressed per mg of DNA were also increased, but to a lesser extent.

Synthetic anabolic-androgenic steroids can act directly on skeletal muscle in view of their capacity to bind to the androgen receptor as shown in the present study. Relative binding affinities of anabolic-androgenic steroids to the androgen receptor were similar in rabbit and rat skeletal muscle and in rat prostate.

The protein/DNA ratio in the muscle samples was used as an estimation of the size of the "functional DNA-unit". The results indicate that slow-twitch fibers have smaller "DNA units", but also that muscle atrophy causes a decrease of the size of the "DNA unit".

In view of these findings, human and rabbit skeletal muscle may be added to known target tissues for androgens, glucocorticoids, and (in rabbits) estrogens. Due to the presence of specific cytosolic receptors for these hormones, human and rabbit skeletal muscle has the potential to respond directly to the hormones in question.

INTRODUCTION

In several physiological conditions as well as in clinical practice, the effects of steroid hormones on skeletal muscle are of major importance. Not until puberty is the difference between the musculature in males and females clearly visible. Pathologically increased or decreased levels of steroid hormones are in many cases linked with changes in skeletal muscle. Medical treatment with steroid hormones can give undesired effects from skeletal muscle.

During the past 20 years the mechanism of action of steroid hormones has become increasingly better understood at the molecular level. Biochemical methods have been developed providing possibilities to study the interaction of steroid hormones with skeletal muscle. A deeper knowledge of this interaction could provide a key for a better understanding of steroid influence on skeletal muscle in states of muscle anabolism or catabolism and atrophy. Increased knowledge in this field could result in an optimation of steroid treatment in clinical practice. This study was undertaken in an attempt to contribute to the knowledge in this area.

Steroid Hormones and Skeletal Muscle

Hormones are secreted from endocrine glands as "chemical messengers" and participate in the regulation of various metabolic processes throughout the body. In the blood the major part of the steroids is transported reversibly bound to plasma proteins, e.g. sex-hormone-binding globulin (SHBG), corticosteroid-binding globulin (CBG) and albumin (Westphal 1971, Andersson 1974, Wagner 1978). Only the relatively small free fraction of steroids in the blood is considered to be biologically active (Catt et al 1981). Changes in the binding capacity of the hormone-binding proteins in blood, accomplished e.g. by the introduction of exogenous steroids or drugs, may lead to alterations in the amount of circulating biologically active hormone (Dunn et al 1981, Pugeat et al 1981). Other important factors participating in the regulation of the active steroid fraction in blood are the rates of steroid metabolism and excretion (Westphal 1971, Wagner 1978, Siiteri et al 1982).

The basic common function of all skeletal muscle is to contract in order to create movement. With respect to contractile and metabolic properties, the cells (fibers) of skeletal muscle in all mammals, including man, can be divided into different types, with different biochemical, metabolic and functional properties (Peter et al 1972, Saltin et al 1977, Barnard et al 1971). In most classifications at least two types of muscle cells are separated according to contraction time and metabolic characteristics (Dubowitz & Brooke 1973, Peter et al 1972). All individual muscles in man are mixed with regard to the distribution of fiber types (Johnson et al 1973), but some muscles in other species consist almost exclusively of one type of fiber (Peter et al 1972, Ariano et al 1973, Wåhlby et al 1978). Several individual muscles with differing relative proportions of fiber types as well as of number and size of fibers have been extensively studied over the years. Changes in muscle due to various types of exercise, immobilization and disuse, aging and various other physiological or pathological conditions have been reported in a vast number of publications. Protein-anabolic effects in skeletal muscle are indicated morphologically by hypertrophy (i.e. increase in size) of fibers in cross-section preparations, whereas a decrease of the cross-section area of the fibers (hypotrophy) indicates protein-catabolic effects. An increase (hyperplasia) or a decrease (hypoplasia) in number of fibers have been less well investigated. This is also true for changes in the length (i.e the number of sarcomeres in a row) of a muscle fiber. Thus, estimations of fiber diameters or areas only partially describe the changes in muscle or fiber mass. Protein synthesis in skeletal muscle can be studied by uptake and incorporation of radiolabeled amino acids, whereas the protein degradation is more difficult to study directly (Millward & Waterlow 1978). Other methods used to study the anabolic or catabolic actions in skeletal muscle include nitrogen-retention studies (see Krüskemper 1968, Kochakian 1976), excretion of 3-methylhistidine (Young & Munro 1978) and antropometric measurements (Heymsfield et al 1982).

The effects of steroid hormones upon skeletal muscle have been recognized clinically since a long time (see e.g. Frohman et al 1981). The changes in muscle composition occurring at puberty as well as the difference in musculature between males and females suggest a relationship between sex steroids and skeletal muscle. Hypersecretion of steroid hormones from testicular, ovarian or adrenal tumors can lead to enhanced or impaired somatic growth. Castration of males causes changes towards a female phenotype with a less prominent musculature. Catabolic states with increased glucocorticoid production, such as burns, trauma or severe infections, are accompanied by losses in body weight and muscle tissue (Dolecek 1969, Cuthbertsson 1979). In farm animal breeding, treatment with anabolic steroids (anabolic-androgenic compounds and/or estrogens) have been used with the aim to increase the efficiency of meat production (Lu & Rendel 1975, Heitzman 1979, Jasiorowski 1982).

Androgens cause growth of several tissues including skeletal muscle, and lead to an increased nitrogen retention in parallel with an increased body weight (Kochakian 1964, 1976). In clinical practice today, however, the indication for androgen treatment is limited mainly to replacement therapy of hypogonadal men (Wilson & Griffin 1980). Androgens and anabolic steroids have also been tried as therapy in several other conditions, such as malnutrition (especially protein malnutrition), diseases of the skeleton and musculature, and diseases of kidney, liver, blood etc. (Krüskemper 1968). Attempts have been made to reverse the increased protein catabolism in burns (Doleček 1969) or trauma using treatment with anabolic steroids (Tweedle et al 1973, Michelsen et al 1982). Although the results of this therapy have often been beneficial, these indications for therapeutical use have not become generally accepted. "Anabolic-androgenic" steroids are modified androgens synthesized in the search of a molecule that could stimulate protein synthesis in extragenital tissues (e.g. skeletal muscle) without or with only minor masculinizing effects, e.g. in the accessory sex organs. Androgens increase the incorporation of amino acids into muscle protein in vitro (Nowak 1957, Breuer & Florini 1965, Buresová & Gutmann 1971), and stimulate the RNA-synthesis in this tissue (Rogozkin 1979a,b). Besides their effects on protein turnover, androgens also regulate e.g. the metabolism of glycogen in muscle (Ciccoli & Bergamini 1974, Chainy & Kanungo 1978, Lamb 1975), modify the neural action at the neuromuscular junction (Hanzliková & Gutmann 1978) etc.

In addition to their effects on carbohydrate and energy metabolism, glucocorticoids are considered to be the main protein catabolic hormones in skeletal muscle (Thompson & Lippman 1974, Ramey 1975, Baxter 1976). Muscle wasting is a well-recognized clinical feature of glucocorticoid excess,

occurring during pathological (Cushing 1932, Nelson 1979) or
iatrogenical conditions (Faludi et al 1964, David et al
1970, Tyrell & Baxter 1981), or as a "stress" reaction in
other clinical states, such as burns (Doleček 1969), trauma
(Hume & Egdahl 1959, Wilmore et al 1976, Cuthbertson 1979),
surgery (Hume et al 1962) or in critically ill patients
(Dahn & Lange 1982). The net protein catabolism due to
glucocorticoids is accomplished in a complex way by changes
in both protein synthesis and breakdown (Young & Munro 1978,
Tomas et al 1979). In endogenous glucocorticoid excess, as
in Cushing´s syndrome (see e.g. Nelson 1979), the proximal
muscles of the lower extremity (i.e. pelvic girdle muscles)
seem to be most profoundly affected by weakness and signs of
myopathy (Müller & Kugelberg 1959). In experimentally
accomplished excess of glucocorticoids (Afifi & Bergman
1969), in particular the fast-twitch (white, phasic, type
II) (Peter et al 1972, Dubowitz & Brooke 1973) muscle fibers
seem to be affected, and develop the most severe myopathic
changes (Smith 1964, Clark & Vignos Jr. 1979). The mechanism
of glucocorticoid-induced catabolism in skeletal muscle has
been suggested to be a reduced uptake of amino acids into
the muscle cells (Kostyo 1965), inhibition of amino acid
incorporation into proteins (Shoji & Pennington 1977b) or
increased activity of proteolytic enzymes (e.g. Mayer et al
1976). A direct effect of glucocorticoids on skeletal muscle
tissue has been indicated by in vitro studies on the regulation of uptake of radiolabeled amino acids (Tomas et al
1979, McGrath & Goldspink 1982, Odedra & Millward 1982).

The effects of estrogen on skeletal muscle have been
studied less extensively. Estrogens have for long time been
used as anabolics in meat production with the purpose to
increase the carcass weight of the animals and the efficiency
of food utilization (Lu & Rendel 1975, Heitzman 1979). The
differences in musculature between males, females and
castrates are well-recognized. Estrogens can act indirectly
by influencing the levels of androgens and glucocorticoids
(Peterson et al 1960) as well as of other anabolic hormones
such as growth hormone (Mode et al 1982). However, a direct
action of estrogens on skeletal muscle was suggested by the
uptake of these steroids in skeletal muscle (Larson et al
1972).

The influence of progestins or mineralocorticoids on
skeletal muscle has been studied very little.

Steroid Hormone Receptors

It is now widely accepted that the effect of a steroid hormone in a target cell is initiated by the binding of the steroid molecule to a specific receptor protein in the cytoplasm. The steroid-receptor complex then enters the cell nucleus, where it interacts with the genome. This inter-action results in the synthesis of mRNA which will serve as template for the subsequent protein synthesis on ribosomes. The newly formed proteins can then alter the cellular meta-bolism (for reviews, see e.g. Chan & O'Malley 1978, Chan & Tindall 1981, Grody et al 1982). Hence, steroid receptors are cellular mediators of hormone action.

The presence of an androgen receptor in skeletal muscle was first proposed about 10 years ago (Jung & Baulieu 1972). Since then, several groups have detected, partially character-ized and quantitated the androgen receptor in mammalian skeletal muscle (Michel & Baulieu 1974, Gustafsson & Pousette 1975, Dubé et al 1976, Krieg 1976, Tremblay et al 1977, Snochowski et al 1980, Dahlberg et al 1981, Snochowski et al 1981a). Hence, skeletal muscle can be included among the target tissues for androgens, and a direct effect of these steroids on skeletal muscle can be expected.

Both Ballard et al (1974) and Giannopoulos et al (1974) reported on the presence of a cytosolic glucocorticoid receptor in most tissues including skeletal muscle, of rat and rabbit. Roth (1974) described changes in specific gluco-corticoid binding with age in rat skeletal muscle. Since then several other groups have confirmed the presence of glucocorticoid receptors in skeletal muscle (Mayer et al 1974, Shoji & Pennington 1977a, Snochowski et al 1980, Dahlberg et al 1981, Snochowski et al 1981a).

Recently, a specific estrogen receptor has been identi-fied in skeletal muscle (Dubé et al 1976, Dahlberg 1982a), indicating the possibility of a direct action of estrogens on this tissue. Whether progestins or mineralocorticoids can act directly on skeletal muscle is not clear at the present time. Attempts to identify a progestin receptor in rat skeletal muscle using similar techniques as in studies on e.g. the androgen receptor have not been successful (Snochowski et al 1980).

Steroid Hormones in Sports

Physical exercise causes changes in almost all endocrine systems of the body (Galbo 1981, Galbo 1983, Frey 1982). Intensive training of girls before puberty can delay menarche and cause menstrual dysfunction after puberty (Warren 1980, Baker 1981, Frisch et al 1981). Serum levels of androgens tend to increase early during exercise (probably due to decreased hormone degradation), but with a higher intensity and/or a longer duration of the physical activity testosterone levels decrease and remain low for a prolonged period (Aakvaag 1978, Kuoppasalmi 1981). Plasma cortisol increases during exercise and the hormone levels are related to the intensity of activity (Kuoppasalmi 1981). Hence, the fluctuations in blood levels of androgens and glucocorticoids resemble the changes seen in other situations of stress. Although banned by sport organizations and medical authorities (American College of Sports Medicine 1977, Ljungqvist et al 1982), anabolic steroids are misused by athletes with the purpose to increase muscle mass and strength (Wilson & Griffin 1980, Ryan 1981). Although biochemical studies imply protein-anabolic effects (Krüskemper 1968, Kochakian 1976, Rogozkin 1979b, Hervey et al 1981), the putative beneficial effect of anabolic-androgenic steroids in sports is still unproven (American College of Sports Medicine 1977, Ljungqvist et al 1982).

Scope of the Present investigation

A common characteristic of target tissues for steroid hormones seems to be their content of specific steroid receptors. These receptors are cellular mediators of steroid hormone action. The capacity of a tissue to respond to a particular steroid seems to be dependent on the amount of steroid receptors present in the tissue (Chan & Tindall 1981).

The purpose of this study was to investigate at a molecular level, steroid hormone interaction with skeletal muscle. The specific aim was to study the following issues:

1. Can androgens and glucocorticoids act directly on skeletal muscle in man? The presence of specific cytosolic receptors for these hormones in human muscle could indicate that this is indeed the case.

2. Can different types of fibers in skeletal muscle be expected to respond differently to direct actions of steroid hormones?

3. Is it possible that the protein-catabolic effect of glucocorticoids is involved in the atrophy of tenotomized or denervated muscle and do protein-anabolic androgens have the potential to prevent this muscle disorder?

4. Can the commercially available synthetic anabolic-androgenic steroids be expected to have a direct effect on skeletal muscle?

MATERIALS AND METHODS

Patients and Experimental Animals

Human muscle samples were taken as open biopsies at surgery for other reasons (Snochowski et al 1981b). An informed consent was obtained from each patient and the studies were approved by the Ethical Committee at the Karolinska Hospital in Stockholm.

Analysis of steroid receptors in skeletal muscle with the in vitro methods used (cf. below) requires about 2-4 g of muscle tissue for a single receptor quantitation. An animal model was hence needed for providing sufficient quantities of tissue for certain experiments. The rabbit yielded enough tissue for analysis of individual muscles (Saartok 1983, Saartok et al 1983b).

After sacrifice of the animals the muscle samples were dissected, cleaned from visible fat and connective tissue and frozen in liquid nitrogen, within 3 min. The intact samples were stored at -70°C, usually for less than 6 weeks before analysis. Whereas minced muscle stored at -20°C loses binding capacity of receptors by about 4% per week, intact samples stored at lower temperature (as in the studies presented in this investigation) show less reduction in specific ligand binding (Dahlberg et al 1981).

Steroid Receptor Identification and Measurement

Preparation of cytosol. Frozen muscle samples were powderized in liquid nitrogen (Dahlberg et al 1981). One volume of buffer (50 mM Tris-HCl, pH 7.4 at 22°C, 1 mM EDTA, 0.1 mM 2,3-dihydroxy-1,4-dithiol-butane, 10% (v/v) glycerol) was added and the homogenate was centrifuged at 105,000 g_{av} for 60 min $(0-4^{\circ})$. The supernatant was used as cytosol, and the cytosolic pH was measured at $0-4^{\circ}$C. The pellet and a portion of the cytosol were saved at -20°C for subsequent determination of DNA and protein, respectively (cf. below).

Assessment of equilibrium. The criteria for steroid-receptor binding include "low" ligand-binding capacity, "high" binding affinity and "high" ligand specificity (see e.g. Chan & Tindall 1981). Furthermore, quantitation of steroid receptors using Scatchard plots (cf. below) require equilibrium conditions. Therefore assessment of the suitable incubation time was first performed.

Methyltrienolone (MT, R 1881) was used as a ligand for the androgen receptor, dexamethasone (DEX) for the gluco-corticoid receptor and moxestrol (R 2858) for the estrogen receptor. These synthetic steroids are advantageous to use as ligands in steroid receptor assays since they have a high receptor affinity, do not bind to plasma steroid-binding proteins and have a slow metabolism (Bonne & Raynaud 1975, Baxter & Tomkins 1970, Raynaud et al 1971, Ojasoo & Raynaud 1978). When measuring the androgen receptor, ^{3}H-MT was used with a 100-fold molar excess of DEX (to block the steroid-binding site of the glucocorticoid receptor, since MT has a slight affinity also for that receptor (Snochowski et al 1980, Ho-Kim et al 1981)). This does not influence the androgen receptor quantitation (Dahlberg et al 1981). For the measurements of glucocorticoid and estrogen receptors, similar incubations were performed with ^{3}H-DEX or ^{3}H-moxestrol, respectively. All incubations were performed at $0-4^{\circ}$C, since the association, dissociation and degradation are highly temperature dependent (Snochowski et al 1980). After various periods of time the protein-bound radioactivity was counted (Dahlberg 1982b) and the specific binding and association rate constants were calculated (Snochowski et al 1980, Snochowski et al 1981b).

Saturation and Scatchard analysis. The appropriate ligand concentrations were estimated by saturation analyses, in which six concentrations of ^{3}H-labelled ligands were incubated (in duplicates) with cytosol for 20-24 h (cf. below) at 0-4°C (for a detailed procedure, see Snochowski et al 1980). The non-specific binding was estimated from a parallel set of incubations with the three highest doses of ^{3}H-ligand, additionally containing a 100-fold molar excess of unlabeled ligand. The protein-bound and unbound radioactivity were separated by charcoal treatment. The total ligand concentrations were determined from a parallel series of incubations where cytosol was substituted with buffer.

Using equilibrium conditions for the incubations and an interactive computer program, the apparent maximum number of binding sites (B_{max}) and equilibrium dissociation constant K_d (or association constant, K_a) were calculated according to Scatchard (1949) after corrections for non-specific binding (Chamness & McGuire 1975), as described earlier (Snochowski et al 1980). The Scatchard analysis was used as a standard method in the receptor quantitations.

The within-assay coefficient of variation was estimated by analyzing a pool of rat muscle cytosol, which was divided into 4 samples for Scatchard analysis of androgen and glucocorticoid receptors, respectively. The mean within-assay coefficient of variation for the K_d of both receptors was 11%. The corresponding value for the B_{max} of the androgen receptor (mean 65 fmol/g of tissue wet weight) was 8% and for the B_{max} of the glucocorticoid receptor (mean 1,060 fmol/g) 9%.

Specificity studies. To incubation mixtures of cytosol and ^{3}H-ligand, solutions of a single (100-fold) or several (1-128-fold) concentrations of competitors were added (Snochowski et al 1980). The capacity of a compound to compete for ligand binding sites on the receptors was estimated by the specific ligand-binding remaining in the presence of competing steroid (as compared to that in the absence of competing steroid) (Snochowski et al 1981a, 1981b). The relative binding affinity (RBA) of each steroid was calculated from logit-log plots (Rodbard et al 1968, Snochowski et al 1980). The RBA was defined as the ratio between the molar concentration of unlabeled ligand and that of competitor required to obtain 50% displacement of the ^{3}H-labeled ligand from its binding sites (Snochowski et al 1980).

Metabolism of steroids in cytosol. The metabolism of ^{3}H-MT, ^{3}H-DEX, ^{3}H-testosterone and 5α-^{3}H-dihydrotestosterone (DHT) was studied under conditions used for incubations at receptor analyses. The conversion of these steroids to metabolites was studied by thin-layer chromatography.

Determinations of Protein DNA

Protein was estimated in the cytosol preparations according to Lowry et al (1951) with modifications described by Peterson (1977) and Dahlberg et al (1981), using bovine serum albumin as the standard.

The pellets stored (cf. above) were ground to a powder in liquid nitrogen and an aliquot was taken for estimations of DNA (Dahlberg et al 1981). DNA was estimated according to Burton et al (1956), with modifications described by Giles and Myers (1965), Richards (1974) and Dahlberg et al (1981), using calf thymus DNA as the standard.

The ratio of protein/DNA was used as an expression of the size of the "functional DNA-unit" or the "cell size" (Cheek et al 1971) as was the ratio muscle wet weight/DNA (Enesco & Leblond 1962, Winick & Noble 1965, van Buul-Offers et al 1982).

Statistical Methods

The precision of the B_{max} and K_d (or K_a) values obtained by Scatchard analysis was described by the 95% confidence interval and the standard deviation (S.D.), respectively. The receptors were considered as detectable only when the slope of the plot was different from zero with 95% confidence (Snochowski et al 1980). Statistical analyses (paired and grouped t-test, analysis of variance, linear correlation, Spearman's rank correlation, Fischer's exact test) have been described in standard texts (e.g. Brownlee 1965, Snedocor & Cochran 1967).

RESULTS AND DISCUSSION

Identification of Steroid Receptors

In both human and rabbit skeletal muscle cytosol, a plateau of maximum specific binding was obtained after about 10-20 h for all receptors at $0-4^{\circ}$C. This maximum level showed only a minor decrease up to 48 h of incubation. The time necessary to reach equilibrium conditions in further experiments was thus regarded to be about 20 h for all ligands. The incubation temperature was chosen as $0-4^{\circ}$C since both degradation and dissociation rates of the ligand-receptor complexes increase considerably at higher temperatures (Snochowski et al 1980). Under the same assay conditions, equilibrium conditions for the ligand-receptor complexes in human and rabbit muscle were similar to those in rat and porcine skeletal muscle (Snochowski et al 1980, 1981a). The association rate constant was higher for MT than for DEX in man and rabbit as well as in the other mammals (Snochowski et al 1980, 1981a). The second-order association rate constant for the estrogen receptor in cytosol from rabbit muscle was similar to that of the estrogen receptor in rat skeletal muscle cytosol (Dahlberg 1982a).

The range of concentrations for the ligands in saturation analyses was $0.05-5$ nM for ^{3}H-MT, $0.5-20$ nM for ^{3}H-DEX and $0.05-2$ nM for ^{3}H-moxestrol (final concentrations, respectively). At the equilibrium conditions used and at these concentrations, cytosolic binding was saturable in all cases. Hence, the use of Scatchard analysis of the specific binding was justified (Scatchard 1949, Chamness & McGuire 1975, Snochowski et al 1980).

Ligand specificity studies showed that androgens were the main competitors for the MT-binding sites, and glucocorticoids for the DEX-binding sites (Snochowski et al 1981b, Saartok 1983). In rabbits, the estrogens were the main competitors for the moxestrol binding sites (Saartok 1983). As in rat and porcine skeletal muscle (Snochowski et al 1980, 1981), progestins and estrogens showed only minor competition for either MT-binding or DEX-binding sites.

In summary, the binding of the ligands to human and rabbit skeletal muscle cytosol was of low capacity and high specificity. Furthermore, Scatchard analysis indicated that the binding was of high affinity. Thus the binding of ^{3}H-MT,

^{3}H-DEX and ^{3}H-moxestrol to cytosol shows the same characteristics as the androgen, glucocorticoid and estrogen receptors,
respectively, in "classical" hormone target tissues (Grody
et al 1982). Thus, human and rabbit skeletal muscle can be
regarded as target tissues for androgens and glucocorticoids,
and rabbit skeletal muscle also for estrogens. The characteristics of the receptor binding are apparently similar in
human, rat, mouse, pig and rabbit skeletal muscle (Snochowski
et al 1980, 1981a, Dahlberg et al 1981).

In rat (Dahlberg 1982a) and rabbit (Saartok 1983)
skeletal muscle, a specific estrogen receptor was identified.
Using the same assay conditions as for the estrogen receptor
in rat (Dahlberg 1982a) and rabbit muscle (Saartok et al
1983b), we have identified estrogen receptors in skeletal
muscle from a young boy (prepubertal, 12 years of age,
operated for osteosarcoma). The K_d of this receptor was 1.30
nM (S.D. 0.37) and the B_{max} was 109 (95% confidence limit,
75-263) fmol/g of tissue wet weight, 2.14 fmol/mg of protein
or 128 fmol/mg of DNA. These are values in agreement with
those expected from data in animals. However, further
studies are needed to confirm the presence of, characterize
and quantitate estrogen receptors in human skeletal muscle
cytosol.

Using ^{3}H-promegestone (R 5020) as a ligand, unsuccess-
ful attempts have been carried out to identify a progestin
receptor in skeletal muscle cytosol (Snochowski et al 1980,
1981b).

Receptor Quantitation

To e.g. facilitate comparisons between the receptor
data and those of other tissues or in other investigations,
the maximum number of binding sites (B_{max}) was always
expressed per g of tissue wet weight, per mg of cytosolic
protein and per mg of DNA.

The levels of glucocorticoid receptors were usually
about ten times higher than those of androgen and estrogen
receptors. In agreement with previous data (e.g. Dahlberg et
al 1981), the glucocorticoid receptor concentration did not
appear to be sexually differentiated. However, males had
lower levels of cytosolic androgen receptor than females
(Dahlberg et al 1981, Snochowski et al 1981a, 1981b, Saartok

et al 1983b). The presence of endogenous steroids leads to translocation of the steroid-receptor complexes to the nuclear compartment (Grody et al 1982), and is therefore associated with low or non-detectable levels of cytosolic receptors (Dahlberg et al 1981, Snochowski et al 1981a).

Decreased exposure to steroid hormones following e.g. castration, or adrenalectomy increases the number of cyto-solic androgen, estrogen and glucocorticoid receptors, respectively (Dahlberg et al 1981, Snochowski et al 1981a). Furthermore, the regulation of the levels of cytosolic steroid receptors seems to be relatively complex. For example, castration causes an increase in the concentration of both androgen and glucocorticoid receptors (Dahlberg et al 1981) and estrogen treatment causes an increase in the concentration of androgen receptor (Bouton et al 1981). Others have reported that estrogen treatment increases androgen, estrogen and progestin receptors (Frenette et al 1982).

Steroid Receptors in a Fast-Twitch and a Slow-Twitch Rabbit Muscle

Metabolic and functional differences in various muscles under different conditions, e.g. scoliotic back muscle (Spencer & Eccles 1976) and muscle atrophy (Booth & Kelso 1973, Häggmark et al 1981), can be due to a different rela-tive distribution of fiber types in the muscles. Human as well as most other mammalian muscles are mixed with regard to the different fiber types (Johnson et al 1973, Ariano et al 1973). In order to compare steroid receptor concentrations in slow-twitch and fast-twitch muscles, respectively, an animal model was needed. The rabbit provides sufficient quantities of muscle tissue for receptor analyses and has certain muscles with mainly one fiber type (Peter et al 1972, Wählby et al 1978).

The rabbit gastrocnemius/plantaris muscle complex (about 90% fast-twitch (FT) fibers) was compared to the soleus muscle (about 90% slow-twitch (ST) fibers) (Wählby et al 1978). The K_d values for the androgen, glucocorticoid and estrogen receptor were similar in the two types of muscles. When expressed per mg of DNA, the concentrations of androgen and glucocorticoid receptors were similar in the two muscle types, whereas the concentration of estrogen receptors was

higher in the slow-twitch than in the fast-twitch muscle.
When expressed per mg of protein, all receptor concentrations
were lower in the gastrocnemius/plantaris complex than in
the soleus, as an effect of the higher protein concentration
in the former muscle. The tissue concentrations (per g of
wet weight) of glucocorticoid and estrogen receptors were
higher in the soleus than in the gastrocnemius muscle,
whereas the difference was not significant for the androgen
receptor. Since the concentration of androgen and glucocorticoid receptors per mg of DNA (i.e. related to the
nuclear concentration, cf. Cheek et al 1971) is similar in
FT- and ST-muscles, the tissue concentration of receptors
(per g of muscle wet weight) will be a function of the
number of cell nuclei in the muscle. However, as mentioned
above, the situation was different for the estrogen receptor,
as the concentration of this molecule per mg of DNA was
higher in the ST- than in the FT-muscle (Saartok 1983).

The higher concentration of glucocorticoid receptors in
ST- when compared to FT-muscles when expressed per mg of
protein, with no difference when the concentration was
expressed per mg of DNA, is in agreement with results for
the glucocorticoid receptor published by Shoji & Pennington
(1977a). In addition, these authors showed that the difference in pH between cytosols from an ST-muscle and an FT-
muscle, respectively, did not change the ratio between
glucocorticoid receptor concentrations of the two muscles.
At low pH (below 6.1) steroid receptors were not detectable
in porcine skeletal muscle (Snochowski et al 1981a). The
difference in pH between the soleus and the gastrocnemius/
plantaris muscles (about 0.3-0.4 units higher in the soleus)
is probably due to the higher glycolytic capacity of the
fast-twitch gastrocnemius/plantaris muscles (Baldwin &
Tipton 1972).

Effects of Atrophy on Androgen and Glucocorticoid Receptors

One or three weeks following tenotomy or denervation of
rabbit gastrocnemius muscle, the K_a values of both androgen
and glucocorticoid receptors showed a similar small increase
to those of the corresponding receptors in the gastrocnemius
muscle of the contralateral, non-operated leg of the rabbit.
Both types of atrophy caused an increase in the concentration
of both androgen and glucocorticoid receptors, when expressed
as tissue concentration (per g of muscle wet weight) or per

mg of cytosolic protein. However, when expressed per mg of
DNA or as the total muscle content, the levels in atrophic
muscle were increased compared to the contralateral side but
unchanged with time. Thus, although there was a decrease in
the muscle content of cytosolic protein (cf. below), the
content of cytosolic receptors was even increased. This
indicates that the loss in cytosolic protein did not include
androgen or glucocorticoid receptors (Saartok et al 1983b).

These findings are similar to those of DuBois & Almon
(1980, 1981), who found an increased concentration of the
glucocorticoid receptor (per mg of protein) after immobilization or denervation of rat leg muscle. These authors suggested
that an increased muscle tissue sensitivity to glucocorticoids, as indicated by the change in receptor concentration,
could be of etiological significance in muscle atrophy
(DuBois & Almon 1981). However, the present study strongly
indicates that the increase in glucocorticoid receptor
concentration in atrophied muscle is mostly due to a concentration effect, since the total muscle content of receptors
and the concentration of receptors per mg of DNA was considerably less than when related to weight or protein.

The Capacity of "Anabolic-Androgenic" Steroid to Act Directly
on Skeletal Muscle

To investigate if anabolic-androgenic steroids may act
directly on skeletal muscle via androgen receptors in this
tissue, the relative binding affinities (RBA:s) of such
steroids to the androgen receptor in skeletal muscle of
rabbit and rat were estimated. To see whether the receptor
in muscle has different properties from that in the "classical"
androgen target tissue the prostate, the estimated RBA:s for
the receptor in skeletal muscle were compared to the RBA:s
determined for the androgen receptor in rat prostate (Saartok
et al 1983a). The binding of the compounds was calculated
relative to that of methyltrienolone. The RBA:s for the
different steroids were very similar in both tissues, indicating that the androgen receptor in skeletal muscle has a
ligand specificity similar to that in the prostate, the
"classical" target organ for androgens. Hence, it was not
possible to identify a specific "anabolic" muscle receptor
different from the androgen receptor. Only the RBA of 5α-
dihydrotestosterone (DHT) was different in the tissues,
being about 10 times lower in skeletal muscle than in the

prostate. This is due to the rapid metabolism of DHT in muscle tissue (Snochowski et al 1980, 1981b).

Whereas only a few synthetic anabolic-androgenic steroids bound better or as well as testosterone to the androgen receptor, most compounds bound less efficiently. Some anabolic-androgenic steroids had RBA values less than 0.01, indicating very low affinity for the androgen receptor. However, it cannot be excluded that these steroids might act via the androgen receptor, if administered at very high doses or if they become metabolized to "active" derivatives, with better receptor binding capacity. Furthermore, the anabolic-andro-genic steroids with low affinity for the androgen receptor may act via indirect mechanisms. One possibility could be an influence on androgen metabolism, another an influence on the levels of other anabolic hormones, such as growth hor-mone (Mode et al 1982). Alternatively, they could displace endogenous androgens from steroid-binding proteins in blood, thereby increasing the free (biologically active) steroid fraction (cf. below) (Pugeat et al 1981).

The RBA:s of anabolic-androgenic steroids were also investigated for serum SHBG, using ^{3}H-DHT as the ligand. The binding pattern of the compounds for SHBG was different from that of the androgen receptor. One synthetic steroid (mestero-lone) was highly efficient in binding to SHBG, whereas most other synthetic steroids had low RBA values for this protein. This latter group included e.g. methyltrienolone, the most active competitor for the androgen receptor (Saartok et al 1983a).

Estimation of the "DNA-Unit"

Even if the muscle fiber is a multinucleated cell, each cell nucleus within the fiber is considered to have juris-diction over a finite mass of cytoplasm. This is the concept of the "functional DNA-unit" and the size of this unit can be estimated by the protein/DNA-ratio (Cheek et al 1971). Tissue growth can be accomplished by increments in the number or size of the cells, or a combination of both (Cheek & Hill 1970, Cheek et al 1971). The cell number is indicated by the DNA content, whereas "cell size" can be estimated by e.g. the "functional DNA-unit" (i.e. the ratio protein/DNA (cf. above)) or weight/DNA (Enesco & Leblond 1962, Winick & Noble 1965). Each of these factors ("cell size" and nuclear

number) is under the influence of e.g. nutritional and
hormonal factors (Cheek & Hill 1970).

In rabbit skeletal muscle, the protein/DNA-ratio was
smaller in the slow-twitch soleus muscle compared to the
fast-twitch gastrocnemius/plantaris complex (Saartok 1983).
In these younger animals, the protein/DNA-ratio of the
gastrocnemius muscle was smaller than in the older rabbits
(Saartok et al 1983b). Furthermore, atrophy caused a decrease in the protein/DNA-ratio (Saartok et al 1983b).

In view of the above findings, knowledge of the distribution of fiber types is necessary in order to interpret
changes in the protein/DNA-ratio.

GENERAL DISCUSSION

Whereas muscle atrophy due to immobilization seems to
affect the slow-twitch fibers selectively (Häggmark et al
1981), glucocorticoid excess seems to predominantly affect
the fast-twitch fibers (for references, see Saartok 1983).
It may therefore be suggested that other factors than glucocorticoid action are more important in the etiology of
disuse atrophy. Since higher levels of endogenous steroids
are associated with lower cytosolic concentrations of steroid
receptors (see e.g. Dahlberg et al 1981), the increase in
glucocorticoid receptor levels in disuse atrophy (Saartok et
al 1983b) is also in agreement with this contention.

In view of the capacity of anabolic/androgenic steroids
to bind to the androgen receptor in skeletal muscle, there
exists a rationale for using these hormones in attempts to
induce muscle growth. The postulated effect of these compounds is that they induce protein anabolism in muscle, i.e.
that they cause a net increase in muscle protein (Krüskemper
1968, Kochakian 1976). Since long, these steroids have been
used as anabolic agents in meat production to increase the
carcass weight of the animals (Lu & Rendel 1975, Heitzman
1979). In human medicine, their use has been limited owing
to their side effects, e.g. hepatic abnormalities (Wright
1980). Also, these compounds would be expected to have more
pronounced effects in tissues containing higher levels of
androgen receptors than skeletal muscle, e.g. the male
reproductive organs. On the other hand, effects of glucocorticoid treatment on skeletal muscle, e.g. weakness and

myopathic or atrophic changes, are mostly unwanted side effects of this therapy. In both cases, there is a practical need for manipulating the specific steroid effects on skeletal muscle when compared to other tissues. Further achievements within the field of steroid hormone action in skeletal muscle may provide a basis for more selective steroid therapy.

Use of Steroids in Sports

As shown in this investigation, anabolic-androgenic steroids can bind to the androgen receptor in skeletal muscle. These results indicate that the molecular basis exists for a direct local effect of these compounds on skeletal muscle. The relatively low receptor affinities characterizing most of the anabolic-androgenic steroids may explain why high doses of these drugs have been reported to be necessary to obtain a "doping" effect (Wright 1980). However, high doses will also increase the incidence of unwanted effects from other organs. Also indirect mechanisms for the actions of the anabolic-androgenic steroids must be considered. The compounds that bind to the transport-proteins in blood (e.g. mesterolone) may by competition increase the free, biologically active portion of endogenous steroids (Pugeat et al 1981). The metabolism of endogenous steroids in the liver or other tissues may be affected by the administration of exogenous steroids (Mode et al 1982). Furthermore, androgens can act directly on the central nervous system and change e.g. the behavioural pattern (Martini 1982). Sex steroids regulate the secretory pattern of growth hormone (Mode et al 1982), which has been suggested to regulate somatic growth and protein metabolism in muscle (Albertsson-Wikland et al 1980, Jansson et al 1982). With these considerations in mind, it is therefore logical to question the suggested lack of effect of the anabolic-androgenic steroids (American College of Sports Medicine 1977, Ljungqvist et al 1982).

These studies were supported by grants from the Swedish Sports Research Council (Idrottens Forskningsråd) and the Swedish Medical Research Council (grant No. 13X-2819).

REFERENCES

Aakvaag A, Bentdal Ø, Quigstad K, Walstad P, Rønningen
H, Fonnum F (1978). Testosterone and testosterone binding globulin (TeBG) in young men during prolonged stress.
Int. J. Andrology 1:22.
Afifi AK, Bergman RA (1969). Steroid myopathy. Johns
Hopkins Med. J. 124:66.
Albertsson-Wikland K, Edén S, Isaksson O (1980). Analysis
of early responses to growth hormone on amino acid
transport and protein synthesis in diaphragms of young
normal rats. Endocrinology 106:291.
American College of Sports Medicine (1977). Position
statement on the use and abuse of anabolic-androgenic
steroids in sports. Med. Sci. Sports 9:xi.
Anderson DC (1974). Sex-hormone-binding globulin. Clin.
Endocr. 3:69.
Ariano MA, Armstrong RB, Edgerton VR (1973). Hindlimb
muscle fiber populations of five mammals. J. Histochem.
Cytochem. 21:51.
Baker ER (1981). Menstrual dysfunction and hormonal status
in athletic women: a review. Fertil. Steril. 36:691.
Baldwin KM, Tipton CM (1972). Work and metabolic patterns
of fast and slow twitch skeletal muscle contracting in
situ. Pflüg. Arch. 334:345.
Ballard PL, Baxter JD, Higgins SJ, Rousseau GG, Tomkins
GM (1974). General presence of glucocorticoid receptors
in mammalian tissues. Endocrinology 94:998.
Barnard RJ, Edgerton VR, Furukawa T, Peter JB (1971).
Histochemical, biochemical, and contractile properties
of red, white, and intermediate fibers. Am. J. Physiol.
220:410.
Baxter JD, Tomkins GM (1970). The relationship between
glucocorticoid binding and tyrosine aminotransferase
induction in hepatoma tissue culture cells. Proc. Nat.
Acad. Sci. 65:709.
Baxter JD (1976). Glucocorticoid hormone action. Pharmacol.
Ther. B 2:605.
Beach RK, Kostyo JL (1968). Effect of growth hormone on
the DNA content of muscles of young hypophysectomized
rats. Endocrinology 82:882.
Bonne C, Raynaud J-P (1975). Methyltrienolone, a specific
ligand for cellular androgen receptors. Steroids 26:227.

Booth FW, Kelso JR (1973). Effect of hindlimb immobilization on contractile and histochemical properties of skeletal muscle. Pflügers Arch. 342:231.

Bouton MM, Pornin C, Grandadam JA (1981). Estrogen regulation of rat prostate androgen receptor. J. Steroid Biochem. 15:403.

Breuer CB, Florini JR (1965). Amino acid incorporation into protein by cell-free systems from rat skeletal muscle. 4. Effects of animal age, androgens, and anabolic agents on activity of muscle ribosomes. Biochemistry 4:1544.

Brownlee KA (1965). Statistical Theory and Methodology in Science and Engineering. Ed. 2. Wiley, New York, p. 1.

Buresová M, Gutmann E (1971). Effect of testosterone on protein synthesis and contractility of the levator ani muscle of the rat. J. Endocr. 50:643.

Burton K (1956). A study of the conditions and mechanism of the diphenylamine reaction for the colorimetric estimation of deoxyribonucleic acid. Biochem. J. 62:315.

van Buul-Offers S, van den Brande JL (1982).: Cellular growth in several organs of normal and dwarfed Snell mice. Acta Endocr. 99:141.

Chainy GBN, Kanungo MS (1978). Effects of estradiol and testosterone on the activity of pyrivate kinase of the cardiac and skeletal muscles of rats as a function of age and sex. Biochim. Biophys. Acta 540:65.

Chamness GC, McGuire WL (1975). Scatchard plots: common errors in correction and interpretation. Steroids 26:538.

Chan L, O'Malley BW (1978). Steroid hormone action: recent advances. Ann. Int. Med. 89:694.

Chan L, Tindall DJ (1981). Steroid hormone action. In Collu R, Ducharme JR, Guyda H (eds): Pediatric Endocrinology - Comprehensive Endocrinology. Raven Press, New York, p. 63.

Cheek DB, Hill DE (1970). Muscle and liver cell growth: role of hormones and nutritional factors. Fed. Proc. 29:1503.

Cheek DB, Holt AB, Hill DE, Talbert JL (1971). Skeletal muscle cell mass and growth: the concept of the deoxyribonucleic acid unit. Ped. Res. 5:312.

Ciccoli L, Bergamini E (1974). Interactions between testosterone and insulin in the regulation of glycogen metabolism in rat perineal muscles. Ster. Lip. Res. 5:321.

Clark AF, Vignos Jr PJ (1979). Experimental corticosteroid myopathy: effect on myofibrillar ATPase activity and protein degradation. Muscle Nerve 2:265.

Cushing H (1932). The basophil adenomas of the pituitary body and their clinical manifestations. Bull. Johns Hopkins Hosp. 50:137.

Cuthbertson DP (1979). The metabolic response to injury and its nutritional implications: retrospect and prospect. J. Parent. Ent. Nutr. 3:108.

Dahlberg E, Snochowski M, Gustafsson J-Å (1980a). Androgen and glucocorticoid receptors in rat skeletal muscle. Acta Chem. Scand. B 34:141.

Dahlberg E, Snochowski M, Gustafsson J-Å (1981). Regulation of the androgen and glucocorticoid receptors in rat and mouse skeletal muscle cytosol. Endocrinology 108:1431.

Dahlberg E (1982a). Characterization of the cytosolic estrogen receptor in rat skeletal muscle. Biochim. Biophys. Acta 717:65.

Dahlberg E (1982b). Quench correction in liquid scintillation counting by a combined internal standard-samples channels ratio technique. Anal. Chem. 54:2082.

Dahn MS, Lange P (1982). Hormonal changes and their influence on metabolism and nutrition in the critically ill. Intensive Care Med. 8:209.

David DS, Grieco MH, Cushman P (1970). Adrenal glucocorticoids after twenty years. A review of their clinically relevant consequences. J. Chron. Dis. 22:637.

Dolecek R (1969). Metabolic Response of the Burned Organism (Ed by Nowinski WW). Charles C Thomas, Springfield, p. 1.

Dubé JY, Lesage R, Tremblay RR (1976). Androgen and estrogen binding in rat skeletal and perineal muscles. Can. J. Biochem. 54:50.

DuBois DC, Almon RR (1980). Disuse atrophy of skeletal muscle is associated with an increase in number of glucocorticoid receptors. Endocrinology 107:1649.

DuBois DC, Almon RR (1981). A possible role for glucocorticoids in denervation atrophy. Muscle Nerve 4:370.

Dunn JF, Nisula BC, Rodbard D (1981). Transport of steroid hormones: binding of 21 endogenous steroids to both testosterone-binding globulin and corticosteroid-binding globulin in human plasma. J. Clin. Endocr. Metab. 53:58.

Enesco M, Leblond CP (1962). Increase in cell number as a factor in the growth of the organs and tissues of the young male rat. J. Embryol. Exp. Morph. 10:530.

Faludi G, Mills LC, Chayes ZW (1964). Effect of steroids on muscle. Acta Endocr. 45:68.

Frenette G, Dubé JY, Tremblay RR (1982). Effect of hormone injections on levels of cytosolic receptors for estrogen, androgen and progesterone in dog prostate. J. Steroid Biochem. 17:271.

Frey H (1982). The endocrine response to physical activity. Scand. J. Social Med. Suppl. 29:71.

Frisch RE, Gotz-Welbergen AV, McArthur JW, Albright T, Witschi J, Bullen B, Birnholz J, Reed R, Hermann H (1981). Delayed menarche and amenorrhea of college athletes in relation to age of onset of training. J. Am. Med. Assoc. 246:1559.

Frohman LA, Felig P, Broadus AE, Baxter JD (1981). The clinical manifestations of endocrine disease. In Felig P, Baxter JD, Broadus AE, Frohman LA (eds) Endocrinology and Metabolism. McGraw-Hill Book Co, New York, p. 3.

Galbo H (1981). Endocrinology and metabolism in exercise. Int. J. Sports Med. 2:203.

Galbo H (1983). Hormonal and Metabolic Adaption to Exercise. Thieme Verlag, Stuttgart, p. 1.

Giannopoulos G, Hassan Z, Solomon S (1974). Glucocorticoid receptors in fetal and adult rabbit tissues. J. Biol. Chem. 249:2424.

Giles KW, Myers A (1965). An improved diphenylamine method for the estimation of deoxyribonucleic acid. Nature (London) 206:93.

Grody WW, Schrader WT, O'Malley BW (1982). Activation, transformation, and subunit structure of steroid hormone receptors. Endocr. Rev. 3:141.

Gustafsson J-Å, Pousette Å (1975). Demonstration and partial characterization of cytosol receptors for testosterone. Biochemistry 14:3094.

Hanzliková V, Gutmann E (1978). Effect of castration and testosterone administration on the neuromuscular junction in the levator ani muscle. Cell Tiss. Res. 189:155.

Heitzman RJ (1979). The efficiacy and mechanism of action of anabolic agents as growth promotors in farm animals. J. Steroid Biochem. 11:927.

Hervey GR, Knibbs AV, Burkinshaw L, Morgan DB, Jones PRM, Chettle DR, Vartsky D (1981). Effects of methandienone on the performance and body composition of men undergoing athletic training. Clin. Sci. 60:457.

Heymsfield SB, Stevens V, Noel R, McManus C, Smith J, Nixon D (1982). Biochemical composition of muscle in normal and semistarved human subjects: relevance to anthropometric measurements. Am. J. Clin. Nutr. 36:131.

Ho-Kim MA, Tremblay RR, Dubé JY (1981). Binding of methyltrienolone to glucocorticoid receptors in rat muscle cytosol. Endocrinology 109:1418.

Hume DM, Egdahl RH (1959). The importance of the brain in the endocrine response to injury. Ann. Surg. 150:697.

Hume DM, Bell CC, Bartter F (1962). Direct measurement of adrenal secretion during operative trauma and convalescence. Surgery 52:174.

Häggmark T, Jansson E, Eriksson E (1981). Fibre type area and metabolic potential of the high muscle in man after knee surgery and immobilization. Int. J. Sports Med. 2:7.

Jansson J-O, Albertsson-Wikland K, Edén S, Thorngren K-G, Isaksson O (1982). Circumstantial evidence for a role of the secretory pattern of growth hormone in control of body growth. Acta Endocr. 99:24.

Jasiorowski H (ed) (1981). International Symposium: Steroids in Animal Production. Warsaw Agricultural University SGGW-AR/Roussel-UCLAF, Warsaw, p. 1.

Johnson MA, Polgar J, Weightman D, Appleton D (1973). Data on the distribution of fiber types in thirty-six human muscles. An autopsy study. J. Neurol. Sci. 18:111.

Jung E, Baulieu E-E (1972). Testosterone cytosol "receptors" in the rat levator ani muscle. Nature 237:24.

Kochakian CD (1964). Protein anabolic property of androgens. Alab. J. Med. Sci. 1:24.

Kochakian CD (1966). Regulation of muscle growth by androgens. In Physiology and Biochemistry of Muscle as a Food. University of Wisconsin Press, Madison/ Milwaukee/London, p. 81.

Kochakian CD (ed) (1976). Anabolic-Androgenic Steroids. Springer Verlag, Berlin/ Heidelberg/New York, p. 1.

Kostyo JL (1965). In vitro effects of adrenal steroid hormones on amino acid transport in muscle. Endocrinology 76:604.

Krieg M (1976). Characterization of the androgen receptor in the skeletal muscle of the rat. Steroids 28:261.

Kuoppasalmi K (1981). Effects of exercise stress on human plasma hormone levels with special reference to steroid hormones. Thesis, University of Helsinki.

Lamb DR (1975). Androgens and exercise. Med. Sci. Sports 7:1.

Larsson LL, Spilman CH, Foote RH (1972). Uterine uptake of progesterone and estradiol in young and aged rabbits. Proc. Soc. Exp. Biol. Med. 141:463.

Ljungqvist A, Björkhem I, Eriksson BO, Sjöqvist F, Elwin C-E, Ek H, Lantto O, Garle M, Krievins S (1982). "Doping - ett medicinskt och etiskt problem". (In Swedish). Läkartidningen 79:1237.

Lowry OH, Rosebrough NJ, Farr AL, Randall RJ (1951). Protein measurement with the Folin phenol reagent. J. Biol. Chem. 193:265.

Lu FC, Rendel J (eds) (1975). Anabolic Agents in Animal Production. Thieme Verlag, Stuttgart, p. 1.

Mainwaring WIP (1977). The Mechanism of Action of Androgens. Springer Verlag, New York, p. 1.

Martini L (1982). The 5α-reduction of testosterone in the neuroendocrine structures. Biochemical and physiological implications. Endocr. Rev. 3:1.

Mayer M, Kaiser N, Milholland RJ, Rosen F (1974). The binding of dexamethasone and triamcinolone acetonide to glucocorticoid receptors in rat skeletal muscle. J. Biol. Chem. 249:5236.

Mayer M, Shafir E, Kaiser N, Milholland RJ, Rosen F (1976). Interaction of glucocorticoid hormones with rat skeletal muscle: catabolic effects and hormone binding. Metabolism 25:157.

McGrath JA, Goldspink DF (1982). Glucocorticoid action on protein synthesis and protein breakdown in isolated skeletal muscles. Biochem. J. 206:641.

Michel MG, Baulieu E-E (1974). Recepteur cytosoluble des androgens dans un muscle strie squelettique. C.R. Acad. Sci., 279:421.

Michelsen CB, Askanazi J, Kinney JM, Gump FE, Elwyn DH (1982). Effect of an anabolic steroid on nitrogen balance and amino acid patterns after total hip replacement. J. Trauma 22:410.

Millward DJ, Waterlow JC (1978). Effect of nutrition on protein turnover in skeletal muscle. Fed. Proc. 37:2283.

Mode A, Gustafsson J-Å, Jansson J-O, Edén S, Isaksson O (1982). Association between plasma level of growth hormone and sex differentiation of hepatic steroid metabolism in the rat. Endocrinology 111:1692.

Müller R, Kugelberg E (1959). Myopathy in Cushing's syndrome. J. Neurol. Neurosurg. Psychiat. 22:314.

Nelson DH (1979). Cushing's syndrome. In deGroot LJ, Cahill Jr GF, Odell WD, Martini L, Potts Jr JT, Nelson DH, Steinberger E, Winegrad AI (eds): Endocrinology, Vol. 2, Grune & Stratton, New York, p. 1179.

Nowak A (1957). Effects of androgenic hormones on the rate of incorporation of labelled amino acids in male adult mice. Am. J. Physiol. 191:306.

Odedra BR, Millward DJ (1982). Effect of corticosterone treatment on muscle protein turnover in adrenalectomized rats and diabetic rats maintained on insulin. Biochem. J. 204:663.

Ojasoo T, Raynaud J-P (1978). Unique steroid congeners for receptor studies. Cancer Res. 38:4186.

Orten JM, Neuhaus OW (1975). Human Biochemistry, 9th Ed. CV Mosby Co, St. Louis, p. 1.

Pertschuk LP, Gaetjens E, Eisenberg KB (1981). Steroid hormone receptor proteins. Histochemical markers of potential hormone-dependence. Meth. Achiev. Exp. Pathol. 10:162.

Peter J, Barnard R, Edgerton V, Gillespie A, Stempel K (1973). Metabolic profiles of three fiber types of skeletal muscle in guinea pigs and rabbits. Biochemistry 11:2627.

Peterson GL (1977). A simplification of the protein assay method of Lowry et al. which is more generally applicable. Analyt. Biochem. 83:346.

Peterson RE, Nokes G, Chen Jr PS, Black RI (1960). Estrogens and adrenocortical function in man. J. Clin. Endorinol. Metab. 20:495.

Pugeat MM, Dunn JF, Nisula BC (1981). Transport of steroid hormones: interaction of 70 drugs with testosterone-binding globulin and corticosteroid-binding globulin in human plasma. J. Endocr. Metab. 53:69.

Ramey ER (1975). Corticosteroids and skeletal muscle. In Blaschko H, Sayers G, Smith AD (eds): Handbook of Physiology. American Physiol. Soc., Washington DC, Sect. VII, Vol. VI, p. 245.

Raynaud JP, Mercier-Bodard C, Baulieu E-E (1971). Rat estradiol binding plasma protein (EBP). Steroids 18:767.

Richards GM (1974). Modifications of the diphenylamine reaction giving increased sensitivity and simplicity in the estimation of DNA. Analyt. Biochem. 57:369.

Rodbard D, Rayford PL, Cooper JA, Ross GT (1968). Statistical quality-control of radioimmunoassays. J. Clin. Endocrinol. Metab. 28:1412.

Rogozkin VA (1979a). Anabolic steroid metabolism in skeletal muscle. J. Steroid Biochem. 11:923.

Rogozkin VA (1979b). Metabolic effects of anabolic steroid on skeletal muscle. Med. Sci. Sports 11:160.

Roth GS (1981). Age-related changes in specific glucocorticoid binding by steroid-responsive tissues of rats. Endocrinology 94:82.

Ryan AJ (1981). Anabolic steroids are fool´s gold. Fed. Proc. 40:2682.

Saartok T (1983). Steroid receptors in two types of rabbit skeletal muscle. Int. J. Sports Med., accepted for publication.

Saartok T, Dahlberg E, Gustafsson J-Å (1983a). Relative binding affinity of anabolic/androgenic steroids: comparison of the binding to the androgen receptors in skeletal muscle and in prostate, as well as to sex hormone-binding globulin. Submitted for publication.

Saartok T, Häggmark T, Dahlberg E, Snochowski M, Eriksson E, Gustafsson J-Å (1983b). Changes in androgen and glucocorticoid receptors, cytosolic protein and tissue DNA in rabbit gastrocnemius muscle following tenotomy or denervation. Manuscript.

Saltin B, Henriksson J, Nygaard E, Andersson P, Jansson E (1977). Fiber types and metabolic potentials of skeletal muscles in sedentary man and endurance runners. Ann. N.Y. Acad. Sci. 301:3.

Scatchard G (1949). The attractions of proteins for small molecules and ions. Ann. N.Y. Acad. Sci. 51:660.

Shoji S, Pennington JT (1977a). Binding of dexamethasone and cortisol to cytosol receptors in rat extensor digitorum longus and soleus muscles. Exp. Neurol. 57:342.

Shoji S, Pennington RJT (1977b). The effects of cortisone on protein breakdown and synthesis in rat skeletal muscle. Mol. Cell. Endocr. 6:159.

Siiteri PK, Murai JT, Hammond GL, Nisker JA, Raymore WJ, Kuhn RW (1982). The serum transport of steroid hormones. Rec. Progr. Horm. Res. 38:457.

Smith B (1964). Histological and histochemical changes in the muscles of rabbits given the corticosteroid triamcinolone. Neurology 14:857.

Snedocor GW, Cochran WG (1967). Statistical Methods. Iowa State University Press, Ames, Iowa, 6th Ed.

Snochowski M, Dahlberg E, Gustafsson J-Å (1980). Characterization and quantification of the androgen and glucocorticoid receptors in cytosol from rat skeletal muscle. Eur. J. Biochem. 111:603.

Snochowski M, Lundström K, Dahlberg E, Peterson H, Edqvist L-E (1981a). Androgen and glucocorticoid receptors in porcine skeletal muscle cytosol. J. Anim. Sci. 53:80.

Snochowski M, Saartok T, Dahlberg E, Eriksson E, Gustafsson J-Å (1981b). Androgen and glucocorticoid receptors in human skeletal muscle cytosol. J. Steroid Biochem 14:765.

Spencer GSG, Eccles MJ (1976). Spinal muscle in scoliosis. Part 2. The proportion and size of type 1 and type 2 skeletal muscle fibres measured using a computer-controlled microscope. J. Neurol. Sci. 30:143.

Thompson EB, Lippman ME (1974). Mechanism of action of glucocorticoids. Metabolism 23:159.

Tomas FM, Munro HN, Young VR (1979). Effect of glucocorticoid administration on the rate of muscle protein breakdown in vivo in rats, as measured by urinary excretion of N -methylhistidine. Biochem. J. 178:139.

Tremblay RR, Dubé JY, Ho-Kim MA, Lesage R (1977). Determination of rat muscles androgen-receptor complexes with methyltrienolone. Steroids 29:185.

Tweedle D, Walton C, Johnston IDA (1973). The effect of an anabolic steroid on postoperative nitrogen balance. Br. J. Clin. Pract. 27:130.

Tyrrell JB, Baxter JD (1981). Glucocorticoid therapy. In Felig P, Baxter JD, Broadus AE, Frohman LA (eds): Endocrinology and Metabolism. McGraw-Hill Book Co, New York, p. 599.

Wagner RK (1978). Extracellular and intracellular steroid binding proteins. Propertis, discrimination, assay and clinical applications. Acta Endocr. Suppl. 218, 88:1.

Walker RA, Cove DH, Howell A (1980). Histological detection of oestrogen receptor in human breast carcinomas. Lancet 1:171.

Warren MP (1980). The effects of exercise on pubertal progression and reproductive function in girls. J. Clin. Endocrinol. Metab. 51:1150.

Westphal U (1971). Steroid-Protein Interactions. Springer Verlag, Heidelberg, p. 1.

Williams-Ashman HG (1979). Biochemical features of androgen physiology. In DeGroot LJ et al (eds): Endocrinology. Vol. 3. New York/San Fransisco/London, Grune & Stratton, p. 1527.

Wilmore DW, Long JM, Mason AD, Pruitt BA (1976). Stress in surgical patients as a neurophysiologic reflex response. Surg. Gyn. Obst. 142:257.

Wilson JD, Griffin JE (1980). The use and misuse of androgens. Metabolism 29: 1278.

Winick M, Noble A (1965). Quantitative changes in DNA, RNA and protein during prenatal and postnatal growth in the rat. Dev. Biol. 12:451.

Wright JE (1980). Anabolic steroids and athletics. In Hutton RS, Miller DI (eds): Exercise and Sports Sciences Reviews, Vol. 8. Franklin Institute Press, p. 149.

Wählby L, Dahlbäck L-O, Sjöström M (1978). Achilles tendons injury. II. Structure of tenotomized rabbit crural muscles after primary and delayed tendon suture. Acta Chir. Scand. 144:359.

Young VR (1970). The role of skeletal and cardiac muscle in the regulation of protein metabolism. In Munro HN (ed): Mammalian Protein Metabolism, Vol. 4. Academic Press, New York, p. 586.

Young VR, Munro HN (1978). N -Methylhistidine (3-methyl-histidine) and muscle protein turnover: an overview. Fed. Proc. 37:2291.

Hormones and Cancer, pages 291–316
© **1984 Alan R. Liss, Inc., 150 Fifth Avenue, New York, NY 10011**

ECTOPIC HORMONE PRODUCTION--BIOLOGICAL AND CLINICAL
IMPLICATIONS

Geoffrey Mendelsohn, M.D., Stephen B. Baylin, M.D.

Departments of Pathology, Medicine and The Oncology Center, The Johns Hopkins Medical Institutions
Baltimore, Maryland 21205

It is 60 years since the earliest recognition of inappropriate (ectopic) endocrine activity in patients with neoplasia (Klemperer 1923). Although, during ensuing years,
inappropriate endocrine syndromes were noted in patients with
a wide variety of non-endocrine tumors, it was not until 1956
that conclusive evidence for ectopic hormone production by
tumors was presented (Connor et al 1956; Plimpton, Gellhorn
1956).

The foundation for our current understanding of ectopic
endocrine activity in tumors was the development of highly
sensitive and specific bioassay, immunological, and receptor
assay techniques which permitted identification of circulating peptide hormones which were responsible for these syndromes. Over the past 10-15 years, refinement of these assay
techniques has permitted identification of peptide hormone
production by tumors even in the absence of clinically overt
syndromes; most recently, development of tissue extraction,
cell culture, and highly sensitive and specific immunological
staining methods, such as immunofluorescence and immunoper-
oxidase techniques, has allowed us to directly identify the
cells responsible for hormone production. These same techniques have shown that ectopic hormones are often secreted
in multiple forms, many of which lack biological activity,
and that tumors frequently contain large molecular weight
precursor forms (Steiner et al 1967; Berson, Yalow 1968).
Such studies have been pivotal, not only in the understanding
of ectopic hormone production, but also in elucidating normal pathways of peptide hormone synthesis.

This review will focus on patterns and proposed mechanisms of ectopic hormone production; and, in considering certain human tumors as models for the study of ectopic hormone production, biological and clinical implications will be addressed.

DEFINITION AND DOCUMENTATION OF ECTOPIC HORMONE PRODUCTION

Ectopic hormone production is classically defined as the synthesis, by a tumor, of polypeptide hormones which are not synthesized by the parent tissue from which the tumor putatively derives. Although the advent of newer culture, immunoassay, immunohistochemical, and receptor binding techniques has indicated that our current definition is inaccurate as applied to many hormones and other tumor markers, the term "ectopic" has important biological and clinical connotations and is well established. Several validation criteria exist for documenting that a particular tumor is responsible for an endocrine syndrome and/or the inappropriate secretion of a hormonal substance (Table 1).

TABLE 1 - VALIDATION CRITERIA FOR CONFIRMING ECTOPIC HORMONE PRODUCTION

1. Evidence of abnormal endocrine activity in a patient with a tumor

   - clinical endocrine syndrome and/or
   - elevated circulating hormone levels

2. Elimination of endocrine activity following the ablation of the tumor

3. Demonstration of an arteriovenous gradient of the hormone across the tumor vascular bed

4. Presence of greater concentrations of hormone in tumor tissue than in adjacent normal tissue

5. Documentation of hormone synthesis by tumor cells

   - cell culture
   - extraction of mRNA from tumor cells

Demonstration of a significantly greater amount of hormone in tumor tissue than in adjacent non-neoplastic tissue, using either assay or immunohistochemical methods, and the demonstration of hormone secretion by tumor cells in culture provide the most convincing evidence for ectopic hormone production. *In vitro* studies of hormone production by tumor cells using labeled amino acids, provide a most powerful tool for documenting hormone production. Similarly, careful and properly controlled immunohistochemical techniques can often document the intracellular location of the peptide hormones in question.

These same studies which have provided our best domumentation of ectopic hormone production have also provided evidence indicating that our current definition of ectopic hormone production is not entirely adequate. The major problem with our current definition relates to proving that the parent tissue from which a given tumor derives in fact lacks the capacity for synthesizing the hormone regarded as "ectopic". During recent years, refinement of sensitive assay and immunohistochemical techniques has demonstrated that a large number of peptide hormones may be synthesized in tissues other than the tissue classically regarded as the sole source of the hormone. One of the most notable examples of this phenomenon is the recent documentation of polypeptide hormones in neural tissues. In this regard, the initial demonstration of vasoactive intestinal peptide (VIP) in neural tumors (Fausa et al 1973; Swift, Bloom, Harry 1975) was regarded as evidence for ectopic VIP production. Subsequent studies (Said, Rosenberg 1976; Hofelt et al 1977;Mendelsohn et al 1979), however, have shown that VIP is, in fact, a normal peptide product of neuronal cells in the brain and peripheral nervous system. Furthermore, it has also been demonstrated that other "intestinal peptides" such as gastrin and cholecystokinin are normally present in the brain (Vanderhaegen et al 1975).

Recent studies of "oncoplacental" proteins such as placental lactogen and human chorionic gonadotropin (HCG) have highlighted the fact that our current definition of ectopic hormones is inaccurate. Although a wide variety of cancers have been associated with production of placental proteins, high circulating levels are most frequently associated with gonadal tumors containing embryonal and/or trophoblastic components (Braustein et al 1973; Rosen et al 1975). What is most important, particularly in regard to our definition of ectopic hormones, is the recent demonstration of detectable levels of HCG in the serum of normal adults (Borkowski, Muquardt 1979) and in adult liver, intestinal tract, and other

tissues (Yoshimoto, Wolfsen, Odell 1977). Should we then
regard the occurrence of increased circulating HCG levels in
patients with gastric carcinoma (24% of cases), hepatic carcinoma (17% of cases), and pancreatic carcinoma (50% of
cases)(Braunstein et al 1973; Rosen et al 1975) as ectopic?

In considering theories and proposed mechanisms of ectopic hormone production, and in discussing certain types of
tumors which serve as models for the study of ectopic hormone production, this brief review will emphasize how such
studies have enhanced our understanding of ectopic endocrine
activity in tumors and how, in the light of such studies, the
term "ectopic" might be redefined.

THE APUD-NEURAL CREST THEORY OF ECTOPIC HORMONE PRODUCTION

During the past 15-20 years, few topics have been of
more interest to the embryologist, pathologist, endocrinolo-
gist, and oncologist, or have been more controversial, than
the APUD cell-neural crest theory initially developed largely
by Pearse and his colleagues. Pearse (1966; 1969) in elegant
studies showed that peptide hormone producing cells in diverse
tissues shared several cytochemical, ultrastructural, and
functional properties. The most notable of these was their
common ability to synthesize and/or store biogenic amines and
the term APUD (Amine Precursor Uptake and Decarboxylation)
was coined to highlight this phenomenon. Furthermore, Pearse
and others showed that some APUD cells were derived from the
embryonic neural crest from where they migrated into different tissues of the body (Pearse 1969; Pearse et al 1973;
Polak et al 1974; Teillet, LeDouarin 1974). The APUD-neural
crest theory was readily embraced. It provided a most convenient unifying concept; it proposed the existence of a
widespread neuro-endocrine system within the body and facili-
tated the understanding of many tumor-associated endocrine
syndromes and the ability of endocrine and non-endocrine
tumors alike to inappropriately produce polypeptide hormones.
Small (oat) cell carcinoma of the lung, for example, a tumor
not infrequently associated with ectopic hormone production,
was regarded as a malignant tumor of bronchial endocrine
cells (K cells) which, in turn, were considered to be of
neural crest derivation (Bonikos, Bensch 1977).

The terms APUD, polypeptide hormone production, and
neural crest ultimately became synonymous and the list of
APUD cells apparently derived from the neural crest expanded

almost explosively, to include thyroid and ultimobranchial
body C cells, carotid body chief cells, sympathetic ganglion
cells, adrenal medullary cells, pancreatic islet cells, gastrointestinal tract and bronchopulmonary endocrine (Kultsch-
itsky) cells, melanocytes, certain thymic epithelial cells,
mast cells, pituitary corticotrophs, melanotrophs and somato-
trophs, pinealocytes, and others.

During the past 10-15 years, experimental studies have
led us to the realization that the possession of APUD characteristics does not necessarily imply origin from the neural
crest. Certainly, evidence for neural crest derivation of
thyroid and ultimobranchial body C cells remains strong.
Pearse and colleagues (Pearse, Carvalheira 1967; Pearse,
Polak 1971) using the technique of formaldehyde induced
fluorescence (FIF), showed that C cells in the mouse origina-
ted within the neural crest and migrated to the ultimobranchial body which ultimately fused with the developing thyroid.
The ingenious transplant chimera studies of LeDouarin and
her co-workers (LeDouarin, Le Lievre 1971; Polak et al 1974)
substantiated the preceding studies of Pearse and co-workers.
LeDouarin and Le Lievre transplanted the quail rhombenceph-
alic neural crest into an equivalent site in 6-10 somite
chick embryos and showed that the chick ultimobranchial bodies
were populated by quail cells. Immunocytochemical studies
subsequently confirmed the C cell nature of these quail cells
(Polak et al 1974).

Similar avian allograft studies have provided convincing
evidence for the neural crest origin of sympathetic ganglion
cells, adrenal medullary cells, and carotid body type I
(chief) cells (Teillet, LeDouarin 1974; LeDouarin, Le Lievre,
Fontaine 1972; Pearse et al 1973); and have also provided
convincing evidence that the APUD cells of the gut and pancreas are not of neural crest derivation (Andrew 1974; Fontaine, LeDouarin 1977). These and other studies (Cheng,
Leblond 1974) indicate that the APUD cells of the intestinal
tract develop and differentiate within the developing endodermal epithelium. Although Pearse (Pearse, Takor 1979) has
recently speculated that the endodermal APUD cells are "neuro-
endocrine-programmed" during their origin from the embryonic
epiblast, this remains purely speculative.

What is most important from these studies is the appreciation that not all cells with APUD characteristics, capable
of producing polypeptide hormones/biogenic amines are derived

from the neural crest or from any other endocrine progenitor. Rather, APUD cells appear to differentiate within various epithelial tissues during the course of embryogenesis and during epithelial cell renewal in adult tissues.

PROPOSED MECHANISMS OF ECTOPIC HORMONE PRODUCTION

Investigations of the appearance of ectopic hormones in tumors have been intimately associated with studies of the biology of tumor growth and tumor differentiation. Although certain aspects of ectopic hormone production have been elucidated, there continues to be much speculation about this subject and several concepts have arisen in an attempt to explain the mechanisms of ectopic hormone synthesis. Although, at the present time, little if any experimental data is available to support any of the existing theories, it is not unreasonable to believe that with the extraordinary advances which have been made in the field of molecular genetics, insight into the mechanisms of ectopic hormone production will be forthcoming.

The "Sponge" Theory

There is evidence that certain tumor cells can bind specific peptides (Schorr et al 1971) and/or steroid hormones (McGuire 1978) which evoke physiological responses in the normal parent tissue. Furthermore, tumor cells may possess receptors for, and respond to, peptide hormones which do not normally bind to the parent tissue (Schorr et al 1972). The "sponge" theory was proposed to explain increased peptide hormone concentrations in neoplastic tissues on the basis of selective uptake and binding of circulating hormones by the tumors (Unger et al 1974). In proposing the sponge theory, it was suggested that release of bound peptides upon death and necrosis of tumor cells would result in increased circulating levels.

While this theory might explain some instances of increased peptide hormone concentration in tumors, there are numerous instances in which proof of arteriovenous gradients across tumor vascular beds (Silva et al 1974) *in vitro* evidence of hormone synthesis (George et al 1972; Rabson et al 1973),and immunocytochemical localization of peptides in tumor cells have validated the synthesis of the hormones by the neoplastic cells themselves.

Genetic Mechanisms

The process of "genetic mutation" has been proposed to explain the inappropriate appearance of hormones in tumors. According to this theory, "abnormal" genes emerge during and/or after neoplastic transformation and subsequently code for hormone synthesis. Mutation, by its purest definition implies random genetic aberrations. Most evidence, to date, would point away from such a process. More likely would be functional DNA rearrangements such as those underlying immunoglobulin expression - or chromosomal translocations which are increasingly being described in many tumors.

There is much evidence to indicate that ectopic hormone production is often not a random process. In considering bronchogenic carcinoma, for example, ectopic ACTH activity is most characteristically seen with small cell (oat cell) carcinoma, but rarely with bronchogenic squamous carcinoma; on the other hand, inappropriate parathyroid hormone-like activity is most frequently associated with bronchogenic squamous carcinoma and not with small cell carcinoma. Similarly, as mentioned previously, ectopic production of "oncoplacental" hormones such as placental lactogen and human chorionic gonadotropin (HCG) is most frequently seen in patients with gastrointestinal, hepatic, and pancreatic carcinomas (Braunstein et al 1973; Rosen et al 1975). It is unlikely that such patterns of hormone production would result from random mutation.

Next, mutational genetic events would be expected to lead to the production of "abnormal" products. The peptide hormone products of tumor tissues are biochemically indistinguishable from those same products produced by normal cells. In addition, abnormal accumulations of large molecular weight precursor molecules (Gewirtz, Yalow 1974), fragments of peptide hormones (Orth et al 1973), and glycoprotein hormone subunits (Rosen et al 1975) frequently occur in tumors. This evidence indicates that the pathways of peptide hormone production in tumors are orderly and the same as those in normal tissues. There is no experimental evidence from DNA or RNA sequencing studies to support widespread emergence of abnormal DNA sequences in human tumor cells. The statement by Uriel (1975) that "extensive immunological and biochemical studies have failed to demonstrate new antigens, enzymes or molecules which logically would be expressed by the progeny of mutated cells" appear still valid.

According to the concept of "gene derepression", portions of DNA which are not normally available for transcription in parent cell, become available, or are "activated" during the process of neoplastic change (Gellhorn 1969). The mechanisms by which such inactive genes might be unmasked during neoplastic transformation are speculative and there is no experimental data which directly confirms that such a process of derepression actually occurs in tumor cells. Recent data concerning hypomethylation of genes, such as growth hormone in non-endocrine tumors, might suggest mechanisms by which abnormal gene expression may emerge in tumors (Feinberg, Vogelstein 1983). However, as discussed in a recent review (Baylin, Mendelsohn 1980), accumulated evidence points away from a process of significant derepression during neoplastic transformation. Indeed, the number of reports of peptide hormones in adult non-endocrine tissues, for example HCG in extracts of normal gastrointestinal tissue and liver (Yoshimoto, Wolfsen, Odell 1977), has led Odell and others (Odell et al 1977) to suggest that gene transcription for many small peptide hormones, and possibly fetal antigens, is never completely repressed in normal non-endocrine adult tissues; that expression of these genes is amplified or less effectively repressed in neoplastic tissues.

The theory of "dedifferentiation" proposes that during the course of neoplastic transformation, there is a return in the tumor tissue to a more primitive state of gene expression than that seen in the parent tissue. This theory usually implies a reversal of differentiation along the embryological pathway through which the parent tissue differentiated. The neoplastic tissue, then, synthesizes products normally found at earlier stages in the differentiation process. The emergence of carcinoembryonic antigen during the process of carcinogenesis and the relationship of alphafetoprotein to the fetal yoke sac and thus to tumors which derive from tissue embryologically related to yoke sac exemplify this theory (Abelev 1974).

As with other genetic theories to explain ectopic hormone production, little, if any, solid evidence exists to implicate reverse or retrograde differentiation in tumors. What has been suggested, rather, is that neoplastic transformation involves early, pluripotential cell forms; that the tumor which evolves contains the early cell forms in addition to more mature cells which continue to differentiate from the progenitor cells (Pierce 1970; Baylin,Mendelsohn1980).

In discussing various tumors as models for the study of ectopic hormone production, we would like to support the concept that "altered" differentiation or "dysdifferentiation"
may more accurately reflect the dynamics by which ectopic
hormone production results.

HUMAN TUMOR MODELS--IMPLICATIONS FOR ECTOPIC HORMONE PRODUCTION

During the course of this section, we will discuss how
studies of certain human tumors have shed new light on the
relationship between tumor biology and ectopic hormone production. We will focus on the evolution of tumor cell populations during the course of neoplastic transformation and
tumor growth; on the relationship of these tumor cell populations to hormone production; and on the relationship of
hormone production to tumor cell differentiation and maturation.

Neurogenic Tumors

The association of hormonally mediated endocrine syndromes with neurogenic tumors is well known. The occurrence
of Cushing's syndrome in patients with ganglioneuromas and
pheochromocytomas (Kogut, Kaplan 1962) and the association
of the watery diarrhea syndrome with ganglioneuromas and
ganglioneuroblastomas (Fausa et al 1973; Mitchell et al 1976)
are the most frequently encountered. During the past several
years, studies of normal neural tissues and neurogenic tumors
have provided convincing evidence linking the production of
certain peptide hormones to neuronal differentiation.

During the course of embryogenesis neuroblastic cells
migrate to various sites in the body where they give rise
to, among other cell types, ganglion cells and pheochromocytes of the adrenal medulla and extra-adrenal paraganglion
system. We (Mendelsohn et al 1979) have studied normal neural
tissues and a spectrum of neuroblastic tumors including (undifferentiated) neuroblastomas, tumors exhibiting ganglion
cell (neuronal) differentiation (ganglioneuroblastomas and
ganglioneuromas), and tumors with pheochromocytic differentiation (pheochromocytomas); our studies have focused on the
relationships between direction and type of neurogenic differentiation and the appearance of two polypeptide hormones
vasoactive intestinal peptide (VIP) and calcitonin. The constant appearance of VIP and the variable appearance of

calcitonin are associated with ganglion cell differentiation.
We were unable to detect these peptide hormones in the progenitor cell (neuroblast) or in pheochromocytes. The difference between ganglion cells and pheochromocytes was dramatically emphasized by an unusual composite pheochromocytoma-
ganglioneuroma which contained distinct pheochromocytic and
ganglioneuromatous elements. The patient in question presented with watery diarrhea and elevated circulating VIP
levels. Immunoreactive VIP and calcitonin were readily demonstrable within the ganglion cells but not within the pheochromocytes (Figure 1). Conversely an intense chromaffin
reaction indicated a high catecholamine content within the
pheochromocytomatous portion of the tumor. Immunohistochemical studies have also demonstrated VIP within neurons and
nerve fibers of the central and peripheral nervous system
(Hokfelt et al 1977; Mendelsohn et al 1979).

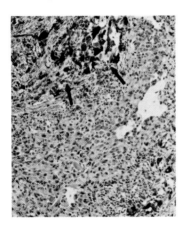

Fig.1. Strongly positive immu-
noperoxidase staining (black)
for VIP in ganglioneuroma component of tumor; no positive
staining is seen in pheochromocytoma component.

Tischler and Greene (1978) have described a rat pheochromocytoma cell line which, when exposed to nerve growth
factor in culture, acquires morphological and cytochemical
properties of neuronal cells. In subsequent studies, Tischler and his co-workers (Tischler et al 1980) demonstrated
the appearance of increased quantities of immunoreactive
VIP occurring concomitantly with the neuronal transformation
of the pheochromocytoma tissue. In stressing the relationship between peptide hormone synthesis and neuronal differentiation in tumors of neuroblastic derivation, it is important to emphasize that assayable immunoreactive VIP, ACTH,
and calcitonin have been reported in pheochromocytoma tissue
(Said, Faloona 1975; Voelkel et al 1973; Heath, Edis 1979).

In an immunohistochemical study of calcitonin in pheochromocytomas from patients with and without medullary thyroid
carcinoma (Mendelsohn et al 1980), we were able to demonstrate immunoreactive calcitonin only in pheochromocytomas
which contained metastatic medullary thyroid carcinoma. The
calcitonin was present within medullary carcinoma cells; we
could not demonstrate immunoreactive calcitonin, at a light
microscopic level, within pheochromocytes. Very recently,
however, O'Connor and co-workers (O'Connor, Frigon, Deftos
1983) have isolated calcitonin within the secretory granules
of human pheochromocytoma tissue.

It is quite likely that the differences which have been
encountered in these various neuroblastic tumors are quantitative rather than purely qualitative; that peptide hormone
synthesis is amplified in neurogenic tumors with neuronal
differentiation while biogenic amine production is amplified
in cells manifesting pheochromocytomatous or paraganglioma-
tous differentiation. What has been clearly demonstrated is
that the appearance of peptide hormone substances in neurogenic tumors is not merely a random phenomenon; that the synthesis of such substances is governed, at least in part, by
the type of differentiation which the cells manifest.

Carcinoma of the Lung

No group of tumors has been more extensively investigated with regard to ectopic hormone production that the spectrum of human lung cancer. Not only are lung carcinomas
among the most common human cancers, they are also, as a
group, the most frequent cause of ectopic endocrine syndromes
and tumor tissues are readily available for biochemical, histochemical and immunocytochemical study. While clinical syndromes such as inappropriate anti-diuretic hormone (ADH) secretion, Cushing's syndrome, and hormonally induced gyneco-
mastia are well described in the setting of lung cancer (for
review see Baylin, Mendelsohn 1980), there is an ever increasing body of information concerning the presence of
multiple polypeptide hormones in the circulation and tumor
tissues of patients with lung cancer. In fact, many of these
ectopically produced peptide hormones are of potential value
as biomarkers for diagnosis and monitoring of clinical course
in patients with lung cancer.

Lung carcinoma is a particularly useful model for studying endocrine-associated tumor activity because the bronchial

epithelium is somewhat unique in giving rise to at least four major histopathologic types of cancer, each having a major clinical impact. The endocrine activity associated with these cancers not only has clinical significance, but also provides a basis for studying the relationship between tumor cell differentiation and the various types of lung cancer.

Small cell (oat cell) carcinoma of the lung has long been recognized as possessing different growth patterns, clinical behavior, and biological behavior from other histologic types of lung cancer (Abeloff et al 1976). The propensity for small cell carcinoma to synthesize small polypeptide hormones and produce ectopic hormone syndromes, together with the presence of dense-core secretory granules within tumor cells has led Pearse (1969) and others (Bonikos, Bensch 1977) to consider small cell carcinoma as a tumor of bronchial endocrine cell (K cell) derivation. It was further speculated that the endocrine cells from which the tumor arose were of neural crest origin. Initially, then, a distinctive cellular origin for small cell carcinoma was thought to explain its propensity for endocrine activity.

During the past several years, however, evidence has accumulated indicating that small cell carcinoma of the lung may, indeed, not be of different origin from the other histological subtypes of lung cancer (adenocarcinoma, squamous cell carcinoma, and large cell undifferentiated carcinoma). It has become apparent during the past several years that histologically typical small cell and non-small cell bronchogenic carcinoma may coexist in the same patient and even within the same tumor lesion (Brereton et al 1978; Abeloff et al 1979). In addition, several investigators have demonstrated abnormally high levels of polypeptide hormones such as calcitonin (Silva et al 1979), ACTH (Gewirtz, Yalow 1974), as well as large molecular weight precursor and biologically inactive forms of peptides such as ACTH (Wolfsen, Odell 1979) in the circulation and/or tumor tissues from patients with all types of lung cancer. Furthermore, in many of these studies, the levels of the peptides did not seem dependent on the histological subtype of the lung cancer.

Studies from our laboratory and from others have indicated a definite histogenetic relationship between small cell and non-small cell lung cancers. Our biochemical studies of lung cancer have focused on the polypeptide hormone calcitonin; the enzyme marker for APUD cells, L-dopa decarboxylase (the "D" in APUD); and the enzyme histaminase (diamine oxidase), an enzyme known to be present in high quantities in certain tumors including small cell carcinoma and medullary thyroid carcinoma (Baylin et al 1978; Baylin et al 1981).

In the context of ectopic endocrine activity, the findings with regard to L-dopa decarboxylase and calcitonin are especially important. The relationship between the different histologic types of lung cancer is demonstrated to great advantage by Figure 2 which depicts the levels of L-dopa de-

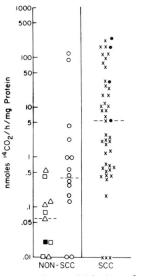

Fig.2. Levels of L-dopa decarboxylase activity in lung cancer. The levels obtained in small cell carcinoma are quantitatively greater than in other types of lung cancer, but there is significant overlap with adenocarcinoma. Note the very high levels in two adenocarcinomas.

△ Squamous Cell Carcinoma - Surgical
□ Large Cell Carcinoma - Surgical
■ Large Cell Carcinoma - Autopsy
○ Adeno Carcinoma - Surgical
x Small Cell Carcinoma - Autopsy
● Small Cell Carcinoma - Surgical

carboxylase activity in the spectrum of human lung cancer. As can be seen, L-dopa decarboxylase, a key element of APUD cells, is not restricted to small cell carcinoma, although differences do exist between the different histologic subtypes. L-dopa decarboxylase activity is clearly highest in small cell carcinoma, but adenocarcinomas can exhibit considerable activity in some cases. Calcitonin has a similar

distribution in these tumors (Berger et al 1981). Furthermore, as shown in Figure 2, we have encountered isolated
cases of adenocarcinoma of the lung in which levels of L-dopa
decarboxylase activity have been as high as the peak values
recorded in small cell carcinomas. Studies of calcitonin
from other groups (Schwartz et al 1979) have also shown highest levels in patients with small cell carcinoma, intermediate levels in patients with adenocarcinoma, and lowest levels
in patients with other histologic subtypes of lung cancer;
studies of ACTH (Yesner 1978) have shown highest levels in
small cell carcinoma, intermediate levels in large cell carcinoma, and lowest levels in other histologic subtypes.

In addition to the known histologic overlap between
different subtypes of bronchogenic carcinoma (Brereton et al
1978; Abeloff et al 1979) and the biochemical evidence of
overlap discussed above, there is a growing body of *in vitro*
data indicating a drift of small cell lung cancer, with time,
towards non-small cell lung cancer. Culture lines of human
small cell carcinoma (Gazdar et al 1980; Luk et al 1981)
have shown a time-dependent change from small cell to large
cell carcinoma. Gazdar and co-workers (1981) noted that
several established culture lines of small cell carcinoma
lost their endocrine features over a two-year period in culture; most importantly, implants of these same tumor cells
in the athymic nude mouse showed concomitant histological
change from small cell to large cell cancer. It is interesting that, as in the patients, the changes in culture have
always involved a shift away from small cell carcinoma towards non-small cell carcinoma. A possibly important clinical implication of this change emerged from recent studies
(Goodwin, Baylin 1982) in which it was shown that the loss
of neuroendocrine biochemistry by small cell carcinoma cells
in culture, even when histological change of the cells was
minimal, was accompanied by a profound development of radiation resistance. It is intriguing to speculate on the
relationship between this change in radiation response in
culture and the known tendency toward therapeutic resistance
in patients with an initial diagnosis of small cell carcinoma.
Recent studies of cell surface markers for the major forms of
human lung cancer (Baylin et al 1982; Goodwin et al 1983)
have provided further evidence that certain forms of large
cell carcinoma of the lung may indeed be of small cell carcinoma lineage.

Studies of experimental bronchial carcinogenesis in the

Syrian golden hamster (Reznik-Shuller 1977) have furnished
additional evidence for a histogenetic link between lesions
with and without endocrine features. Reznik-Schuller showed
that nitrosamine-induced lesions in the bronchus were initially characterized by a proliferation of typical endocrine
(APUD) cells; under the continued influence of nitrosamines,
the APUD cells underwent progressive squamous metaplasia,
Clara cells invaded the lung parenchyma, and the tumors which
developed consisted primarily of Clara-type cells with a few
squamous metaplastic and endocrine cells.

All these studies in humans and animal models indicate
a much closer link between small cell and non-small cell carcinomas than was originally suspected. The differences in
endocrine activity are quantitative rather than purely qualitative; endocrine activity appears to reflect a particular
direction of cellular differentiation within the epithelial
cell system.

Prostatic Carcinoma

While ectopic hormone production by prostatic carcinomas
is admittedly uncommon, the association of ectopic endocrine
activity and prostatic carcinoma has important implications
for the relationship between endocrine activity, tumor cell
differentiation and underlying mechanisms of ectopic hormone production. There are several well documented cases of
Cushing's syndrome in patients with prostatic carcinoma. It
is important to note that although the majority of prostatic
carcinomas associated with ectopic ACTH production have been
small cell carcinomas (Wenk et al 1977; Vuitch, Mendelsohn,
1980), others have been typical adenocarcinomas (Lovern et
al 1975).

As with other non-endocrine tumors associated with inappropriate endocrine function, the APUD-neural crest theory
was incriminated to explain the endocrine activity and it
was suggested that these tumors were derived from argentaf-
fin/argyrophil cells normally present within the prostate
(Wenk et al 1977). Azzopardi and Evans (1971) in reporting
two cases of mixed adenocarcinoma-"carcinoid tumor" implicated "divergent differentiation" to explain this phenomenon
in prostatic carcinomas. We have recently studied a case
(Vuitch, Mendelsohn 1980) which supports this contention of
divergent differentiation. The case in question was a patient with prostatic carcinoma who developed classical

Cushing's syndrome during the course pf progression of his disease. Sequential prostatic biopsies revealed a clear progression from moderately well differentiated adenocarcinoma to a tumor with adenocarcinomatous and small cell components. Immunoreactive ACTH was demonstrable within the small cell component of the tumor but not within the adenocarcinomatous component, suggesting again that APUD characteristics and the capacity for polypeptide hormone synthesis do not necessarily imply origin from an endocrine progenitor cell but rather reflect a particular type of differentiation within the tumor.

It is most likely, then, as illustrated by the above selected tumors, that expression of endocrine activity is at least in part related to mechanisms other than endocrine cell origin; that cells with endocrine characteristics arise through ongoing differentiation processes in normal and/or neoplastic epithelial tissues.

Medullary Carcinoma of the Thyroid

Neurogenic tumors, lung cancer, and cancer of the prostate were used as models for relating inappropriate endocrine activity to tumor cell differentiation. In the above sections, we proposed that endocrine activity was a function available to tumor cells in diverse tumors and that expression of endocrine activity, and hence ectopic hormone production, did not necessarily connote derivation from a particular progenitor cell. What we have also tried to emphasize is that expression of certain hormones, such as VIP and HCG, in certain tumors is not necessarily "ectopic" (inappropriate); that these substances, initially thought to be produced only in tumors, are in fact present in non-neoplastic tissues as well, albeit in lesser concentrations.

In considering medullary thyroid carcinoma (MTC), we will not focus specifically on ectopic hormone production, but on changes which occur in tumor cell populations with time and tumor progression. We will discuss how the cellular characteristics of a tumor can change with time and will consider the biologic and clinical implications of such change. In discussing lung cancer, we noted briefly a time-dependent drift from small cell carcinoma towards large cell carcinoma, both *in vivo* and *in vitro* (Abeloff et al 1979; Gazdar et al 1980; Luk et al 1981). MTC is a particularly useful model for studying the morphological and biochemical

changes which accompany tumor progression because the parent
cell, the C cell, has been identified (Williams 1966), all
stages of tumor evolution from C-cell hyperplasia to advanced carcinoma have been studied (Wolfe et al 1973; Mendelsohn et al 1978), the tumor exhibits a wide spectrum of
clinical behavior (Lippman et al 1982), and the key biochemical characteristics of the thyroid C cell have been identified and can be monitored (Foster, MacIntyre, Pearse 1964;
Pearse 1966). Although calcitonin and L-dopa decarboxylase
are normal rather than "ectopic" components of MTC, a study
of these endocrine substances provides some insight into how
inappropriate endocrine activity might evolve in subpopulations of tumor cells. The changes which occur not only have
important biological implications, but also have considerable impact upon the clinical care of patients.

In its early stages, and throughout the course of disease in most patients, MTC behaves as a rather indolent,
slow growing tumor that maintains a relatively high degree
of cellular differentiation. In such a setting, a rather
precise relationship between increasing tumor size and increasing circulating calcitonin levels is maintained (Wells
et al 1978). In a small cadre of patients, however, MTC
behaves aggressively with widespread dissemination and resultant death from tumor. In our experience (Trump, Mendelsohn, Baylin 1979; Lippman et al 1982), virulent tumor behavior in MTC has been accompanied by a striking diminution
in the efficacy for calcitonin production; in some cases,
this has produced a significant discordance between tumor
burden and circulating calcitonin levels (Trump, Mendelsohn,
Baylin 1979; Lippman et al 1982). The reduction in calcitonin production is manifested not only by an absolute reduction in total calcitonin content in lesions, but also by
a progressive heterogeneity of calcitonin immunostaining
within the lesions. In contrast to the early and localized
lesions where most cells contain significant quantities of
immunoreactive calcitonin (Mendelsohn et al 1978), the lesions from patients with widely disseminated, virulent disease exhibit only focally positive or even negative staining for hormone (Figure 3) (Trump, Mendelsohn, Baylin 1979;
Lippman et al 1982).

Our recent studies of early, localized, and disseminated
MTC have also shown an inverse relationship between the dis-
tribution of calcitonin and the other endocrine marker of
MTC, namely L-dopa decarboxylase (Lippman et al 1982); a loss

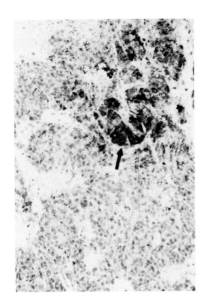

Fig.3. Focal immunostaining for calcitonin (arrow) in a case of aggressive MTC.

of calcitonin content in virulent disease is accompanied by an increase in L-dopa decarboxylase activity in the same lesions. We have considered that this change in endocrine biochemistry may reflect the degree to which the tumor cells are unable to differentiate fully along the endocrine cell maturation pathway (Baylin, Mendelsohn 1982). These findings dramatically emphasize the changes in specific biochemistry which can evolve in a tumor either with the passage of time or with the onset of change in biologic behavior of the tumor. In fact, the biochemistry of tumor cells in virulent lesions, is so different from the biochemistry of the parent cell, that if the parent cell were not known and the stages of neoplastic development were not available for study (as is the case for most human tumors), the presence of calcitonin in the virulent lesions might easily be interpreted as an example of ectopic hormone production by some of the tumor cells.

Just as calcitonin synthesis may be lost in certain populations of tumor cells during tumor progression, so too it is possible that the appearance of other (ectopic) hormones not normally associated with the parent cell, might be related to the evolution of these changing subpopulations of tumor cells. A variety of "ectopic" hormones have been associated with MTC including ACTH, MSH, serotonin, and prosta-

glandins (Williams, Karim, Sandler 1968; Iwanaga et al 1978).
At the present time, conflicting evidence exists concerning
the question of whether one tumor cell type is responsible
for the simultaneous secretion of calcitonin and other polypeptide hormones (Kameya et al 1977; Capella et al 1978).
We have recently demonstrated, using double immunostaining
techniques (Mendelsohn unpublished data), that individual
MTC tumor cells may contain several different substances
including calcitonin, somatostatin, and CEA.

In summary, then, studies of MTC indicate that normal
and inappropriate endocrine activity in tumors should be
viewed as a dynamic process intimately associated with ongoing processes of tumor cell differentiation and tumor progression. The presence of certain peptide hormones and neural properties appears to be associated with ongoing changes
in tumor cell subpopulations. These biochemical findings
may reflect important stages of tumor evolution which are
critically important to the clinical behavior of MTC in a
given patient.

CLINICAL IMPLICATIONS

It is suggested in this review that the current definition of "ectopic hormone production" is not entirely accurate and may need to be revised. This fact has been addressed
by other reviewers as well (Rees 1975; Odell et al 1977). In
fact, Odell and co-workers, based on their finding of hormones such as HCG in virtually all normal tissues and tumors
have suggested that peptide hromone synthesis is a "universal concomitant of neoplasia" (Yoshimoto, Wolfsen, Odell
1977; Odell et al 1977). Certainly, it would appear that at
least some peptide hormones and fetal antigens are elaborated
in normal adult epithelial tissues. The presence, then, of
these proteins in tumors derived from these tissues is not
truly inappropriate. What seems to occur is either an amplification of the ability of tumor cells to produce these
substances or of cell populations which may predominate in
the tumor, but which are present in very low number in the
normal tissues from which the tumors arise. As a definition
for the appearance of endocrine syndromes in patients with
non-endocrine cancers, the term ectopic is most appropriate
and should best be reserved for designating such inappropriate clinical syndromes, rather than describing the actual
presence of hormones in tumor tissue.

The recognition of ectopic endocrine syndromes is an important facet of diagnosis and patient management. Not only do the syndromes have an impact on prognosis and course of disease, but the presence of abnormal quantities of circulating hormones provides the clinician with potentially useful markers for monitoring response to therapy and progression of disease. In this regard, it is crucial to emphasize that tumors are composed of heterogeneous populations of cells; and that shifts in tumor cell populations occur during various stages of tumor evolution and progression. This aspect of tumor biology almost certainly explains how discrepancies between tumor burden and circulating marker levels can occur. It is important to be aware that increases in tumor burden need not necessarily be refelcted by increasing tumor marker levels. Caution should be exercised in tracking the course of disease by circulating marker levels and markers should not be used in isolation for this purpose.

To better understand the mechanisms and dynamics of peptide hormone synthesis in tumors, careful correlative studies of tumor hormone levels, immunohistochemical localization of hormones in tumor cells themselves, and the impact of these on circulating peptide levels are needed.

REFERENCES

Abelev GI (1974). α ~ Fetoprotein as a marker of embryo-specific differentiation in normal and tumor tissues. Transplant Rev 20:3.

Abeloff MD, Eggleston JC, Mendelsohn G, Ettinger DS, Baylin SB (1979). Changes in morphologic and biochemical characteristics of small cell carcinoma of the lung- A clinicopathologic study. Am J Med 66:757.

Andrew A (1974). Further evidence that enterochromaffin cells are not derived from the neural crest. J Embryol Exp Morphol 31:589.

Azzopardi JG, Evans DJ (1971). Argentaffin cells in prostate carcinoma: Differentiation from lipofuscin and melanin in prostate epithelium. J Pathol 104:247.

Baylin SB, Weisburger, WR, Eggleston JC, Mendelsohn G, Beaven MA, Abeloff MD, Ettinger DS (1978). Variable content of histaminase, L-dopa decarboxylase, and calcitonin in small-cell carcinoma of the lung-biologic and clinical implications. N Engl J Med 299:105.

Baylin SB, Mendelsohn G (1980). Ectopic (Inappropriate) hormone production by tumors: Mechanisms involved and the biological and clinical implications. Endocrinol Rev 1: 45.

Berger CL, Goodwin G, Mendelsohn G, Eggleston JC, Abeloff MD, Baylin SB (1981). Endocrine related biochemistry in the spectrum of lung carcinoma. J Clin Endocrinol Metab 53:422.

Berson SA, Yalow RS (1968). Immunochemical heterogeneity of parathyroid hormone in plasma. J Clin Endocrinol Metab 28:1037.

Bonikos DS, Bensch KG (1977). Endocrine cells of bronchial and bronchiolar epithelium. J Pathol 104:247.

Borkowski A, Muquardt C (1979). Human chorionic gonadotropin in the plasma of normal, nonpregnant subjects. N Engl J Med 301:298.

Braunstein GD, Vaitukaitis JL, Carbone PP, Ross GT (1973). Ectopic production of human chorionic gonadotropin by noeplasms. Ann Intern Med 78:39.

Brereton HD, Matthews MM, Costa J, Kent H, Johnson RE (1978). Mixed anaplastic small-cell and squamous-cell carcinoma of the lung. Ann Intern Med 88:805.

Capella C, Bordi C, Monga G, Buffa R, Fontana P, Bonfani S, Bussolati G, Solcia E (1978). Multiple endocrine cell types in thyroid medullary carcinoma. Virch Arch A Path Anat and Hist 377:111.

Cheng H, Leblond CP (1974). Origin, differentiation, and renewal of the four main epithelial cell types in the mouse small intestine .V. Unitarian theory of the origin of the four epithelial cell types. Am J Anat 141:537.

Connor TB, Thomas WC, Howard JE (1956). The etiology of hypercalcemia associated with lung carcinoma. J Clin Invest 35:697.

Fausa O, Fretheim B, Elgjo K, Semb LS, Gjone E (1973). Intractable watery diarrhea, hypokalemia, and achlorhydria associated with non-pancreatic retroperitoneal neurogenous tumor containing vasoactive intestinal peptide (VIP). Scand J Gastroenterol 8:713.

Feinberg AP, Vogelstein B (1983). Hypomethylation distinguishes genes of some human cancers from their normal counterparts. Nature 301:89.

Fontaine J, LeDouarin NM (1977). Analysis of endoderm formation in the avian blastoderm by the use of quail-chick chimeras: Problem of the neuro-ectodermal origin of the cells of the APUD series. J Embryol Exp Morphol 41:209.

Foster GV, MacIntyre I, Pearse AGE (1964). Calcitonin production and the mitochondrion rich cells of the dog thyroid. Nature 203:1029.

Gazdar AF, Carney DN, Russell EK, Sims HL, Baylin SB, Bunn PA, Guccion JG, Minna JD (1980). Establishment of continuous, clonable cultures of small cell carcinoma of the lung which have amine precursor uptake and decarboxylation cell properties. Cancer Res 40:2502.

Gazdar AF, Carney DN, Guccion JG (1981). Small cell carcinoma of the lung: Cellular origin and relationship to other pulmonary tumors. In Greco FA, Oldham RK, Bunn PA Jr. (eds): "Small cell lung cancer", New York: Grune and Stratton, p.145.

Gellhorn A (1969). Ectopic hormone production in cancer and its implication for basic research on abnormal growth. Adv Int Med 15:299.

George JM, Capen CC, Phillips AS (1972). Biosynthesis of vasopression "in vitro" and ultrastructure of a bronchogenic carcinoma. J Clin Invest 51:141.

Gewirtz G, Yalow RS (1974). Ectopic ACTH production in carcinoma of the lung. J Clin Invest 53:1022.

Goodwin G, Baylin SB (1982). Relationships between neuroendocrine differentiation and sensitivity to γ-radiation in culture line O-H-I of human small cell lung carcinoma. Cancer Res 42:1361.

Goodwin G, Shaper JH, Abeloff MD, Mendelsohn G, Baylin SB (1983). Analysis of cell surface proteins delineates a differentiation pathway linking endocrine and non-endocrine human lung cancers. Proc Natl Acad Sci (USA) In Press.

Heath H, Edis AJ (1979). Pheochromocytoma associated with hypercalcemia and ectopic secretion of calcitonin. Ann Int Med 91:208.

Hokfelt T, Elfvin LG, Schultzberg M, Said SI, Mutt V, Goldstein M (1977). Immunohistochemical evidence of vasoactive intestinal peptide-containing neurons and nerve fibers in sympathetic ganglia. Nueroscience 2:885.

Iwanaga T, Koyama H, Uchiyama S, Takahashi Y, Nakano S, Itoh T, Horai T, Wada A, Tateishi R (1978). Production of several substances by medullary carcinoma of the thyroid. Cancer 41:1106.

Kameya T, Shimosato Y, Adachi I, Abe K, Kasai N, Kimura K, Baba K (1977). Immunohistochemical and ultrastructural analysis of medullary carcinoma of the thyroid in relation to hormone production. Am J Pathol 89:555.

Klemperer P (1923). Parathyroid hyperplasia and bone destruction in generalized carcinomatosis. Surg Gynecol

Obstet 36:11.

Kogut MD, Kaplan SA (1962). Systemic manifestations of neurogenic tumors. J Pediatr 60:694.

LeDouarin NM, LeLievre (1971). Sur l'origine des cellules à calcitonine du corps ultimobranchial de l'embryon d' Oiseau. CR Ass Anat 152:558.

LeDouarin NM, LeLievre C, Fontaine J (1972). Recherches experimentales sur l'origine embryologique du corps Earotidien chez les Oiseaux. C R Acad Sci (Paris) 275 D: 583.

Lippman SM, Mendelsohn G, Trump DL, Baylin SB (1982). The prognostic and biological significance of cellular heterogeneity in medullary thyroid carcinoma. J Clin Endocrinol Metab 54:233.

Lovern WJ, Fariss BC, Wettlanfer JN, Hane S (1975). Ectopic ACTH production in disseminated prostatic adenocarcinoma. Urology 5:817.

Luk GD, Goodwin G, Marton LT, Baylin SB (1981). Polyamines are necessary for the survival of human small-cell lung carcinoma in culture. Proc Natl Acad Sci (USA) 78:2355.

McGuire WL (1978). Hormone receptors: Their role in predicting prognosis and response to endocrine therapy. Sem Oncol 5:428.

Mendelsohn G, Eggleston JC, Weisburger WB, Gann DS, Baylin SB (1978). Calcitonin and histaminase in C-cell hyperplasia and medullary thyroid carcinoma. Am J Pathol 32: 35.

Mendelsohn G, Eggleston JC, Olson JL, Said SI, Baylin SB (1979). Vasoactive intestinal peptide and its relationship to ganglion cell differentiation in neuroblastic tumors. Lab Invest 41:144.

Mitchell CH, Sinatra FR, Crast FW, Griffin R, Sunshine P (1976). Intractable watery diarrhea, ganglioneuroblastoma and vasoactive intestinal peptide. J Pediatr 89:593.

O'Connor DT, Frigon RP, Deftos LJ (1983). Immunoreactive calcitonin in catecholamine storage vesicles of human pheochromocytoma. J Clin Endocrinol Metab 56:582.

Odell WD, Wolfsen A, Yoshimoto Y, Weitzman R, Fisher D, Hirose F (1977). Ectopic peptide synthesis: A universal concomitant of neoplasia. Trans Assoc Am Phys 90:204.

Orth DN, Nicholson WE, Mitchell WM, Island DP, Liddle GW (1973). Biologic and immunologic characterization and physical separation of ACTH and ACTH fragments in the ectopic ACTH syndrome. J Clin Invest 52:1756.

Pearse AGE (1966). Common cytochemical properties of cells

producing polypeptide-hormone secretion with particular reference to calcitonin and the thyroid C cells. Vet Rec 79:587.

Pearse AGE (1969). The cytochemistry and ultrastructure of polypeptide hormone-producing cells of the APUD series and the embryologic, physiologic, and pathologic implications of the concept. J Histochem Cytochem 17:303.

Pearse AGE, Carvalheira AF (1967). Cytochemical evidence for an ultimobranchial origin of rodent thyroid C cells. Nature (Lond) 214:929.

Pearse AGE, Polak JM (1971). Cytochemical evidence for the neural crest origin of mammalian ultimobranchial C cells. Histochemistry 27:96.

Pearse AGE, Polak JM, Rost FWD, Fontaine J, LeLievre C, LeDouarin NM (1973). Demonstration of the neural crest origin of type I (APUD) cells in the avian carotid body, using a cytochemical marker system. Histochemistry 34:191.

Pearse AGE, Takor TT (1979). Embryology of the diffuse neuroendocrine system and its relationship to the common peptides. Fed Proc 38:2288.

Pierce GB (1970). Differentiation of normal and malignant cells. Fed Proc 29:1248.

Plimpton CH, Gellhorn A (1956). Hypercalcemia in malignant disease without evidence of bone destruction. Am J Med 21:750.

Polak JM, Pearse AGE, LeLievre C, Fontaine J, LeDouarin NM (1974). Immunocytochemical confirmation of the neural crest origin of avian calcitonin-producing cells. Histochemistry 40:209.

Polak JM, Pearse AGE, LeLievre C, Fontaine J, LeDouarin NM (1974). Immunocytochemical confirmation of the neural crest origin of avian calcitonin-producing cells. Histochemistry 40:209.

Rabson AS, Rosen SW, Tashjian AH, Weintraub BD (1973). Production of human chorionic gonadotrophin "in vitro" by a cell line derived from carcinoma of the lung. J Natl Cancer Inst 50:669.

Ratcliffe JG (1972). Tumor and plasma ACTH concentrations in patients with and without the ectopic ACTH syndrome. Clin Endocrinol 1:27.

Reznik-Schuller H (1977). Sequential morphologic alterations in the bronchial epithelium of Syrian golden hamsters during N-nitrosomorpholine-induced pulmonary tumorigenesis. Am J Pathol 89:59.

Rosen SW, Weintraub, BD, Vaitukaitis JL, Sussman HH, Hershman JM, Muggia FM (1975). Placental proteins and their subunits as tumor markers. Ann Intern Med 82:71.

Said SI, Faloona GR (1975). Elevated plasma and tissue levels of vasoactive intestinal polypeptide in the watery-diarrhea syndrome due to pancreatic, bronchogenic and other tumors. N Engl J Med 293:155.

Said SI, Rosenberg RN (1976). Vasoactive intestinal polypeptide: Abundant immunoreactivity in neural cell lines and normal nervous tissue. Science 192:907.

Schorr I, Rathnam P, Saxena BB, Ney RL (1971). Multiple specific hormone receptors in the adenylate cyclase of an adrenocortical carcinoma. J Biol Chem 246:5806.

Schorr I, Hinshaw HT, Cooper MA, Mahafee D, Ney RL (1972). Adenylcyclase hormone responses of certain human endocrine tumors. J Clin Endocrinol Metab 34:447.

Schwartz KE, Wolfsen AR, Forster B, Odell WD (1979). Calcitonin in non-thyroidal cancer. J Clin Endocrinol Metab 49:438.

Silva OL, Becker KL, Primack A, Doppman J, Snider RH (1974). Ectopic secretion of calcitonin by oat cell carcinoma. N Engl J Med 290:1122.

Silva OL, Broder LE, Doppman JL, Snider RH, Moore CF, Cohen MH, Becker KL (1979). Calcitonin as a marker for bronchogenic cancer. Cancer 44:680.

Steiner DF, Cunningham D, Spigelman L, Aten B (1967). Insulin biosynthesis: Evidence for a precursor. Science 157:697.

Swift PGF, Bloom SR, Harry F (1975). Watery diarrhea and ganglioneuroma with secretion of vasoactive intestinal peptide. Arch Dis Child 50:896.

Teillet MA, LeDouarin NM (1974). Determination par la methode des graffes heterospecifiques d'ebauches neurales de caille sur l'embryon de poulet, du niveau du neuraxe dont derivent les cellules medullo-surrenaliennes. Arch Anat Micr Morph Exp 63:51.

Tischler AS, Greene LA (1978). Morphologic and cytochemical properties of a clonal line of rat adrenal pheochromocytoma cells which respond to nerve growth factor. Lab Invest 39:77.

Tischler AS, DeLellis RA, Biales B, Nunnemacher G, Carabba V, Wolfe HJ (1980). Nerve growth factor-induced neurite outgrowth from normal human chromaffin cells. Lab Invest 43:399.

Trump DL, Mendelsohn G, Baylin SB (1979). Discordance between plasma calcitonin and tumor cell mass in medullary thyroid carcinoma. N Engl J Med 301:253.

Unger RH, dev Lochner J, Eisentraut AM (1974). Identification of insulin and glucagon in a bronchogenic metastasis. J Clin Endocrinol Metab 24:823.

Uriel J (1975). Fetal characteristics of cancer. In Becker FF (ed): "Cancer. A comprehensive treatise", Vol 3, "Biology of tumors: Cellular biology and growth", New York: Plenum Press, p.21.

Vanderhaegen JJ, Signeau JC, Gepts W (1975). New peptide in the vertebrate CNS reacting with antigastrin antibodies. Nature (Lond) 257:604.

Voelkel EF, Tashjian AH, Davidoff FF, Cohen RB, Perlia CP, Wurtman RJ (1973). Concentrations of calcitonin and catecholamines in pheochromocytomas, a mucosal neuroma and medullary thyroid carcinoma. J Clin Endocrinol Metab 37:297.

Vuitch MF, Mendelsohn G (1981). Relationship of ectopic ACTH production to tumor differentiation: A morphologic and immunohistochemical study of prostatic carcinoma with Cushing's syndrome. Cancer 47:296.

Wells SA Jr, Baylin SB, Gann DS (1978). Medullary thyroid carcinoma: relationship of method of diagnosis to pathologic staging. Ann Surg 188:377.

Wenk RE, Bhagavan BS, Levy R, Miller D, Weisburger WR (1977). Ectopic ACTH, prostatic oat cell carcinoma and marked hypernatremia. Cancer 40:773.

Williams ED (1966). Histogenesis of medullary carcinoma of the thyroid. J Clin Pathol 19:114.

Williams ED, Karim SMM, Sandler M (1968). Prostaglandin secretion by medullary carcinoma of the thyroid. A possible cause of the associated diarrhea. Lancet 6:22.

Wolfe HJ, Melvin KEW, Cervi-Skinner SJ, AL Saadi AA, Juliar JP, Jackson CE, Tashjian AH Jr (1973). C-cell hyperplasia preceding medullary thyroid carcinoma. N Engl J Med 289:437.

Wolfsen AR, Odell WD (1979). Pro-ACTH: Use for early detection of lung cancer. Am J Med 66:765.

Yesner R (1978). Spectrum of lung cancer and ectopic hormones. Pathol Ann 13:217.

Yoshimoto Y, Wolfsen AP, Odell WD (1977). Human chorionic gonadotropin-like substance in normal human tissues. Science 197:575.

Index

PROGRESS IN CLINICAL AND BIOLOGICAL RESEARCH

Series Editors